WE 460 REN   66.00

D1380557

TELFORD

CB014155

ATLAS OF
Spine Injection

Donald L. Renfrew, MD

Center for Diagnostic Imaging
Winter Park, Florida

ATLAS OF
Spine
Injection

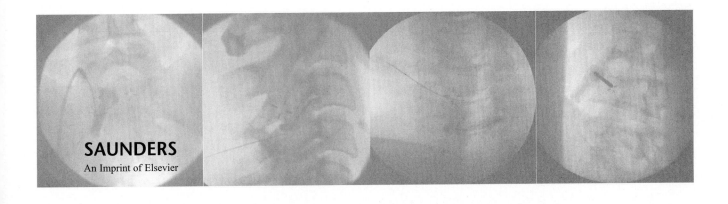

SAUNDERS

An Imprint of Elsevier

SAUNDERS
An Imprint of Elsevier Inc.

The Curtis Center
Independence Square West
Philadelphia, Pennsylvania 19106

ATLAS OF SPINE INJECTION ISBN 0–7216–0420–X

Notice

Radiology is an ever-changing field. Standard safety precautions must be followed but as new research and clinical experience broaden our knowledge, changes in treatment and drug therapy may become necessary or appropriate. Readers are advised to check the most current product information provided by the manufacturer of each drug to be administered to verify the recommended dose, the method and duration of administration, and contraindications. It is the responsibility of the treating physician, replying on experience and knowledge of the patient, to determine dosages and the best treatment for each individual patient. Neither the publisher nor the author assumes any liability for any injury and/or damage to persons or property arising from this publication.

The Publisher

Library of Congress Cataloging-in-Publication Data

Renfrew, Donald L.
    Atlas of spine injection / Donald Renfrew.–1st ed.
        p. ; cm.
    Includes bibliographical references.
    ISBN 0-7216-0420-X
    1. Spine–Puncture–Atlases. 2. Injections, Spinal–Atlases. I. Title.
    [DNLM: 1. Injections, Spinal–Atlases. 2. Spinal Diseases–therapy–Atlases. 3.
    Spine–radiography–Atlases. WE 17 R411ab 2004]
    RC400.R465 2004
    616.8′56–dc22   2003059125

Editor-in-Chief, Surgery: Richard Lampert
Acquisitions Editor: Allan Ross
Project Manager: Tina Rebane
Book Designer: Karen O'Keefe Owens

EH/MVY

Printed in the United States of America.

Last digit is the print number: 9 8 7 6 5 4 3 2 1

To Mother

Contributors

Mark Beckner, MD
Jewett Orthopedic Clinic
Winter Park, Florida

Kent B. Remley, MD
Center for Diagnostic Imaging
Indianapolis, Indiana

Preface

As I noted in the preface to my prior book, *Atlas of Spine Imaging* (Saunders, 2003), I have had a career-long interest in the spine and in back pain. For the past few years, I've had the good fortune to be able to dedicate almost all of my professional time to imaging and diagnostic and therapeutic injection of the spine. After the completion of the *Atlas of Spine Imaging*, I felt that the job was "half done." This book represents the other half of the task: the presentation of diagnostic and therapeutic injections of the spine. This text summarizes diagnostic and therapeutic injection in a concise yet detailed fashion.

This book offers discussion and description of the more commonly performed diagnostic and therapeutic spine injections from a radiologist's perspective. Neuroradiologists and interventional radiologists are demonstrating more and more interest in these procedures, and they may find a text providing a radiologist's perspective useful. In addition, anesthesiologists and physiatrists (as well as others performing diagnostic and therapeutic spine injections) may find a radiologist's approach complementary to their own, and may find valuable information in this volume.

In addition to providing a radiologist's perspective, this volume also offers a few strengths not found in most other books. While books written by multiple authors have the advantage of drawing from expertise not usually found in a single author, they also frequently have the weaknesses of a lack of uniform focus, repetition and self-contradiction. This book, for better or worse, came from a single hand,[1]

and is designed to provide a uniform approach to the field with little repetition and no self-contradiction. With these goals in mind, I organized the book as follows:

Chapter 1 reviews back pain, with sections on definitions, theories of causation, imaging abnormalities, treatment, and the rhetoric of pain. Chapters 2 to 9 address individual procedures. Each chapter has separate sections on definition, literature review, rationale for the procedure, required equipment, informed consent, patient selection, and procedure description. The uniform, modular organization in these chapters will allow the harried injectionist to skip not only the chapters of little or no interest, but the sections of little or no interest.

Speaking of the harried injectionist, it must be noted that no matter how busy said injectionist might be, perusal of this book cannot be construed as adequate training to perform these procedures. These procedures must be learned in residency, or in any of the several courses on spine injection, or by direct experience in an existing practice. This book is meant to be an adjunct to, not a substitute for, this training. However, it was my goal to provide the injectionist with a handy textbook to illustrate the injections and their possible complications, and also to provide at least some insight into the theory and science behind these injections. The reader will be the ultimate judge of whether I've succeeded. I hope that I have, and that you enjoy reading this book as much as I've enjoyed writing it.

Donald L. Renfrew, MD

---

[1]Or "hands," in this era of the word processor. In addition, Drs. Mark Beckner and Kent Remley were kind enough to help me with the chapter on vertebroplasty/kyphoplasty, and Dr. Beckner with the chapter on IDET.

Acknowledgments

Several individuals contributed to the completion of this textbook.

I thank the diagnostic and therapeutic injection physicians Drs. Roberto Ang, Blake Johnson, Steve Pollei, and Kurt Schellhas, who were kind enough to share their knowledge of procedures with me.

I thank my contributors, Drs. Mark Beckner and Kent Remley, for their work on the book.

In addition, I would like to thank the Center for Diagnostic Imaging (CDI). CDI is, on the one hand, a corporation that owns and manages the facilities that allow me a unique radiology practice, and, on the other hand, a collection of exceptional and talented individuals. Technologists who were particularly helpful in the completion of this project included Charmaine Barclay, Janice Blackburn, Shawn Brownell, Joie Dixon, Nita Duncan, Daniel Fernandez, Gina Genovese, Gina Patterson, Cindy Wylie, and Teri Yost. Kellie Ashley, Robert LaDouceur, Tom Kelly, and Shannon Risdon all provided exceptional management. Finally, Dr. Kenneth Heithoff's vision and leadership have not only made CDI possible, but have also created an environment that allows such projects as this book.

My understanding of spine injection would not be the same without the input of orthopaedic spine surgeons. Drs. Mark Beckner, Reginald Tall, Michael Macmillan, and Gregory Munson from the Jewett Orthopedic Center; Drs. Joseph Flynn, Jr. and Geoffrey Stewart from the the Spine and Scoliosis Center; Dr. Richard Smith from the Florida Center for Orthopedics; Dr. Stephane Lavoie from Florida Orthopedic Associates; and Drs. Stephen Goll, Grady McBride, and Steven Weber of Orlando Orthopedics Center have all been kind enough to share their knowledge and insight regarding care of spine patients.

Finally, I would like to thank my wife, Susan, for all her support during the work I did on this book.

Contents

1 Review of Spine Pain

DONALD L. RENFREW

Definitions

Philosophers of the mind maintain that pain is a *quale*, or subjectively experienced state of consciousness (Guzeldere 1997).[1] Although some philosophers still assert what seems to be a dualist stance (Chalmers 1996), most now regard qualia as manifestations of neurophysiologic processes (Searle 1997). Simply stated, mind states (pain) arise from brain states (neuronal firing). If the mind-state of pain is based in the brain-state of neuronal firing, then theories of pain must ultimately address neuronal firing in the brain; such theories are under development (Melzack 2001).

The International Association for the Study of Pain has defined pain as "An unpleasant sensory and emotional experience associated with actual or potential tissue damage, or described in terms of such damage" (Merskey 1994). Thus, spine pain patients typically describe their pain in terms of its location (e.g., "My back hurts." or "I have sciatica.") or in terms of an imaging abnormality ("I have pain from a herniated disc."). Patients never say "I am experiencing the quale of pain, quite possibly from an imbalanced neuromatrix." Discussions of spine pain proceed as if the culprit lesion existed in the spine, and, depending on how "cause" is defined, the "cause" of such pain is indeed the spine. The vocabulary of spine pain has thus developed as if the spine *is* the cause, with the following "types" of pain: *axial pain*, *radicular pain*, and *somatic referred pain*.

Axial pain is pain coming directly from the axial skeleton (Bogduk 1997), such as pain coming from a compression fracture of the vertebral body.

Radicular pain is pain coming from a spinal nerve or its roots (Bogduk 1997), such as pain coming from irritation of the S1 nerve roots from a large disc herniation at L5-S1. Although purists (Bogduk 1997) distinguish *radicular pain* from *radiculopathy* (a neurologic condition in which conduction is blocked), most patients and health care practitioners use the terms interchangeably. From the purist's perspective, radiculopathy is manifested by numbness (from conduction block of sensory neurons) and weakness (from conduction block of motor neurons).

Somatic referred pain is pain wherein the true source is in a skeletal or muscular structure, but the perceived pain is in a region innervated by nerves other than those that serve the true source of the pain (Bogduk 1997). An example is pain in the shoulder secondary to a cervical disc herniation.

Functionally, how does one decide which of the types of pain an individual has? Typically, this is done using a combination of factors, including discussion with the patient and written information obtained either directly from the patient or from the patient's other health care providers.

Patients with radicular pain complain of band-like, shooting pain that is well localized and often runs down an extremity in a narrow strip. Patients with somatic referred pain, on the other hand, describe pain that is much more poorly localized, deep, and with an aching rather than a shooting character (Bogduk 1997). One of the first questions I ask pain patients is, "Do you have mostly leg (or arm) pain or mostly back (or neck) pain?" Patients with mostly back (or neck) pain are presumably suffering from axial pain, whereas those with leg (or arm) pain may be having either radicular pain or somatic referred pain, which requires further questioning regarding the characteristics noted above.

Written information may take several forms. In our clinic, we use an information form (Fig. 1–1) that has an area for a written description of the patient's pain, a check-box for location of the pain, and a pain diagram. The written description may contain spontaneously offered descriptors that favor radicular or somatic referred pain over axial pain, whereas the check-box explicitly solicits input in this regard. The pain diagram may help categorize the patient's pain (Mann 1992): axial pain will be drawn centrally or on the side of an afflicted facet (Fig. 1–2), radicular pain as a narrow strip down the extremity (Fig. 1–3), and somatic referred pain typically as an off-axis, relatively broad area (Fig. 1–4). Some authors (Ransford 1976) have used pain diagrams to evaluate whether further psychological testing might be warranted prior to surgery, when "unreal pain diagrams" not corresponding to any conceivable anatomic lesion or "I hurt here" arrows are added to the diagram (Fig. 1–5).

---

1. Of course, as with anything in philosophy, this is not a universal view (Dennett 1988).

CDI
Center for Diagnostic Imaging

PATIENT INFORMATION SHEET

PLEASE PRINT

Date _____
FL Location _____
Account # _____
F/U Appt w/Ref MD _____

NAME _____
Last, First, Middle

SOCIAL SECURITY # _____

AGE ____ BIRTHDATE _____ HEIGHT _____ WEIGHT _____ SEX: ○ M ○ F

FEMALES: Are you pregnant? ○ YES ○ NO   When was your last menstrual period? _____ Are you breastfeeding? _____

REFERRING PHYSICIAN _____ DR. PHONE # _____

① Briefly describe your problem/pain and how long you have had these symptoms? _____
_____

DATE OF INJURY (IF APPLICABLE) _____

DO YOU HAVE ANY ALLERGIES? ○ YES ○ NO   IF SO, WHAT ARE THEY? _____

HAVE YOU HAD SURGERY IN THE AREA TO BE SCANNED? ○ YES ○ NO

IF YES, DESCRIBE WHAT WAS DONE AND WHEN THE SURGERY WAS PERFORMED_____
_____

IF SURGERY, ARE YOUR SYMPTOMS: BETTER   WORSE   SAME   DIFFERENT (CIRCLE AND DESCRIBE)
_____

Please circle any MEDICAL PROBLEMS you have:

CANCER ASTHMA   BRONCHITIS   DIABETES   PANCREAS   GALLBLADDER LIVER   KIDNEY   FEMALE ORGAN

Comment on any other medical problems: _____

Have you had any of the following: (Please check)

○ Head Surgery   ○ Head Trauma   ○ Headaches   ○ Ringing Sound   ○ Buzzing Sound   ○ Hearing Loss

○ Vertigo   ○ Dizziness   ○ Blurred Vision   ○ Bell's Palsy   ○ TMJ Problems/Surgery

HAVE YOU HAD ANY OF THE FOLLOWING STUDIES PERTAINING TO TODAY'S EXAM? IF SO, INDICATE BELOW.

TEST	WHEN	WHERE	RESULTS
X-rays			
CT Scan			
MRI Scan			
Ultrasound			
Nuclear Medicine			
Therapeutic Injection			
Arthrogram			

INDICATE SYMPTOMS:

Please check: ②

	RIGHT	LEFT	BOTH
Arm Pain			
Neck Pain			
Back Pain			
Leg Pain			
Tingling			
Weakness			
Numbness			

Scan Type_____
Pre-Scan_____
Scan Time_____
Bolus Rad Approved _____
Study # _____
Total # of Images _____

③

C2/3 =
C3/4 =
C4/5 =
C5/6 =
C6/7 =
C7/T1 =
L1/2 =
L2/3 =
L3/4 =
L4/5 =
L5/S1 =

FRONT   LOCATION OF PAIN   BACK

Please shade in painful areas.

Right   Left   Left   Right

T1/2 =
T2/3 =
T3/4 =
T4/5 =
T5/6 =
T6/7 =
T7/8 =
T8/9 =
T9/10 =
T10/11 =
T11/12 =
T12/L1 =

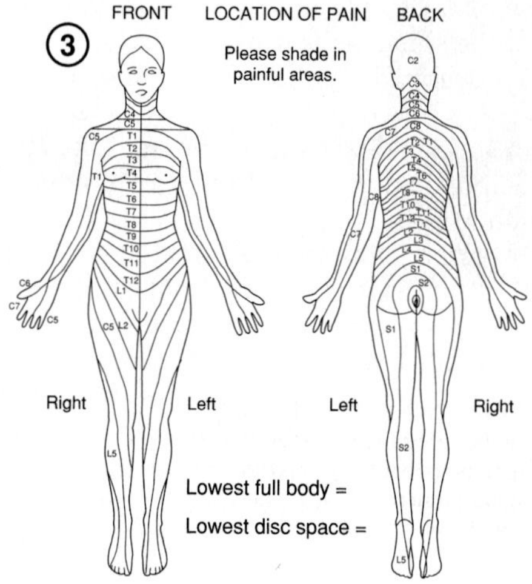

Lowest full body =
Lowest disc space =

FIGURE 1–1

Patient Intake Form. This form has multiple areas. Note that in addition to the usual demographic data, the patient is specifically asked to describe his or her pain (1). Furthermore, there are check-boxes (2) that inquire about arm and leg pain, as well as tingling, weakness, and numbness (findings of radiculopathy). Finally, a body outline (3) is provided so that the patient can draw a pain diagram.

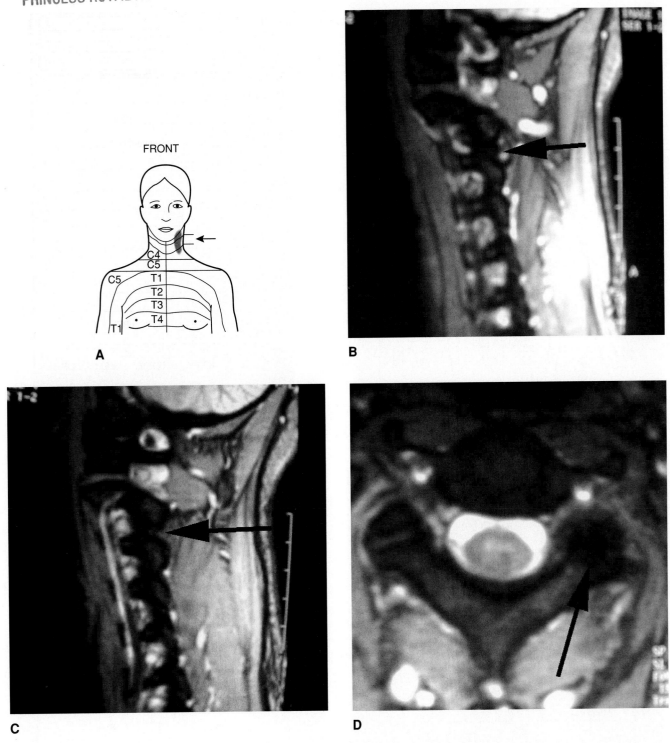

FIGURE 1–2

Pain Diagram for Axial Pain. This 42-year-old woman had persistent, left-sided neck pain. *A,* Pain diagram demonstrating unilateral, left-sided neck pain. *B,* Left parasagittal magnetic resonance imaging examination demonstrates facet arthropathy at the C2-3 level (arrow). *C,* Right parasagittal magnetic resonance imaging examination shown for comparison demonstrates a normal-appearing facet joint on this side (arrow). *D,* Axial magnetic resonance imaging demonstrates marked asymmetry of the C2-3 facet joints, with left-sided facet arthropathy (arrow). Similar findings were apparent on computed tomographic examination (not shown), without other levels of abnormality.

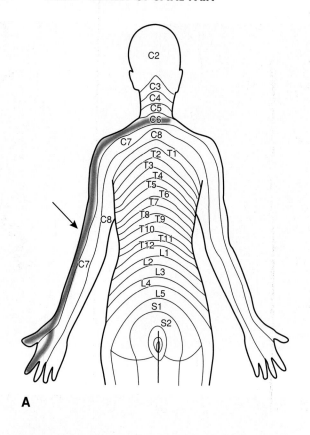

A

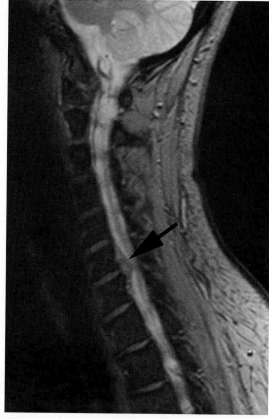

B

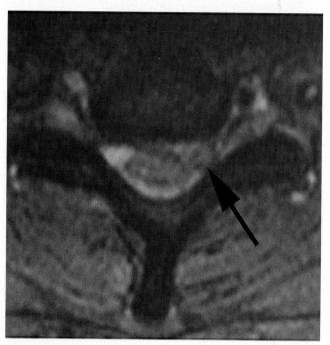

C

FIGURE 1–3

Pain Diagram for Radicular Pain. This 54-year-old woman had neck and left arm pain. *A*, Pain diagram indicating neck and left arm pain in a narrow, band-like distribution (arrow) reaching the hand, suggesting radicular pain. *B*, Left parasagittal T2-weighted gradient echo magnetic resonance imaging study demonstrates a large cranially and caudally dissecting C6-7 disc extrusion (arrow). *C*, Axial T2-weighted gradient echo examination at the level of the C6-7 neural foramina demonstrates a large, left central disc extrusion (arrow) with associated cord compression and C7 nerve root displacement and compression.

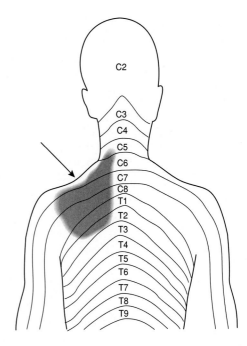

FIGURE 1–4

Pain Diagram for Somatic Referred Pain. This 45-year-old man with single-level C6-7 disc degeneration and a small disc protrusion without neural compression on magnetic resonance imaging scan (not shown) had left trapezius region pain. The pain diagram demonstrates left-sided pain.

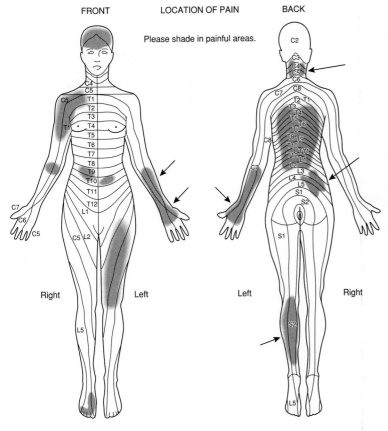

FIGURE 1–5

Unreal Pain Diagram. This 36-year-old woman had a 1-mm disc protrusion at L3-4. The nonanatomic pain diagram and multiple (patient-drawn) arrows indicate sites of pain that are in a nonanatomic distribution and bear no relationship to visualized morphologic abnormalities of the spine.

Theories of Causation

Neurophysiologic classification divides pain into non-nociceptive pain (further divided into psychogenic and neuropathic pain) and nociceptive pain (further divided into somatic and visceral pain) (Kanner 1997). Psychogenic pain, visceral pain, and peripheral neuropathic pain exceed the scope of this text, which leaves radicular pain as the type of non-nociceptive pain, and axial and somatic referred pain as the types of nociceptive pain, for discussion here.

With respect to radicular pain, pressure alone on normal nerves or nerve roots generally causes conduction block (and hence radiculopathy) rather than radicular pain. However, pressure on abnormal nerves or nerve roots, or pressure on the normal dorsal root ganglion, may result in radicular pain (Garfin 1991, Howe 1977, Kelly 1956, Kuslich 1991). Several categories of causes may be responsible for such pressure and inflammation, including foraminal stenosis, epidural disorders, and meningeal disorders, and each of these categories, in turn, may have many causes (foraminal stenosis may result from osteophytic spurring along the disc margin or spondylolisthesis, for example) (Bogduk 1997). Although ubiquitous "dermatome charts" (derived from Keegan and Garret's 1948 paper [Keegan 1948]) map generalities regarding the correspondence of perceived pain and spinal level, the injectionist should realize that generalizations are not universally applicable, and that the location of pain in a given individual may vary one or more levels from the charted "ideal" (van Akkerveeken 1993).

With respect to nociceptive pain, nociceptors are nerve fibers that demonstrate a relatively high threshold of stimulation (Raja 1999). Stimulation of these nociceptors by noxious stimuli (mechanical, thermal, or chemical) results in nociceptive pain. Nociceptors may be sensitized by endogenous chemical stimuli (algogenic substances) such as serotonin, substance P, bradykinin, prostaglandin, and histamine (Kanner 1997). Much of the work on nociceptors involves cutaneous fibers, but virtually every structure (with the exception of the internal aspect of the normal intervertebral disc) of the spine is innervated by nociceptors (Bogduk 1997, Calliet 1991) and thus a possible source of nociceptive pain.

While neurophysiologic classification provides a framework, the exact causes and treatment of spine pain continue to be a source of ongoing research and controversy. For example, consider a young man with the acute onset of low back pain radiating in a narrow band down the posterior aspect of his left leg to his heel (Fig. 1–6). The patient's complaint indicates radicular pain and the imaging findings demonstrate an obvious "cause" of the pain: a large disc extrusion. This leads to the natural question, "What should be done about it?" which leads to another question, "Why do disc extrusions hurt?" If one believes in mechanical compression of neural tissue as the main explanation, as originally proposed by Mixter and Barr in 1934 (Mixter 1934), then the solution is mechanical treatment (removal of the disc). If one believes in chemical irritation of neural tissue as the main explanation (whether from phospholipase A2 [Lee 1998, Saal 1990], matrix metalloproteinases [Roberts 2000], nitrous oxide [Kang 1996], tumor necrosis

factor-α [Olmarker 1998], or free glutamate [Harrington 2000]), then treatment is directed toward this irritation (either systemic or locally applied anti-inflammatory medication). If one is a medical nihilist, one may cite literature demonstrating the spontaneous regression of disc herniations (Bozzao 1992, Mochida 1998, Teplick 1985) and state that the best course of action is to do nothing, since the natural history of the disease is almost invariably benign and self-limiting. Thus, even in the case of a "simple" disc herniation (the patients most practitioners want to treat because they are so "straightforward"), there are several different theories regarding the explanation of the patient's pain, and these different theories result in radically different treatment recommendations. In most cases of patients presenting for evaluation and treatment of spine pain, the situation is even less clear-cut.

Imaging Abnormalities

Imaging studies have evolved rapidly in the past few decades, and the problem of linking findings with spine pain has changed in nature. A mere generation ago, imaging studies (confined to plain films and oil myelography) revealed gross abnormalities (compression fractures, tumors, severe spinal stenosis, large disc extrusions) in a minority of patients while revealing nonspecific degenerative changes or nothing in most patients with spine pain. Now, there is an embarrassment of riches: imaging studies (almost exclusively magnetic resonance imaging, supplemented by myelo-computed tomography on occasion) reveal multiple findings, even in asymptomatic volunteers who deny ever experiencing significant backache (Boden 1990a, Boden 1990b, Jarvik 2001, Jensen 1994, Matsumoto 1998, Stadnik 1998, Teresi 1987, Weinreb 1989, Weishaupt 1998, Wiesel 1984). To dismiss the entire enterprise as worthless, however, flies in the face of hundreds of peer-reviewed journal articles as well as multiple textbooks.[2] To make the most use of magnetic resonance imaging findings in caring for patients with spine pain, placement into one of the following three categories is frequently helpful: (1) There is an abnormality that almost certainly accounts for the patient's symptoms. (2) There are one or more abnormalities that *may* account for the patient's symptoms. (3) There are no abnormalities that could possibly account for the patient's symptoms.

1. There is an imaging abnormality that almost certainly accounts for the patient's symptoms. As in the example given (see Fig. 1–6), there are cases in which any knowledgeable physician reviewing the images would say "The problem here is obvious." The degree of disc extrusion illustrated in Figure 1–6 has never been reported in any "normal" volunteer,[3] and if the provided clinical history

---

2. Might I recommend Renfrew's *Atlas of Spine Imaging* (Philadelphia, Elsevier Press, 2002) in this regard?

3. Claims that some large proportion of the asymptomatic population have disc "herniations" usually somewhat misrepresent the primary literature. While imaging studies of asymptomatic volunteers may reveal small and relatively flat disc contour abnormalities causing no neural impingement, such studies virtually never demonstrate large extrusions or severe neural compression. See Renfrew 2002 for a full discussion.

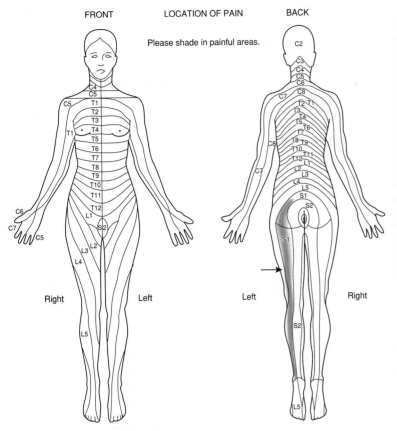

FRONT   LOCATION OF PAIN   BACK

Please shade in painful areas.

Right   Left

Left   Right

A

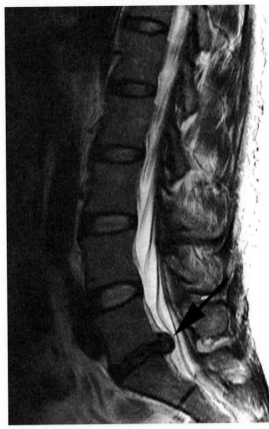

B

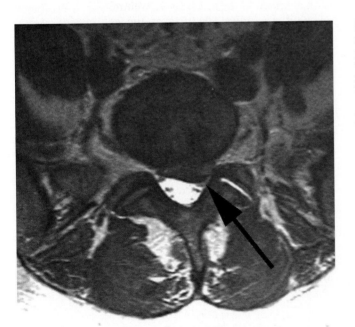

C

FIGURE 1–6

Example of Acute Disc Herniation. This 25-year-old man without any prior history of back or leg pain presented with acute pain radiating down the posterior aspect of his left leg. *A*, Pain diagram demonstrates a pain pattern suggesting left S1 radicular pain (arrow). *B*, Sagittal T2-weighted magnetic resonance imaging scan demonstrates an L5-S1 disc extrusion (arrow). *C*, Axial T2-weighted magnetic resonance imaging scan demonstrates the L5-S1 disc herniation with posterior displacement and compression of the traversing S1 nerve (arrow) between the herniated disc and the L5 lamina.

is neck and arm pain, then either the wrong patient's paperwork is in hand or the patient misunderstood the form. Note that while in Figure 1–6 the finding is obvious, there are many patients in whom the imaging findings are far less obvious but the linkage is still unequivocal (see Fig. 3–1), which underscores the importance of having expert interpretation of imaging in the first place. While having a single abnormality that almost certainly accounts for the patient's symptoms does not constitute the majority of cases, it does represent a large number of patients undergoing imaging. The rare cases of infection and tumor usually fall into this category, although there are occasions when asymptomatic benign nerve sheath tumors are incidentally discovered on imaging. There are also rare cases in which the patient has an extraspinal cause of pain mimicking a spinal cause of pain (Bickels 1999).

2. There are one or more abnormalities that *may* account for the patient's symptoms. Such cases account for the majority of patients undergoing imaging. Studies of many patients demonstrate disc contour abnormalities (either diffuse or focal), disc desiccation, facet arthropathy, and variable degrees of spinal stenosis with little or no neural compression. Given the innervation of almost every structure within the spine, the nonspecificity of the resulting perceived pain, and the ubiquity of such imaging findings (even in the asymptomatic population), linkage between imaging findings and symptoms is difficult or impossible. Indeed, this lack of linkage is one of the reasons for performance of diagnostic and therapeutic injections. If disc morphology were completely predictive of discography results (which it is not [Brightbill 1994, Gibson 1986, Horton 1992, Kornberg 1989, Osti 1992, Schneiderman 1987, Zucherman 1988]), why would discography be necessary? If facet morphology were completely predictive of the response to medial branch blocks (which it is not [Schwarzer 1995]), one could proceed directly to rhizotomy without the diagnostic blocks. However, even if the pain pattern is (as usual) vague and the imaging findings are (as usual) multiple, the imaging should, along with the patient's history and physical examination, help direct the type and location of diagnostic and therapeutic injection.

3. There are no imaging abnormalities that could possibly account for the patient's symptoms. Sacroiliac joint abnormality may be subtle or hard to diagnose, and yet patients may still obtain pain relief upon injection, anesthetization of normal-appearing facet joints may lead to pain relief (Schwarzer 1995), and normal-appearing discs on magnetic resonance imaging examination may still have symptomatic (at least to discography) full-thickness annular fissures (Brightbill 1994, Horton 1992, Kornberg 1989, Osti 1992, Zucherman 1988), particularly in the cervical spine (Schellhas 1996, Schellhas 2000). Patients with normal magnetic resonance imaging study findings are distinctly unusual. It is more frequently the case that the imaging study misleads: it may show degenerative disc disease with normal-appearing facet joints, and yet the patient obtains good pain relief with medial branch blocks and rhizotomy.

The injectionist should review the patient's imaging studies prior to injection. Review of such studies may result not only in a change of approach to a given procedure but also in a complete change of procedure.

Treatment

Treatment of spine pain should be based on the diagnosis. Patients with tumors and infections will not come for therapeutic injection, although they may present for diagnostic biopsy (see Chapter 7). Most patients undergoing diagnostic and therapeutic injections have one of various "degenerative" conditions. In broad brushstrokes, the treatment spectrum in these patients includes the following:

1. Doing nothing. As noted earlier, the natural history of degenerative conditions of the spine is usually benign, and unless there are signs or symptoms of neural compression (along with an accompanying cause on imaging studies), doing nothing is always an option and may be the best option.
2. Physical therapy. There are several schools of physical therapy. One interesting study found three different methods of physical therapy to be better than doing nothing but also found aerobic exercise (not directed at the spine) to be equivalent and less costly (Mannion 1999).
3. Manipulation. Osteopathic medicine was founded on this principle (although it seems to have undergone "convergent evolution" with allopathic medicine), as was chiropractics (which has remained dedicated to, predominantly, manipulation therapy).
4. Oral medication. Nonsteroidal anti-inflammatory drugs are a mainstay of treatment, with analgesics (including narcotics) in relatively common use as well (Lipetz 1998, van Tulder 1997).
5. Acupuncture.
6. Diagnostic and therapeutic injection. See Chapters 2 through 9.
7. Surgery. In broadest possible terms, most procedures involve either decompressing neural tissue (e.g., discectomy, decompression laminectomy, foraminotomy) or fusing motion segments.

Often patients undergo multiple treatments concurrently. The variety of treatments (as well as the variety of causes and explanations) of spine pain emphasizes that it is a complex, poorly understood phenomenon (Shapiro 1997). If any one of these therapies worked well in all cases, the others would go the way of blood-letting. Until something new and clearly superior comes along, however, health care practitioners involved in the care of spine pain patients will likely hear their patients tell them "I've tried everything, and nothing helps." The job of the injectionist is to find (and possibly even provide) something that *does* help.

Assumptions of Diagnostic and Therapeutic Injections

Fundamental assumptions of diagnostic and therapeutic injections (Table 1–1) imply that injections may be per-

TABLE 1-1. Fundamental Assumptions of Diagnostic and Therapeutic Injections

1. Needle placement and injection close to or at the site of a symptomatic structure will stimulate nociceptors and thus reproduce the patient's typical pain.
2. Anesthetic placed through the needle will (at least temporarily) decrease activity within nociceptors and thus relieve the patient's typical pain.
3. Pain may be secondary to inflammation contributing to nociceptor stimulation and may respond to steroid injection.

formed for diagnostic purposes, to help identify the specific site or cause of irritated nociceptors, or for therapeutic purposes, to decrease discharge of irritated nociceptors for prolonged periods. Note that while these fundamental assumptions underlie nearly everything in Chapters 2 through 6, they are not unassailable. Clinicians who forego ordering diagnostic and therapeutic injections may do so on the basis of disagreement with one or more of the assumptions.

The Rhetoric of Back Pain

Aristotle defined *rhetoric* as "The faculty or skill of discovery of the available means of persuasion in a given case." As David Zarefsky has noted, although the term *rhetoric* has taken on pejorative connotations, it has a rich history as the study of how messages influence people (Zarefsky 2001). One can obtain valuable insights into how medicine is practiced, and how medical research is performed and interpreted, by the study of argumentation. Zarefsky states that argumentation should be understood as the study of effective reasoning, and that arguing is reason giving. The application of these tenets to medicine in general, and the diagnosis and treatment of back pain patients in particular, become clear as one listens to "debate" regarding clinical questions. "I would treat this patient with an anti-inflammatory because they have been shown to work." "It's worthless to obtain plain radiographs. These have been shown to not be cost-effective." "I was taught in my fellowship to treat these patients with posterior fusion only." "In my experience, rhizotomy works well."

Evidence can be divided into three broad categories: objective data, social consensus, and credible, authoritative sources. Medical scientists are generally wedded to objective data (at least within their area of expertise), whereas physicians in practice will usually admit that there is simply too much to know to run down the ultimate source of the objective data backing up every detail of diagnosis and treatment. Many times, practicing physicians must accept what was given to them during medical school, residency, and fellowship training as valid, since it comes from an authoritative source. Similarly, at many conferences and meetings, the attendees focus more on the competence, trustworthiness, good will, and dynamism of the presenters (factors contributing to their credibility; see Zarefsky 2001) than on the objective data found in the presented studies. With respect to social consensus, consider that while symptoms, signs, and laboratory data form objective data, how a disease is defined (the reference or criterion standard chosen as the sine qua non of the disease) is determined by the society of physicians.

For centuries, medicine relied on simple observation of the condition of the patient before and after treatment to evaluate treatment efficacy. As Shapiro and Shapiro (1997) have written, "The panorama of treatment since antiquity provides ample support for the conviction that, until recently, the history of medical treatment is essentially the history of the placebo effect." The "placebo effect" (or "meaning response"; see Moerman 2002) has been known since ancient times and became an important methodologic tool in scientific trials in the 20th century (de Oliveira 1995). The power of this method of scientific investigation has resulted, at least in some segments of medicine, in the conviction that "[o]nly independently evaluated (i.e., not by the treating clinicians, and preferably by observers unaware of the treatment assignment) randomized controlled trials can establish an effect of a treatment above and beyond natural history of the condition and nonspecific [placebo] effects" (Turner 1994). Therefore, randomized controlled trials form, for some researchers, the *only* legitimate "available means of persuasion" in the case of medical treatment. Furthermore, the value of the trial is increased if the investigators and patients are both unaware of whether the patients are undergoing the treatment or the control. In addition, the control must "match" the treatment relatively closely, since the "placebo effect" increases from doing nothing, to pills, to injections, to surgery (Turner 1994, Wall 1992). A nonblinded trial is liable to the charge of observer bias, and a trial controlling surgery with natural history or more conservative treatment is liable to the charge of placebo effect (and, often, observer bias as well).

"But wait," a thoughtful reader might object. "Randomized control trials for pills are all well and good. But do we need a randomized control trial for ruptured appendicitis? For dissecting aortic aneurysm? For gangrenous cholecystitis?" Accepted treatment of these diseases has never undergone randomized controlled trials, and it is safe to say that it probably never will. And although treatment of back pain with physical therapy (Mannion 1999), manipulation (Ernst 2001), oral medication (Katz et al, 2003), and acupuncture (Leibing 2002) have all undergone randomized, controlled clinical trials,[4] no randomized controlled trials exist for spine surgery, if by *controlled* we mean that the treatment and control patients are treated with like degrees of intervention.[5] At present there are few such evaluations of *any* type of surgery, but these

---

4. In answer to the question, "Do studies demonstrate unequivocal benefit beyond placebo?" the answers are: for physical therapy, probably not; for manipulation, probably not; for oral medication, yes; for acupuncture, probably not; for injection, yes (see remainder of text).

5. There are studies that compare surgical results to nonsurgical results in (of course) a nonblinded manner. See, for example, Weber 1983 for disc herniation and Fritzell et al 2001 for fusion surgery.

evaluations may be forthcoming in the near future. When and if such studies on spine surgery are published, they could have a profound influence on the practice of such surgery, and hence the treatment of patients with back pain. Randomized controlled trials do exist for spinal injection therapy and rhizotomy; these are reviewed in detail in the appropriate chapters of this book.

A final comment regarding the "placebo effect," "non-specific effect," or "meaning response," however defined. While this salubrious effect might be regarded as a nuisance in the design of clinical research, it results in profound benefit to patients in daily medical practice. As noted by Turner et al (1994): "The quality of the interaction between the physician and patient can be extremely influential in patient outcomes, and, in some (perhaps many) cases, patient and provider expectations and interactions may be more important than specific treatments." A physician may, through enthusiasm, apparent warm feelings for the patient, confidence, and authority provoke a healing response *in addition to* any specific effect of a therapeutic maneuver demonstrated in a randomized, controlled trial (Harrington 1997). Key to the nonspecific effects of the patient-physician interaction is altering the meaning attached to the illness experience in a positive direction, which Brody (Brody 1997) breaks down into three general components: providing an understandable and satisfying explanation of the illness; demonstrating care and concern; and holding out an enhanced promise of mastery or control over symptoms. Thus, in the administration of an epidural steroid injection, the likelihood of obtaining beneficial effects may be greatly increased by allowing the patient to explain his or her pain pattern and circumstances fully and then stating, "In many cases, the pain that you are describing may come from inflammation and irritation of nerve fibers. Usually, your body will heal this inflammation with time and your pain will go away. What we are going to do today is to put a powerful anti-inflammatory drug close to where the inflammation is. For many people, this provides good pain relief." This presentation of the facts (and there are scientific references to studies supporting every statement made, but these are usually irrelevant to the patient) will definitely result in a better outcome than certain alternative presentations. For example, in another context, Thomas (1987) tested the effect of the following statement: "I cannot be certain what is the matter with you. I am not sure that the treatment I am going to give you will have an effect." He demonstrated that a physician providing this statement (which also presents the facts regarding epidural steroid) to patients resulted in those patients doing much more poorly than when an alternative phrasing was used. While deliberate prescription of placebos without patient knowledge may currently be considered dishonest or unethical (de Oliveira 1995), it is neither dishonest nor unethical to present the known facts in a manner known to enhance the likelihood of a beneficial effect.

References

Bickels J, Kahanovitz N, Rubert CK, Henshaw RM, Moss DP, Meller I, Malawer MM. Extraspinal bone and soft-tissue tumors as a cause of sciatica: clinical diagnosis and recommendations—analysis of 32 cases. Spine 1999; 24:1611–1616.

Boden SD, Davis DO, Dina TS, Patronas NJ, Wiesel SW. Abnormal magnetic-resonance scans of the lumbar spine in asymptomatic subjects. J Bone Joint Surg Am 1990a; 72:402–408.

Boden SD, McCowin PR, Davis DO, Dina TS, Mark AS, Wiesel S. Abnormal magnetic-resonance scans of the cervical spine in asymptomatic subjects. J Bone Joint Surg Am 1990b; 72:1178–1184.

Bogduk N. Clinical Anatomy of the Lumbar Spine, 3rd ed. New York, Churchill Livingstone, 1997.

Bozzao A, Gallucci M, Masciocchi C, Aprile I, Barile A, Passariello R. Lumbar disc herniation: MR imaging assessment of natural history in patients treated without surgery. Radiology 1992; 185:135–141.

Brightbill TC, Pile N, Eichelberger RP, Whitman M. Normal magnetic resonance imaging and abnormal discography in lumbar disc disruption. Spine 1994; 19:1075–1077.

Brody H. The doctor as therapeutic agent: a placebo effect research agenda. In Harrington A. The Placebo Effect: An Interdisciplinary Exploration. Cambridge, MA, Harvard University Press, 1997.

Calliet R. Neck and Arm Pain. Philadelphia, F.A. Davis Company, 1991.

Chalmers D. The Conscious Mind. Oxford, Oxford University Press, 1996.

Dennett DC. Quining qualia. In: Bisiach E, Marcel AJ (eds). Consciousness in Contemporary Science. New York, Oxford University Press, 1988.

de Oliveira GG. The placebo effect: a review. Am J Ther 1995; 2:216–224.

Ernst E, Harkness E. Spinal manipulation: a systematic review of sham-controlled, double-blind, randomized clinical trials. J Pain Symptom Manage 2001; 22:879–889.

Fritzell P, Hagg O, Wessberg P, Nordwall A. Lumbar fusion versus nonsurgical treatment for chronic low back pain. A multicenter randomized controlled trial from the Swedish lumbar spine study group. Spine 2001; 26:2531–2534.

Garfin SR, Rydevik BL, Brown RA. Compressive neuropathy of spinal nerve roots: a mechanical or biological problem? Spine 1991; 16:162–166.

Gibson MJ, Buckley J, Mawhinney R, Mulholland RC, Worthington BS. Magnetic resonance imaging and discography in the diagnosis of disc degeneration. J Bone Joint Surg Br 1986; 68:369–373.

Guzeldere G. The many faces of consciousness: a field guide. In Block N, Flanagan O, Guzeldere G (eds). The Nature of Consciousness: Philosophical Debates. Cambridge, MA, MIT Press, 1997.

Harrington A. Introduction. In Harrington A (ed). The Placebo Effect. Cambridge, MA, Harvard University Press, 1997.

Harrington JF, Messier AA, Bereiter D, Barnes B, Epstein MH. Herniated lumbar disc material as a source of free glutamate available to affect pain signals through the dorsal root ganglion. Spine 2000; 25:929–936.

Horton WC, Daftari TK. Which disc as visualized by magnetic resonance imaging is actually a source of pain? A correlation between magnetic resonance imaging and discography. Spine 1992; 17:S164–S171.

Howe JF, Loeser JD, Calvin WH. Mechanosensitivity of dorsal root ganglia and chronically injured axons: a physiological basis for the radicular pain of nerve root compression. Pain 1977; 3:25–41.

Jarvik JJ, Hollingworth W, Heagerty P, Haynor DR, Deyo RA. The longitudinal assessment of imaging and disability of the back (LAIDBack study). Spine 2001; 26:1158–1166.

Jensen MC, Brant-Zawadski MN, Obuchowski N, Modic MT, Malkasian D, Ross J. Magnetic resonance imaging of the lumbar spine in people without back pain. N Engl J Med 1994; 331:69–73.

Kang JD, Georgescu HI, McIntyre-Larkin L, Stefanovic-Racic M, Donaldson WF, Eans CH. Herniated lumbar intervertebral discs spontaneously produce matrix metalloproteinases, nitric oxide, interleukin-6, and prostaglandin E(2). Spine 1996; 21:271–277.

Kanner R. Pain Management Secrets. Philadelphia, Hanley and Belfus, 1997.

Katz N, Ju WD, Krupa D et al. Efficacy and safety of rofecoxib in patients with chronic low back pain. Results from two 4-week randomized, placebo-controlled, parallel-group, double-blind trials. Spine 2003; 28:851–859.

Keegan JJ, Garret FD. The segmental distribution of the cutaneous nerves in the limbs of man. Anat Rec 1948; 102:409–437.

Kelly M. Is pain due to pressure on nerves? Neurology 1956; 6:32–36.

Kornberg M. Discography and magnetic resonance imaging in the diagnosis of lumbar disc disruption. Spine 1989; 14:1368–1372.

Kuslich SD, Ulstrom CL, Michael CJ. The tissue of origin of low back pain and sciatica: a report of pain response to tissue stimulation during operations on the lumbar spine using local anesthesia. Orthop Clin North Am 1991; 22:181–187.

Lee HM, Weinstein JN, Meller ST, Hayashi N, Spratt KF, Gebhart GF. The role of steroids and their effects on phospholipase A2: an animal model of radiculopathy. Spine 1998; 23:1191–1196.

Leibing E, Leonhardt U, Koster G, Goerlitz A, Rosenfeldt JA, Hilgers R, Ramadori G. Acupuncture treatment of chronic low-back pain—a randomized, blinded, placebo-controlled trial with 9-month follow-up. Pain 2002; 96:189–196.

Lipetz JS, Malanga GA. Oral medications in the treatment of acute low back pain. Occup Med 1998; 13:151–166.

Mann NH, Brown MD, Enger I. Expert performance in low-back disorder recognition using patient pain drawings. J Spinal Disorders 1992; 5:254–259.

Mannion AF, Muntener M, Taimela S, Dvorak J. A randomized clinical trial of three active therapies for chronic low back pain. Spine 1999; 24:2435–2448.

Matsumoto M, Fujimura Y, Suzuki N, Nishi Y, Nakamura M, Yabe Y, Shiga H. MRI of the cervical intervertebral discs in asymptomatic patients. J Bone Joint Surg Br 1998; 80:19–24.

Melzack R. Toward a new concept of pain for the new millennium. In Waldman SD (ed). Interventional Pain Management, 2nd ed. Philadelphia, W.B. Saunders, 2001.

Mersky N, Bogduk N (eds). Classification of Chronic Pain: Task Force of Taxonomy, 2nd ed. Seattle, IASP Press, 1994.

Mixter WJ, Barr JS. Rupture of the intervertebral disc with involvement of the spinal canal. N Engl J Med 1934; 211:210–214.

Mochida K, Kormori H, Okawa A, Muneta T, Haro H, Shinomiya K. Regression of cervical disc herniation observed on magnetic resonance images. Spine 1998; 23:990–997.

Moerman DE, Jonas WB. Deconstructing the placebo effect and finding the meaning response. Ann Intern Med 2002; 136:471–476.

Olmarker K, Larsson K. Tumor necrosis factor alpha and nucleus-pulposus-induced nerve root injury. Spine 1998; 23:2538–2544.

Osti OL, Fraser RD. MRI and discography of annular tears and intervertebral disc degeneration: a prospective clinical comparison. J Bone Joint Surg Br 1992; 74:431–435.

Raja SN, Meyer RA, Ringkamp M, Campbell JN. Peripheral neural mechanisms of nociception. In Wall PD, Melzack R (eds). Textbook of Pain, 4th ed. Philadelphia, Churchill Livingstone, 1999.

Ransford AO, Cairns D, Mooney V. The pain drawing as an aid to the psychologic evaluation of patients with low-back pain. Spine 1976; 1:127–134.

Renfrew DL. Atlas of Spine Imaging. Philadelphia, Elsevier Press, 2002.

Roberts S, Caterson B, Menage J, Evans EH, Jaffray DC, Eisenstein SM. Matrix metalloproteinases and aggrecanase: their role in disorders of the human intervertebral disc. Spine 2000; 25:3005–3013.

Saal JS, Franson RC, Dobrow R, Saal JA, White AH, Goldthwaite N. High levels of inflammatory phospholipase A2 activity in lumbar disc herniations. Spine 1990; 15:674–679.

Schellhas KP, Smith MD, Gundry CR, Pollei SR. Cervical discogenic pain. Prospective correlation of magnetic resonance imaging and discography in asymptomatic patients and pain sufferers. Spine 1996; 21:300–312.

Schellhas KP, Garvey TA, Johnson BA, Rothbart JP, Pollei SR. Cervical diskography: analysis of provoked responses at C2-3, C3-4, and C4-5. Am J Neuroradiol 2000; 21:269–275.

Schneiderman G, Flannigan B, Kingston S, Thomas J, Dillin WH, Watkins RG. Magnetic resonance imaging in the diagnosis of disc degeneration: correlation with discography. Spine 1987; 12:276–281.

Schwarzer AC, Wang SC, O'Driscoll D, Harrington T, Bogduk N, Laurent R. The ability of computed tomography to identify a painful zygapophyseal joint in patients with chronic low back pain. Spine 1995; 20:907–912.

Searle J. The Mystery of Consciousness. New York, New York Review, 1997.

Shapiro AK, Shapiro E. The placebo: is it much ado about nothing? In Harrington A (ed). The Placebo Effect. Cambridge, MA, Harvard University Press, 1997.

Stadnik TW, Lee RR, Coen HL, Neirynck EC, Buisseret TS, Osteaux MJC. Annular tears and disk herniation: prevalence and contrast enhancement on MR images in the absence of low back pain or sciatica. Radiology 1998; 206:49–55.

Teplick JG, Haskin ME. Spontaneous regression of herniated nucleus pulposus. AJR 1985; 145:371–375.

Teresi LM, Lufkin RB, Reicher MA, Moffit BJ, Vinuela FV, Wilson GM, Bentson JR, Hanafee WN. Asymptomatic degenerative disk disease and spondylosis of the cervical spine: MR imaging. Radiology 1987; 164:83–88.

Thomas KB. General practice consultations: is there any point in being positive? Br Med J 1987; 294:1200–1202.

Turner JA, Deyo RA, Loeser JD, Von Korff M, Fordyce WE. The importance of placebo effects in pain treatment and research. JAMA 1994; 271:1608–1614.

van Akkerveeken PF. On pain patterns of patients with lumbar nerve root entrapment. Neuro-Orthopedics 1993; 14:81–102.

van Tulder MW, Koes BW, Bouter LM. Conservative treatment of acute and chronic nonspecific low back pain: a systematic review of randomized controlled trials of the most common interventions. Spine 1997; 22:2128–2156.

Wall PD. The placebo effect: an unpopular topic. Pain 1992; 51:1–3.

Weber H. Lumbar disc herniation: A controlled, prospective study with ten years of observation. Spine 1983; 8:131–139.

Weinreb JC, Wolbarsht LB, Cohen JM, Brown CEL, Maravilla KR. Prevalence of lumbosacral intervertebral disk abnormalities on MR images in pregnant and asymptomatic nonpregnant women. Radiology 1989; 170:125–128.

Weishaupt D, Zanetti M, Hodler J, Boos N. MR imaging of the lumbar spine: prevalence of intervertebral disk extrusion and sequestration, nerve root compression, end plate abnormalities, and osteoarthritis of the facet joints in asymptomatic volunteers. Radiology 1998; 209:661–666.

Wiesel SW, Tsourmas N, Feffer HL, Critrin CM, Patronas N. A study of computer-assisted tomography I. The incidence of positive CAT scans in an asymptomatic group of patients. Spine 1984; 9:549–551.

Zarefsky D. Argumentation: The Study of Effective Reasoning. Chantilly, VA, The Teaching Company, 2001.

Zucherman J, Derby R, Hsu K, Picetti G, Kaiser J, Schofferman J, Goldthwaite N, White A. Normal magnetic resonance imaging with abnormal discography. Spine 1988; 13:1355–1359.

2 Epidural Steroid Injection

DONALD L. RENFREW

Definition

Epidural steroid injection is placement of steroids into the epidural space. This space separates the dura internally from the peridural membrane (the homologue of the periosteum on the interior of the vertebral canal) externally (Wiltse 1993). The epidural space extends from the base of the skull to the middle of the sacrum and continues along the spinal segmental nerves as the circumneural sheath (Wiltse 1993).

Literature Review

Thousands of patients undergo epidural steroid injections every year. Orthopedic spine surgeons, neurosurgeons, and other physicians from multiple specialties routinely request these injections. Patients allow and even seek epidural steroid injections. Many algorithms for treatment of sciatica and back pain include epidural steroid injection (Boden 1996). Epidural steroid injection has a role in the conservative management of many patients with sciatica and low back pain.

There is, however, some controversy regarding the efficacy of epidural steroid injection. There have been studies and studies of studies; one of the latter concludes that there is no conclusion (Koes 1995). Critics claim that the efficacy of epidural steroid injection has never been proven. How can the seemingly straightforward issue of whether epidural steroid injection improves pain generate such controversy? In this section, I review the existing literature and give my opinions regarding the merits and conclusions of published studies.

Early studies of epidural injection used saline (Davidson 1961), saline and anesthetic (Daly 1970, Evans 1930, Kelman 1944), and anesthetic and steroids (Burn 1970, Goldie 1968, Heyse-Moore 1978, Swerdlow 1970, Warr 1972). These studies usually measured self-reported pain response days, weeks, or months after injection. These studies reported success rates of 23% (Goldie 1968) to 81% (Heyse-Moore 1978), and many of the experimenters expressed enthusiasm about their results. However, there is a legitimate criticism of these studies. Although exceptions abound, most of the time back pain, even chronic back pain, will improve regardless of treatment. One way to overcome this shortcoming when designing a study is to compare epidural steroid injection with another treatment. For

example, Coomes (1961) compared epidural injection of anesthetic (50 mL of procaine) with bedrest. He found that patients treated with epidural anesthetic recovered more quickly and more often demonstrated improvement of neurologic signs. Coomes did not inject the bedrest group of patients with any substance, however, so both the patients and Coomes knew which treatment the patients received. This study suffers from both possible bias on the part of the evaluator and the placebo effect on the part of the patients. Double-blind studies eliminate these problems.

Dilke, Burry, and Grahame published the first double-blind study of epidural steroid injection in 1973 (Dilke 1973). They reported the results of injecting 100 patients with sciatica with either 80 mg of methylprednisolone and 10 mL of saline in the epidural space (the experimental group) or with 1 mL of saline in the supraspinatus ligament (the control group). The experimental group requested less analgesic while in the hospital, self-reported less pain, and had significantly more members return to work at 3 months. The authors concluded, "This treatment seems to be a valuable adjunct to the management of lumbar nerve root compression syndromes associated with degenerative disc disease."

Snoek, Weber, and Jorgensen published a double-blind study in 1977 with a different conclusion (Snoek 1977). They state, "Our results indicate that a single extradural injection of methylprednisolone (80 mg) is no more effective than a placebo injection in relieving chronic symptoms due to myelographically demonstrable lumbar disc herniation." Scrutiny of their paper leads me to disagree. The investigators randomly assigned patients to a control group, injected with 2 mL of saline, and an experimental group, injected with 80 mg of methylprednisolone. The investigators evaluated response to injection "48 ± 24 hours" after injection. Twenty-four hours is too soon for maximal effect from epidural steroid injection, and one cannot tell from reading the paper how many patients were evaluated at 24 hours versus 72 hours after injection. Furthermore, the investigators considered only dramatic improvements as any improvement at all: only if low back pain *disappeared* was it considered improved. Similarly, the investigators considered "impulse pain" (pain worsening with cough or sneeze) improved only if it disappeared, and analgesic consumption improved only if entirely eliminated. The investigators treated only radiating pain with some degree of leniency: they considered it improved if it disappeared *or* if it did not extend as far after injection. Using these extremely rigid criteria, the investigators report that there was "no statistically significant difference" between the control and experimental groups. Reviewing Table 2 of their paper, which reports the actual data from the study, it can be seen that relief of low back pain, relief of radiating pain, relief of impulse pain, relief of pain interfering with sleep, discontinuation of analgesic consumption, improvement noted by the physiotherapist, and improvement subjectively reported by the patient *all show a higher percentage in the treated group than in the control group.* Indeed, in the experimental group, patients were 1.53 to 3.53 times as likely to demonstrate improvement. Most categories showed at least twofold improvements, and the greatest difference was in the one category that did not require complete eradication of the symptom to be recorded as an improvement, namely relief of impulse pain. In other words, even using strict criteria and evaluating many patients before the optimal effect from steroids could be detected, this study shows that patients treated with steroid are twice as likely to demonstrate improvement of pain as patients receiving placebo. These differences were judged not "statistically significant." This study demonstrates a classic type II statistical error, or failure to reject the null hypothesis because of insufficient numbers of patients included in the study (Riegelman 1989). Virtually any of the comparisons between control and experimental groups presented in the data table, if increased by more patients and maintaining the same trends in data, would become statistically significant in favor of the group of patients treated with epidural steroid injection.

Cuckler and colleagues (1985) published another double-blind study that critics of epidural steroid injection frequently cite. The authors studied 73 patients; they injected 41 patients with 5 mL of 1% procaine and 80 mg of methylprednisolone in 2 mL of saline (the experimental group) and 32 patients with 5 mL of 1% procaine and 2 mL of saline (the control group). They measured short-term success at 24 hours and defined success as 75% or greater improvement in patient pain. However, not only is 24 hours too soon to measure the success of steroids (as noted earlier), but epidural local anesthetics alone may be associated with long-term pain relief (to *at least* 24 hours), and local anesthetics were given to both groups. Furthermore, although better than the complete pain relief required by the previously cited study, 75% improvement of pain is probably still too stringent a criterion: patients may be delighted with 50% reduction of pain. The authors recognized this problem themselves: they injected steroids in *any* patient who had achieved less than 50% pain relief at 24 hours. Long-term evaluation in this study is also perplexing. The authors again chose 75% relief as the criterion of "success" for injection, even though many patients would be pleased with lesser degrees of pain relief. Even raising the bar this high, injection succeeded for 26% of the experimental group and 15% of the "placebo" group at 13 to 30 months later, so members of the experimental group were 1.73 times more likely to have marked pain relief an average of 21 months after injection. There is no way to tell from the paper whether many additional patients achieved lesser but subjectively significant pain relief.

Ridley and colleagues published an additional double-blind study in 1988 documenting the effectiveness of epidural steroid injection in patients with sciatica (Ridley 1988). The investigators injected patients with either 10 mL of saline and 80 mg of methylprednisolone or 2 mL of saline. They found, using much less stringent criteria than the two other studies discussed, 17 of 19 or 90% of patients treated with steroid reported at least some improvement of pain, whereas only 3 of 16 or 19% of placebo patients improved.

Bush and Hillier published yet another double-blind prospective study in 1991 (Bush 1991). In this study, patients were randomized into groups receiving either 25 mL of saline or 25 mL of a solution containing 0.5% procaine hydrochloride and 80 mg of triamcinolone. The investigators measured subjective patient symptoms with a specially designed questionnaire and a visual analogue pain scale and objective signs with a straight-leg-raising test. They found all three aspects of patient evaluation significantly improved in the experimental group at 4 weeks.

Of the five double-blind, prospective studies just reviewed, then, the authors of three state that epidural injection provides significant patient benefit, measured by either subjective pain relief or objective measures of decreased analgesic consumption, decreased time of bedrest, return to work, or improved straight-leg raising. In the other two studies, the authors maintain that epidural steroid is of no benefit; however, as I have noted, the studies have significant design flaws, *despite which* data from the papers demonstrate at least some efficacy of epidural steroid injection. Why do many critics continue to claim that epidural steroid injection "does not work"? I believe that two factors make evaluation of epidural steroid injection (and hence, of epidural steroid injection studies) difficult.

First, back pain and sciatica is a symptom and not a specific diagnosis. Just as there are myriad causes of chest pain, many different entities cause back pain. A given patient may have three or four lesions, making correct assignment of a diagnosis challenging for even the most astute of clinicians and the most diligent of radiologists working in concert. If different lesions respond differently to epidural steroid injection (which we would expect), then unless patients are sorted prior to inclusion in a study, patients with nonresponding lesions will dilute out the salubrious effects on patients with responding lesions. We will find that some, but not all, patients improve after epidural steroid injection. In this regard, Rivest and colleagues have shown that only 38% of patients with spinal stenosis demonstrated improvement in pain scores at 2 weeks, compared with 61% of patients with herniated discs (Rivest 1998), and Ridley and colleagues noted that patients with "signs suggesting complete root palsy with motor, sensory, and reflex deficit" were more likely to demonstrate long-term benefit from epidural steroid injection (Ridley 1988). Furthermore, a given lesion may respond better earlier in its course, so that more patients achieve acceptable results if injected sooner rather than later. Heyse-Moore (1978) reported 81% success with acute pain versus 44% with chronic pain; Ridley and colleagues noted that patients with repeated episodes of sciatica tended to show a poorer long-term response; and Berman and colleagues (1984) found more favorable results in patients with pain of less than 3 months' duration.

Second, drug delivery is a problem: White and colleagues (1980) documented 25% to 30% inaccuracy in epidural placement when not using fluoroscopic guidance, and my colleagues and I (Renfrew 1991) have published results demonstrating that even experienced physicians confident of correct needle placement are inaccurate 15% of the time without use of fluoroscopy and contrast, and that less experienced physicians or difficult patients (or both) result in far less accuracy. This state of affairs may be responsible for an old rule of thumb suggesting a trial of three epidural steroid injections: with three injections, at least one should be correct in 90% to 99% of patients.[1] If epidural steroid injection is successful only for a subset of all patients, *and* if a substantial portion of those patients do not receive correct placement of the steroids, very few indeed may benefit from the procedure, and this could account for some minimization of differences between control and experimental groups noted in the referenced studies. In this regard, note that only Bush's study routinely used two injections, and that this study demonstrated statistically significant differences between the control and experimental groups despite having only 23 patients in the entire study. McNeill and colleagues (1995) published a prospective blinded study, which documented epidural placement of steroids in a special set of patients. They placed epidural steroids at the time of operation; patients operated on for lumbar spinal stenosis needed less analgesia after the operation, although patients operated on for a herniated disc did not. Similarly, Debi and colleagues (2002) found that patients with a steroid-soaked collagen sponge placed at the site of discectomy had statistically significantly less back pain in the postoperative period than those with a saline-soaked collagen sponge. Other controlled (Karppinen 2001a, Riew 2000) and uncontrolled (Wang 2002) studies of epidural steroid injection using fluoroscopic guidance and contrast injection have demonstrated a decreased necessity for surgery in the steroid group.

Considering all these factors, it is my conclusion that existing studies adequately document the efficacy of epidural steroid injection, and that additional studies on whether epidural steroid injections "work" or not are not necessary.

Placement of drugs within the epidural space is better than placement outside of the epidural space, and specific placement in proximity to the symptomatic lesion should be better yet. Most of the literature regarding the efficacy of epidural steroid injection (reviewed earlier) is based on blinded caudal or interlaminar injections. However, the transforaminal approach (Johnson 1999, Link 1998, Lutz 1998, Vad 2002) provides an alternative to caudal and interlaminar injections, which has the advantage of better targeting of foraminal and anterior lesions. Recently, directed controlled trials evaluating transforaminal epidural steroid injection (Karppinen 2001a, Karppinen 2001b, Riew 2000) showed a significant difference between patients treated with bupivacaine alone versus those treated with bupivacaine and

betamethasone who had radiographic findings of nerve root compression, using the outcome measure of whether the patient proceeded to surgery. Karppinen and colleagues (2001b), in another controlled trial, found a steroid/bupivacaine mixture superior to saline at avoiding operations, at least for what they termed "contained" disc herniations.

To summarize the literature regarding epidural steroid injection:

1. Multiple studies have demonstrated efficacy of epidural steroid injection. Studies that claim to disprove the efficacy of epidural steroid injection have many flaws, but even these studies, when closely analyzed, show benefit to those patients treated with epidural steroids.
2. Not all patients benefit from epidural steroid injection. Patients with short-term pain and who have not undergone operation tend to show more benefit, whereas patients with long-term pain are less likely to benefit. Some studies show patients with disc herniation demonstrating more benefit, whereas others show patients with lumbar stenosis demonstrating more benefit.
3. Despite possible measurable differences between *groups* of patients, it is very difficult to predict whether any *particular* patient may benefit from an epidural steroid injection. The best, and perhaps the only, way to determine whether a given patient with back or leg pain will benefit from epidural steroid injection is to perform epidural steroid injection on that patient. Having said this, if a single injection has been correctly performed (as described later) and is of no benefit, there is little reason to perform additional injections in the same manner unless the pain pattern or symptom-producing lesion is thought to have changed.
4. Optimal injection technique includes fluoroscopic guidance and nonionic contrast administration (Renfrew 1991, Stojanovic 2002, White 1980). The correct site and level must be approached based on the pain pattern, imaging studies, and results of prior injections. Documentation of the epidural needle tip (and hence drug) location via fluoroscopy is mandatory, and injection of nonionic contrast material should be performed unless there is a strong contraindication. Distribution of injected materials in the epidural space varies depending on needle position, contrast volume (Hogan 1999), and whether the patient has undergone prior surgery (Fredman 1999).
5. Correctly performed epidural steroid injections require a high level of knowledge, skill, and interest.

Rationale for Procedure

As noted in Chapter 1, Table 1–1, we assume, when performing diagnostic and therapeutic injection, that pain may be secondary to inflammation in proximity to nociceptors, and that such inflammation (and therefore associated pain) may respond to steroid injection. In addition to the clinical trials noted, there are animal data to support this concept (Hayashi 1998, Lee 1998). Innervated structures that may be reached by epidural steroid injection include the dorsal disc margin, dura, nerve roots, ganglia, spinal segmental nerves, pars interarticularis, laminae, and the anteromedial margins of the facet joints. Identification of the specific culprit lesion (based on the patient's pain pattern, imaging,

---

[1]Making the unreasonable assumption of independent assortment for the three tries, one would get $0.75 + 0.75 \times 0.75 + 0.75 \times 0.75 \times 0.75 = 98.4375\%$. Making the more reasonable assumption that if you did not get in the first time, you are only 50% likely to get in the second time, and if you fail in both the first two tries, you are only 25% likely to succeed on a third attempt, you will succeed at least once in 90.625% of cases.

and response to prior injections), and injection in proximity to that lesion (via an interlaminar, caudal, or transforaminal approach) maximizes the likelihood of success for epidural steroid injection.

Equipment and Supplies

Table 2–1 lists equipment required for epidural steroid injection.

A standard fluoroscope can be used for epidural steroid injection in a pinch, but this is usually a clumsy and inadequate substitute. A laser aiming device (an attachment that shows a cross-hair on the fluoroscopic screen corresponding in position to a red dot on the skin surface) is extremely helpful for proper needle placement. Selection of needle type varies with the operator; a 22-gauge spinal needle for most lumbar injections and a 25-gauge spinal needle for thoracic and cervical injections work well. These needles are inexpensive, are readily available, and can usually be inserted without prior local anesthetic. Some injectionists use glass syringes, but these are not required for the techniques described in this book. Everything injected into the patient must be as safe as possible and preferably safe for intrathecal use, since there will be occasions when, despite the utmost diligence on the part of the operator, some of the injected materials will reach the thecal sac. For this reason, nonionic contrast material approved for intrathecal injection, anesthetic approved for intrathecal injection (consult the package insert), and the most benign steroid obtainable should be used. In addition, if the contrast injection pattern suggests that the injection is intrathecal, it is usually best to stop injecting, abandon the procedure, and reschedule the patient for another day.

In addition to the equipment listed in Table 2–1, a crash cart should be readily available to handle medical emergencies (e.g., contrast and drug reactions).

Informed Consent Issues

For the purposes of discussion here, I divide informed consent issues into three sections: description of the procedure, warning the patient about possible drug side effects, and delineation of material risks. Informed consent also implies that a description of alternatives to the proposed treatment have been described; for a general description of such alternatives, see Chapter 1.

Either the performing physician or a trained subordinate should completely explain the entire procedure in detail to the patient prior to performance of the procedure. Patients who know what to expect are much less anxious than those fretting over what is coming next. A step-by-step description, including reassurance that the procedure takes only a few minutes, that many patients undergo a similar such procedure every day, and that the amount of pain caused by needle insertion is similar to that caused by drawing blood or starting an intravenous access line, provides a considerable calming effect on most patients.

The performing physician or a trained subordinate should also explain that local anesthetic may cause numbness of the buttocks or lower extremities or both (with interlaminar or caudal injections) or numbness and weakness of the leg (with transforaminal injection). I do not inject any anesthetic for cervical epidural steroid injections, because in my opinion the risks of injection outweigh the benefits. Patients should be warned that the injection may recreate or exacerbate their pain. While this side effect typically relents within moments of injection of local anesthetic, occasionally it will persist and even lead to patients declining further injections. Steroid side effects include changes in mood (usually mild euphoria but occasionally anxiety), appetite (usually increased), insomnia, sweating, hot flashes, facial flushing, rash, and gastrointestinal upset. We usually warn patients that they may "feel different" because of the steroids, and that this will usually go away in 1 to 3 days. Some patients benefit from medications to relieve anxiety or insomnia.

I divide complications into two categories: occasional (but inevitable) and rare but reported in the literature. Vasovagal reactions (treated with time, intravenous fluids, and atropine as necessary) and inadvertent thecal puncture constitute the first category. As noted earlier, any recognized thecal puncture should result in immediate removal of the needle and rescheduling of the procedure. Inadvertent injection of local anesthetic into the lumbar thecal sac usually results in a spinal block, urinary incontinence, and inability to move the lower extremities for the duration of the block. Inadvertent injection of steroid into the thecal sac will probably not result in such obvious immediate problems but carries the risk of arachnoiditis (Benzon 1986, Nelson 1973). Some patients who have had an inadvertent thecal puncture, as well as some who undergo myelography or diagnostic lumbar puncture, may develop a "post-tap headache." Treatment of such headaches includes bedrest, caffeine, pain killers, and an epidural "blood patch" (or saline injection) (Raskin 1990). The epidural blood patch is applied as indicated for an interlaminar epidural steroid injection, with injection of 10 to 15 mL of freshly drawn venous blood from the patient injected into the epidural space.

Less frequent but either reported or theoretical complications of epidural steroid injection are listed in Table 2–2. Patients should be off all anticoagulants and other agents that might increase the risk of epidural hematoma formation prior to performance of epidural injection. Note that cord injection with paralysis occurred when epidural steroid injection was performed in sedated patients (a practice I do not recommend), and that cervical cord infarction resulted from transforaminal injection in the cervical spine (another practice that I do not recommend). With respect to anaphylactic reaction, patients should be screened for

---

TABLE 2–1. Equipment and Supplies for Epidural Steroid Injection

C-arm fluoroscope
Surgical scrub
Needles
Syringes
Connecting tube
Nonionic contrast material
Anesthetic
Steroid (see Appendix 2)

TABLE 2–2. Reported or Theoretical Complications of Epidural Steroid Injection

Reported
Transient hypercorticism (Stambough 1984)
Epidural lipomatosis (Roy-Camille 1991)
Transient paralysis (McLain 1997)
Epidural abscess (Knight 1997, Mamourian 1993)
Epidural hematoma (Williams 1990)
Cord injection with paralysis in cervical injection (Hodges 1998)
Cord infarction and death from cervical transforaminal injection (Brouwers 2001)
Retinal hemorrhage with transient blindness (Victory 1991)
Paraplegia following transforaminal lumbar injection (Houten 2002)

Theoretical (but reported for other procedures)
Anaphylactic reaction to contrast material
Anaphylactic reaction to anesthetic
Anaphylactic reaction to steroid
Anaphylactic reaction to latex, surgical scrub solution, etc.

contrast sensitivity. If a patient has had a prior minor reaction to intravenous contrast material, either reassurance or oral prednisone prior to the procedure is advised. For prior major contrast reactions, the best option is probably to forego the procedure, since contrast is essential to avoid intrathecal injection, and since intrathecal injection of steroids may result in adhesive arachnoiditis, which is essentially incurable (Guyer 1989). Non-latex gloves and surgical scrubs without iodine can be used as appropriate.

After hearing of possible complications (however rare), patients may wish to reconsider or decline epidural steroid injection. In the interests of balancing these infrequent complications with the usual course of events, the performing physician or a trained subordinate may wish to review with the patient one or more of three large series in the literature. Waldman and colleagues (1989) reported on 790 consecutive cervical epidural steroid injections with six complications: two dural punctures requiring blood patches, three vasovagal reactions, and one delayed infection requiring incision and drainage. Johnson and colleagues (1999) reported on 5334 epidural steroid injections with 4 (0.07%) resulting in hospital or emergency room visits: one each for vasovagal response, transient hypotension, and epidural hematoma (not requiring surgical drainage), and one for transient tachycardia with hypertension; no patients suffered any permanent sequelae. Botwin and colleagues (2000) reported on 322 transforaminal injections with one vasovagal reaction, one case of intraoperative hypertension, and one transient elevation of blood sugar in an insulin-dependent diabetic patient, without any serious or permanent ill effects.

Patient Selection

In some clinics, physicians refer for pain management, and in these clinics the injecting physician must make the initial decision regarding whether to use diagnostic and therapeutic injection (including epidural steroid injection). In other clinics, patients will come with a prescription for epidural steroid injection in hand. In either scenario, the injectionist must take ultimate responsibility for the decision to undertake, and the performance of, the injection. As

discussed in Chapter 1 and in the above section on Literature Review, however, the indications for epidural steroid injection are vague and broad (back and/or leg pain; neck and/or arm pain), and the variability of human response patterns complicates evaluation of pain severity.

Once the decision to perform epidural steroid injection has been made, the decision to perform lumbar, thoracic, or cervical injection is relatively straightforward and based on the location of the dominant complaints.

For lumbar injections, possibilities include caudal, interlaminar, and transforaminal injection. To choose among these options, one must first establish, on the basis of available evidence, the most likely culprit lesion (e.g., herniated disc, degenerative disc disease, facet arthropathy, stenosis, pars defect). Distinction between axial, somatic referred, and radicular pain patterns (see Chapter 1) will refine the diagnosis. In some practices, a single injection is routinely performed; in others, it is routine to have patients return at weekly intervals until either the pain is adequately relieved or three injections have been performed, whichever comes first.

In those cases in which a single injection is to be performed, the injection should be chosen to deliver the maximal amount of drug to the putative culprit lesion. Generally, if there is midline backache or bilateral lower extremity symptoms and multilevel disease, broad-based anterior disc abnormality, or bilateral facet abnormality, the single injection will be interlaminar. In postoperative cases in which multilevel decompression has been done, injection directed at the site of prior laminectomies usually results in a wet tap because of either removal of the peridural membrane or scarring of the epidural membrane and adjacent tissue to the dura, so an interlaminar approach above or below the level of the surgery or a caudal approach below the level of the surgery is preferred. If there is a predominance of leg symptoms and a subarticular or foraminal disc herniation or subarticular or foraminal stenosis in the anatomically appropriate location, a transforaminal injection may be more appropriate.

In clinics where patients are scheduled for a series of visits, starting with an interlaminar injection offers the following benefits: (1) Patients often find transforaminal injections significantly more painful than interlaminar

TABLE 2–3. Step-by-Step Description of Lumbar Interlaminar Epidural Steroid Injection

1. Position the C-arm fluoroscope so that a clear view of the chosen interlaminar space is visualized.
2. Insert the needle along the course of the x-ray beam far enough so that it is anchored. Insertion should be through a skin site that has been prepped and draped in a sterile fashion.
3. Check position with the C-arm fluoroscope.
4. Adjust as necessary.
5. Move to lateral position and check position with the C-arm fluoroscope.
6. When the needle is just behind the spinal canal, inject 0.1 to 0.2 mL of nonionic contrast material and confirm position.
7. Unhook the connecting tube and draw 1 to 2 cm of air into the tube.
8. Reattach the connecting tube and advance the needle until the meniscus quivers.
9. Inject 2.0 to 3.0 mL of nonionic contrast material under fluoroscopic control.
10. Inject steroid and anesthetic agents and take frontal and lateral images.
11. Monitor for pain response and record percentage of pain relief at 30 minutes.
12. Release patient when stable. Provide patient with a telephone number to call if there is persistent or increased pain or numbness or if fever, swelling, or redness develops.

injections, and convincing the patient to return for a second injection is easier following an interlaminar injection than a transforaminal injection. (2) Some patients with predominant leg symptoms and associated appropriate culprit lesions still benefit more from interlaminar injections than transforaminal injections. (3) A transforaminal injection may be performed if an interlaminar injection offers little pain relief. (4) There is the remote risk of paraplegia with transforaminal injections (Houten 2002) (this has not been reported with interlaminar injections).

For thoracic injections, selection of the level and route of injection is more difficult. Identification of the culprit lesion, even with good imaging, is usually more difficult than in the lumbar spine. Enumeration of levels is complicated, particularly in the mid-thoracic region, where repeated fluoroscopy with markers is often necessary to document the level. Relatively broad laminae decrease the space available for interlaminar injections, whereas overlying ribs complicate transforaminal injection. In many patients, an interlaminar injection using a relatively steep angle of approach may form the best route of access.

For cervical injections, I currently use the interlaminar approach for all injections. I once used transforaminal injections and have performed many such injections without

complication, but after learning of multiple cases (more than 15 at present count) of quadriplegia or death (including one in my own community), I abandoned this procedure. Note that at least some of these complications do not appear to be the result of faulty needle placement: even with needle position in the posterior cervical neural foramen lateral to the vertebral canal, catastrophic consequences have ensued. This may be the result of small, unnamed radicular arteries within the posterior foramen that feed the spinal cord: injection of any of these end arteries would result in, at best, transient paralysis (with anesthetic) or permanent cell death (with particulate matter such as is found in steroid-containing solutions). While Hodges and colleagues (1998) have reported cervical spinal cord injection with the posterior approach, I believe that it would be virtually impossible to inject a damaging amount of material into the cord using the technique described in the following section.

Procedure Description

LUMBAR INTERLAMINAR EPIDURAL STEROID INJECTION

Table 2–3 describes and Figures 2–1, 2–2, and 2–3 illustrate lumbar interlaminar epidural steroid injection. Figure 2–2

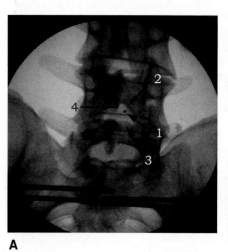

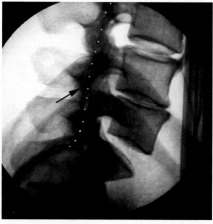

A   **B**

FIGURE 2–1

Skeletal Specimen Radiograph Demonstrating Target Position for Interlaminar Lumbar Epidural Steroid Injection. *A*, Frontal specimen radiograph with a metallic bead (arrow 1) taped between the inferior aspect of the right L4 lamina (arrow 2) and the superior aspect of the L5 lamina (arrow 3). The spinous process (arrow 4) is medial to the bead. Note that the C-arm has been rotated approximately 15 degrees to the right. This approach allows passage of the needle without traversing the interspinous ligament. There are two advantages to avoiding this structure: (1) It is more innervated than the adjacent musculature and soft tissues, and avoiding it decreases the patient's pain; and (2) tactile feedback is extremely blunted once the needle is in the interspinous ligament. With the needle off midline, the difference between the dorsal musculature, fat, and perifascial tissues and the ligamentum flavum is (at least with experience) easily palpable, decreasing the likelihood of inadvertent puncture of the thecal sac. (The metallic bars through the pelvis hold the sacrum and pelvis together in this specimen.) Note that by convention, radiographs will be viewed as if "from the rear" so that the right side of the specimen (or patient) will be to the viewer's right and the left will be to the viewer's left. The opposite prevails for cross-sectional imaging studies: on axial computed tomography or magnetic resonance imaging studies, the patient's right side is displayed on the viewer's left and vice versa. *B*, Lateral view with the metallic bead (arrow) faintly seen posteriorly. The posterior margin of the spinal canal is marked with a series of white dots.

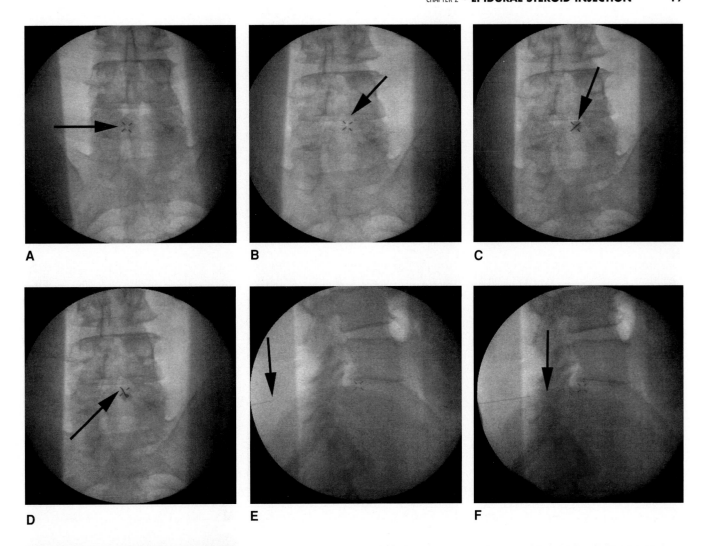

A   B   C

D   E   F

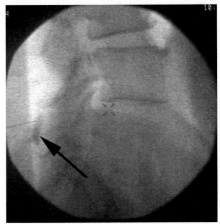

G

FIGURE 2–2

Step-by-Step Lumbar Interlaminar Epidural Steroid Injection. The patient was a 50-year-old man with right-sided low back pain and degenerative disc disease at the L4-5 level. *A,* Frontal fluoroscopic view as the fluoroscopic monitor is first turned on. The cross-hairs of the laser aiming device (arrow) is on the left L5 laminae. *B,* The fluoroscope has been moved so that the laser-aiming device is between the inferior margin of the L4 lamina (arrow) and the superior margin of the L5 lamina. *C,* A 22-gauge spinal needle has been placed into the patient's body using the dot of light created by the laser-aiming device as a target. The needle tip was placed on the patient's skin and the hub positioned to intercept the light so that the needle was ideally positioned down the central ray of the C-arm. The hub of the needle shows up as a faint radiopacity (arrow), whereas the metallic portion of the needle lines up with the cross-hairs. *D,* The needle has been advanced. The tip (arrow) is tracking toward midline. *E,* The fluoroscope has been moved to a lateral position. The needle tip (arrow) is well posterior to the posterior-most aspect of the spinal canal. *F,* The needle has been advanced anteriorly. However, the needle tip is still posterior to the estimated posterior aspect of the spinal canal (arrow). *G,* A small amount (0.1–0.2 mL) of contrast material has been injected, which pools around the needle tip (arrow) and which is clearly not within the epidural space. At this point, the connecting tube is unhooked from the needle and 1 to 2 cm of air is drawn into the connecting tube. The tube is then reattached and the needle is advanced. Careful attention is paid to the tactile sensation on the end of the needle, which will feel like it is entering the rubber stopper of a bottle upon engaging the ligamentum flavum. A slight quiver of the meniscus at the interface between the air and the contrast material in the connecting tube will occur as the needle tip enters the epidural space. With each advance of 0.5 to 1.0 mm of the needle, gentle pressure on the syringe plunger should result in the meniscus "bouncing," or returning to its original position following release of pressure. Loss of this bouncing indicates probable location in the epidural space.

(figure continues on following page)

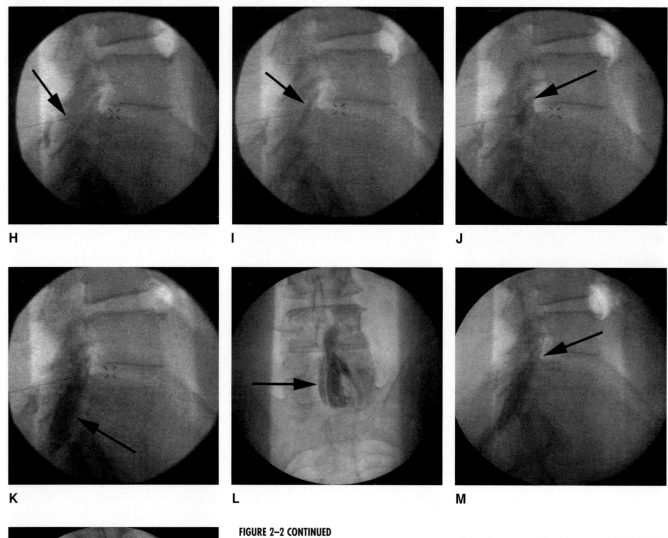

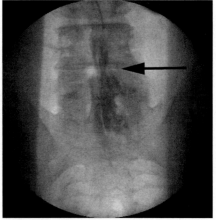

FIGURE 2–2 CONTINUED

H, Position of the needle tip (arrow) at the time of slight motion of the contrast-air interface. *I*, Injection of 0.1 to 0.2 mL of contrast material shows flow within the epidural space (arrow). *J*, Additional injection demonstrates more anterior flow within the epidural space (arrow). *K*, Yet more injection demonstrates inferior flow within the epidural space (arrow). *L*, Return to frontal fluoroscopic position demonstrates contrast within the epidural space (arrow) inferior to the needle location at L4-5. *M*, Lateral view taken after injection of contrast, steroid, and anesthetic demonstrates contrast material along the dorsal margin of the target L4-5 intervertebral disc (arrow). *N*, Frontal view taken after injection of contrast material, steroid, and anesthetic demonstrates contrast material both superior and inferior to the target L4-5 intervertebral disc (arrow).

illustrates an epidural injection with particularly successful results. For such an injection, our typical case report includes several sections. After demographics and examination information, including a list of specific procedures performed for coding purposes, the report consists of an introduction, technical information, interpretation, and conclusion sections. The introduction presents a brief summary of the patient's symptoms and related imaging abnormalities. The technical information section includes a description of the procedure, including a description of specific injected materials. The conclusion section includes a listing of what was done and what is planned.

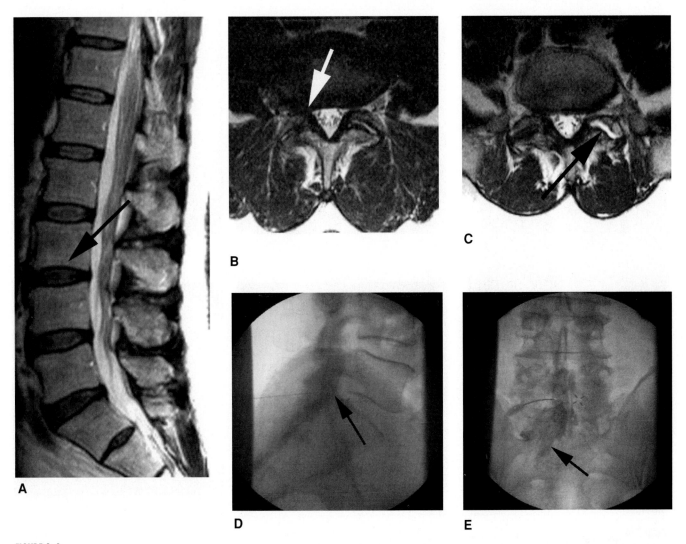

FIGURE 2–3

Interlaminar Epidural Steroid Injection with Excellent Relief of Pain Following a Single Injection. This 64-year-old man had low back and left leg pain. *A*, Sagittal T2-weighted magnetic resonance imaging scan demonstrates mild disc dehydration and disc bulging of the lower lumbar discs and most pronounced at L3-4 (arrow), without disc extrusion or neural compression. *B*, Axial T1-weighted magnetic resonance imaging scan shows degenerative disc bulging. There is a 2 to 3 mm disc protrusion along the right subarticular and foraminal aspect of the disc margin (arrow), with associated right subarticular recess narrowing. *C*, Axial T2-weighted image at the L5-S1 level shows asymmetric facet joint arthropathy with a right joint effusion. No associated synovial cyst or neural compression is seen. *D*, Lateral examination taken during epidurography shows contrast material in the epidural space centered at the L5-S1 level (arrow). *E*, Frontal examination demonstrates a needle placed from the left side to the L5-S1 level, with more flow along the left L5 and S1 (arrow) nerves than along the same structures on the right. For a complete report on this injection, see text.

For the epidural steroid injection illustrated in Figure 2–3, the report reads as follows:

INTRODUCTION

The patient describes relatively typical left S1 radicular pain with buttock, posterior thigh, and posterior calf and heel pain. Magnetic resonance imaging examination demonstrates multilevel degenerative disease with no large disc extrusion or severe neural compression. There is subarticular recess narrowing at L5-S1, but this appears to be more pronounced on the right (asymptomatic) side.

TECHNICAL INFORMATION

Informed consent was obtained. Using sterile technique and fluoroscopic guidance, a 22-gauge spinal needle was placed into the epidural space at the left L5-S1 level via an interlaminar approach. Confirmation of needle tip position within the epidural space was established via loss of resistance to flow and fluoroscopic visualization of contrast material in the epidural space. A total of 2 mL of nonionic contrast material was injected. This was followed by 2 mL of triamcinolone 40 mg/mL and 2.0 mL of 0.5% bupivacaine. The needle was removed. The patient tolerated the procedure well.

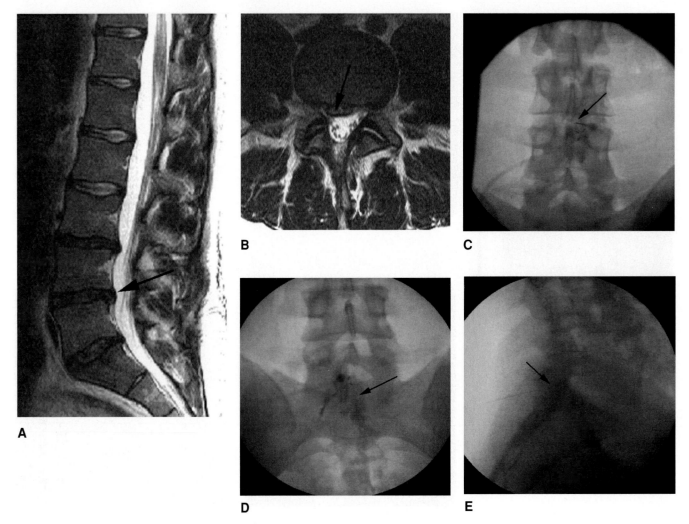

FIGURE 2–4

Interlaminar Injection Below the Level of Prior Surgery Resulting in No Pain Relief, with Subsequent Injection Above the Level of Surgery Providing Excellent Pain Relief. This 30-year-old man was 2 years status post L4-5 microdiscectomy. The patient's right leg pain was relieved following surgery but he had ongoing and increasing central low back pain. *A*, Sagittal T2-weighted magnetic resonance imaging scan demonstrates L3-4, L4-5, and L5-S1 disc dehydration. There is a 6 mm disc protrusion at L4-5 (arrow). *B*, Axial T2-weighted magnetic resonance imaging scan demonstrates the 6 mm protrusion (arrow) in a central and right-central subarticular position. *C*, Frontal view from initial interlaminar lumbar epidural steroid injection demonstrates the needle tip (arrow) to be at the L3-4 level, above the postoperative site. Contrast flows in the epidural space both superior and inferior from the needle tip. The patient received little pain relief from this injection. *D*, Frontal view from a subsequent interlaminar lumbar epidural steroid injection done at the L5-S1 level. Because of concern for scarring at the L4-5 level and an associated inadvertent lumbar puncture and the lack of response to the L3-4 injection, an L5-S1 injection was performed. Contrast flows predominantly inferiorly within the epidural space (arrow). *E*, Lateral view shows the needle tip at the L5-S1 level, with contrast material flowing proximally and distally from the injection site within the epidural space. The patient had good relief of pain with the L5-S1 injection.

INTERPRETATION

Frontal and lateral films demonstrate contrast distribution within the epidural space. There is proximal and distal, circumferential, and bilateral contrast distribution. Contrast material appears to have reached the target location. The patient experienced reproduction of typical symptoms upon injection. Immediate response to injected local anesthetic was 100% pain relief.

CONCLUSION

1. Technically successful lumbar interlaminar epidurography with injection of nonionic contrast material, local anesthetic, and steroid.

2. The interlaminar approach appears to work well for this patient based on the contrast distribution pattern, reproduction of typical pain, and complete relief of pain with local anesthetic. If he does not get good relief of pain from the interlaminar approach, however, a left S1 transforaminal injection could be performed. This would be done more on the basis of symptoms than on the basis of imaging abnormality, since no dominant lesion along S1 is identified on a recent MRI examination.

Figure 2–4 shows an example of a patient who achieved little pain relief from an initial interlaminar injection performed above the level of prior surgery, with good relief following injection below the level of prior surgery. Figure 2–5 shows an example of asymmetric flow, with poor pain relief from a right-sided injection followed by much better relief of pain from a left-sided injection.

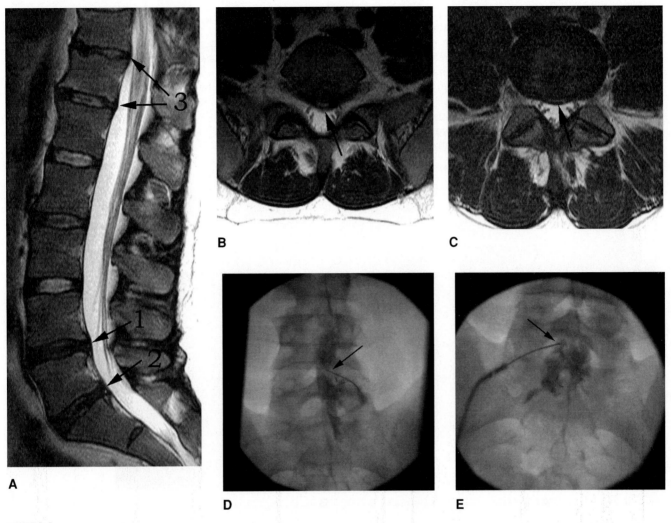

FIGURE 2–5

Asymmetric Flow of Injected Materials, with Better Pain Relief by Contralateral Injection. This 26-year-old man had low back and left leg pain. *A,* Sagittal T2-weighted magnetic resonance imaging scan demonstrates degenerative dehydration and bulging with a small disc protrusion at L4-5 (arrow 1) and L5-S1 (arrow 2). In addition, there is disc narrowing and irregularity of the endplates at the T11-12 and T12-L1 levels. The term *juvenile discogenic disease* has been applied to the coexistence of Scheuermann's disease and lower lumbar degenerative changes (Heithoff 1994). *B,* Axial T2-weighted magnetic resonance imaging scan at the L5-S1 level shows a central disc protrusion mildly indenting the thecal sac (arrow), along with T2 prolongation of the dorsal disc annulus (high intensity zone). *C,* Axial T2-weighted magnetic resonance imaging scan at the L4-5 level shows a similar appearance with a small central disc protrusion (arrow) and accompanying T2 prolongation. No significant neural compression is identified on the magnetic resonance imaging study. *D,* Frontal view following injection at the L4-5 level on the right. Contrast flows from the needle tip (arrow) in both cranial and caudal directions but is predominantly right-sided within the spinal canal. The patient achieved little pain relief following this injection. *E,* Frontal view during subsequent injection performed one week later from the left side at L5-S1 shows the needle tip (arrow) and excellent flow bilaterally within the epidural space. The patient had much better pain relief following this injection.

TABLE 2–4. Problems Encountered During Lumbar Interlaminar Epidural Steroid Injection

Definite intrathecal injection (see Fig. 2–6)
Possible intrathecal injection (see Fig. 2–7)
Posterior injection (see Fig. 2–8)
Venous injection (see Fig. 2–9)
Inadvertent discogram (see Fig. 2–10)
Epimembranous injection (see Figs. 2–11 and 2–12)
Pars defect injection (see Fig. 2–13)
Intra-articular facet joint injection (see Fig. 2–14)
Plica mediana dorsalis (see Fig. 2–15)
Lack of flow past an area of stenosis (see Fig. 2–16)
Peculiar flow pattern along the circumneural sheaths (see Fig. 2–17).

Table 2–4 lists difficulties that may be encountered during lumbar interlaminar epidural steroid injection. With regard to these various difficulties, note the following:

DEFINITE INTRATHECAL INJECTION

See Figure 2–6. The best course of action, as noted previously, is to terminate the procedure and reschedule for another day.

POSSIBLE INTRATHECAL INJECTION

In young patients, the epidural space may have a particularly smooth and even flow pattern (Fig. 2–7). Generally,

intrathecal injections show a thin line of very dense contrast along the anterior-most aspect of the thecal sac (see
Fig. 2–6). Contrast material in a young person's epidural
space tends to blur out over a wider area. If there is any
doubt, refrain from injecting anesthetic or steroid agents. If
available, a computed tomography scan done following
injection (see Fig. 2–7) will document the exact location of
contrast material, and if the patient returns for additional
injections, these may be performed with confidence that the
injected material is within the epidural space.

POSTERIOR INJECTION

Occasionally, contrast material will flow readily away
from the tip of the needle even though one is not within
the vertebral canal (Fig. 2–8). When this happens, the
pattern will usually be recognized as incorrect once 1.0 to
1.5 mL of nonionic contrast material has been injected,
at which time advance of the needle tip will usually bring
it into the epidural space for an otherwise uneventful
injection.

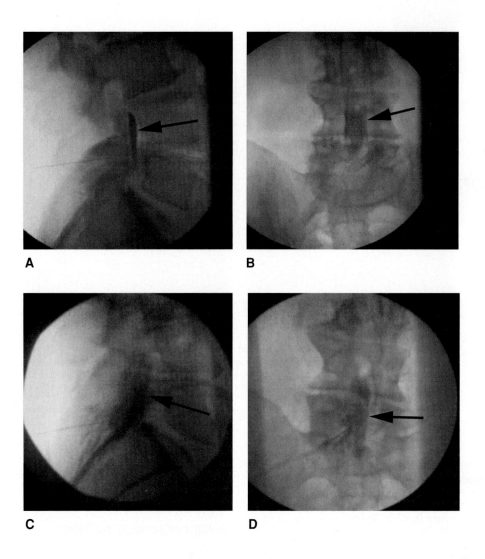

A

B

C

D

FIGURE 2–6

Wet Tap with Procedure Repeated 1 Week Later. This 62-year-old man had low back and bilateral leg pain with multilevel degenerative disc disease and
L5-S1 degenerative spondylolisthesis on magnetic resonance imaging. *A,* Lateral view demonstrates intrathecal contrast (arrow). Note that the contrast
material flows well away from the needle tip (in the posterior spinal canal). B. Frontal view also demonstrates intrathecal contrast material (arrow),
although on this view it is more difficult to make a distinction between intrathecal and epidural injection. The procedure was terminated at this time, and
the patient was informed that a spinal tap headache might result. He was instructed to remain relatively horizontal for the next 24 hours. No headache
resulted. He returned 1 week later for injection. C. Lateral view taken 1 week later shows typical epidural injection pattern (arrow). *D,* Frontal view shows
epidural contrast material. While the distinction between intrathecal and epidural injection is more difficult to make on the frontal view, note that a
relatively complete plica mediana dorsalis stops contrast material from flowing past the midline (arrow), something that would not happen with an
intrathecal injection.

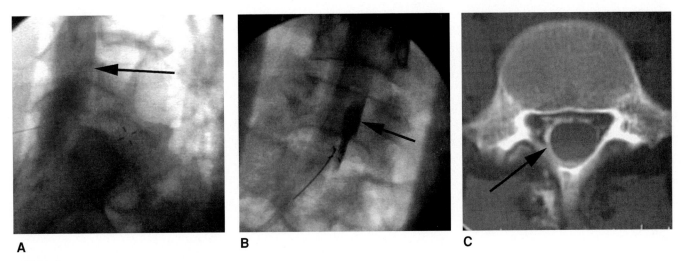

A   B   C

FIGURE 2–7

Possible Intrathecal Injection on Fluoroscopic Imaging. This 25-year-old woman with an L5-S1 disc extrusion and back and right leg pain underwent lumbar interlaminar injection at the L5-S1 level. *A,* Lateral view demonstrates the needle projecting in the posterior aspect of the vertebral canal and very even distribution of contrast material (arrow). *B,* Frontal view also shows a very uniform distribution of contrast material within the vertebral canal. Such an appearance is worrisome for an intrathecal injection, although no nerve roots are visualized. Note the particular density of contrast material near the needle tip (arrow), which favors an epidural location for at least some of the contrast material. *C,* Computed tomographic scan obtained immediately after the procedure confirms that the contrast material is peripherally located (arrow), external to the thecal sac and within the epidural space.

FIGURE 2–8

Initially Posterior Injection Corrected into an Epidural Location. This 38-year-old man had low back and intermittent leg pain and underwent lumbar interlaminar epidural steroid injection at L5-S1. *A,* Lateral view demonstrates contrast projecting along the posterior margin of the vertebral canal (arrow). The contrast material appears to be relatively free flowing. *B,* Frontal view demonstrates a right-sided, relatively loculated collection of contrast material with somewhat "feathered" edges, suggesting a soft tissue or perifascial injection (arrow). *C,* Repeat lateral view after needle advancement and additional contrast injection demonstrates a much more typical appearance of contrast within the epidural space (arrow). *D,* Repeat frontal view also demonstrates a much more typical appearance of epidural contrast flow (arrow). The initially injected and more posteriorly located contrast material is seen near the needle tip.

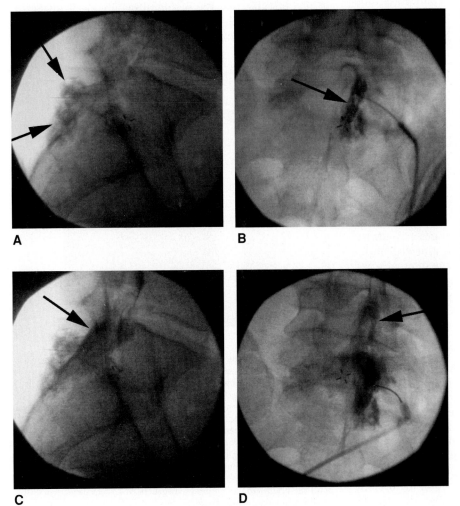

A   B

C   D

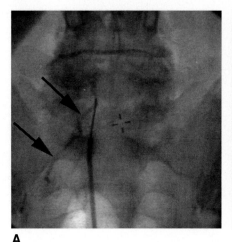

A

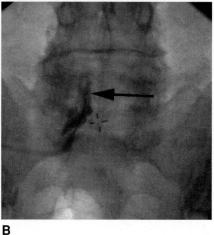

B

FIGURE 2–9

Venous Injection. This 77-year-old man had low back pain and degenerative spondylolisthesis. *A,* Frontal view demonstrates flow of contrast material along a tubular structure (arrows). This collection of contrast material was evanescent. *B,* Repeat frontal view after adjustment of needle tip and further injection of contrast material shows a typical epidural injection pattern (arrow).

VENOUS INJECTION

Venous injection occurs in interlaminar injections, with rates ranging from 2% (Sullivan 2000) to 8% (Furman 2000). Such injection is not necessarily accompanied by venous backflow into the needle hub or connecting tube. The typical evanescent tubular filling within the venous system, however, is usually readily recognized (Fig. 2–9).

INADVERTENT DISCOGRAM

It is difficult, but possible, to inadvertently perform discography when performing interlaminar epidural steroid injection (Fig. 2–10). This is unlike the case with transforaminal epidural steroid injection when there is a large foraminal disc extrusion, wherein inadvertent discography occurs much more frequently (see later).

EPIMEMBRANOUS INJECTION

Explanation of this particular problem requires a somewhat lengthy aside. The term *epimembranous* is a neologism for that space between the peridural membrane internally and the inner aspect of the vertebral canal (vertebral body, laminae, facet joints, and ligamentum flavum) externally. The peridural membrane was described by Wiltse and colleagues (1993) and is the homologue of the periosteum on the interior of the vertebral canal. Wiltse and colleagues recommend that the epidural space be defined as between the peridural membrane and the dura. Analogous to separate compartments between the dura and arachnoid (subdural) and arachnoid and pia (subarachnoid), we have compartments between the peridural membrane and dura (epidural) and vertebral canal margins and peridural membrane (epimembranous). This space is the location of the anterior fluid collections that occasionally accompany disc herniations (Chiba 2001, Gundry 1993). The anatomy of this space, which includes a central septum in the midline and which is tethered at the level of the disc, dictates the

radiographic appearance of disc herniations and tumors (Schellinger 1996). While Wiltse and colleagues imply that the peridural membrane is continuous along the interior of the vertebral canal around its circumference, Hogan (1991) states that the peridural membrane only exists anteriorly. It is also possible that the peridural membrane is always or nearly always well developed anteriorly but inconstantly developed posteriorly.

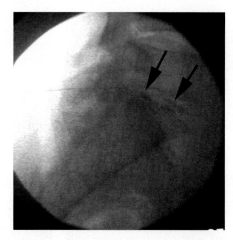

FIGURE 2–10

Inadvertent Discogram. This 60-year-old, 320-pound man with degenerative disc disease and spinal canal stenosis presented for epidural steroid injection. *A,* Lateral view during injection. When advancing the needle, it was very difficult to see the needle tip even with maximum radiographic technique. The usual "meniscal quiver" did not occur when the needle was advanced. When the needle appeared as if it was certainly within the posterior spinal canal, pressure was applied to the syringe and the needle was slowly advanced. The first flow of contrast material, surprisingly, was not within the posterior epidural space, nor the thecal sac, nor even the anterior epidural space, but within the disc. The patient's combination of spinal stenosis and degenerative disc bulging caused a lack of contrast flow until the needle tip was within the degenerated L5–S1 intervertebral disc, resulting in a discogram (arrows).

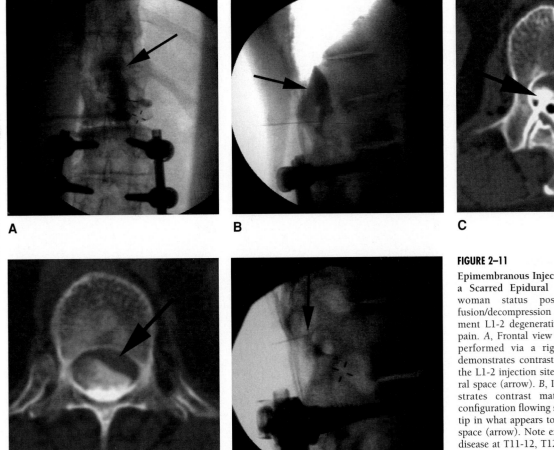

FIGURE 2–11

Epimembranous Injection versus Injection into a Scarred Epidural Space. This 70-year-old woman status post L2 through sacral fusion/decompression surgery had adjacent segment L1-2 degenerative disc disease and back pain. *A,* Frontal view from the initial injection performed via a right-sided L1-2 approach demonstrates contrast tracking superiorly from the L1-2 injection site, apparently in the epidural space (arrow). *B,* Initial lateral view demonstrates contrast material in a lens-shaped configuration flowing superiorly from the needle tip in what appears to be the posterior epidural space (arrow). Note extensive degenerative disc disease at T11-12, T12-L1, and L1-2. Following the injection, the patient had exacerbation of her usual back pain that persisted for more than 2 hours. At that point, repeat fluoroscopic examination demonstrated persistence of contrast material at the injection site, and a computed tomographic scan was obtained. *C,* Axial computed tomographic study at the level of the L1 pedicles demonstrates loculated contrast material along with a small air bubble along the posterolateral, right aspect of the spinal canal (arrow). The thecal sac is compressed anterolaterally. *D,* Axial computed tomography study at the level of the T12 pedicle demonstrates even more compression of the thecal sac (arrow). At this point, the patient was returned to the fluoroscopy unit, with aspiration of the injected material. *E,* Lateral view at the end of aspiration of injected material. The needle tip projects into the spinal canal (arrow). Approximately 3 mL of material was aspirated, with little or no visible contrast remaining after aspiration. The patient had immediate pain relief of the new pain that accompanied the initial injection.

Figure 2–11 illustrates an "epidural injection," wherein the injected material collected in a loculated bolus and did not spread to the anterior aspect of the vertebral canal. Whether this injection indeed represents injectate splitting the bony and soft tissue walls of the vertebral canal and the peridural membrane, or a subdural injection between the dura and arachnoid, or even simply represents a pronounced loculation within the epidural space, is not possible to say (even with computed tomographic examination). The clinical consequences of the injection illustrated in Figure 2–11, however, were unfavorable: the patient had persistent severe back pain at the site of the injection for 2 hours despite narcotics. The patient's pain relented within seconds of aspiration of the injected material. Figure 2–12 demonstrates a different case in which the initial contrast material flow suggested a sharply defined, loculated pocket and where advancing the needle 1 to 2 mm resulted in a typical epidural injection pattern, presumably resulting from changing the position of the needle tip from epimembranous to epidural.

PARS DEFECT INJECTION

If the existence of a posterior epimembranous space is questionable, then its relationship to pars defects is even more so. However, a space is occasionally encountered that may connect to one or both pars defects (Fig. 2–13). McCormick and colleagues (1989) described this space as "retrodural," and it does appear to be at least partially within the spinal canal but not epidural, leaving the epimembranous space (as defined above) as the only option. However, while part of the contrast material injected in these cases flows into the pars defects and part flows along the inner margin of the vertebral canal, material also appears to flow into a confined space posterior to the spinal canal.

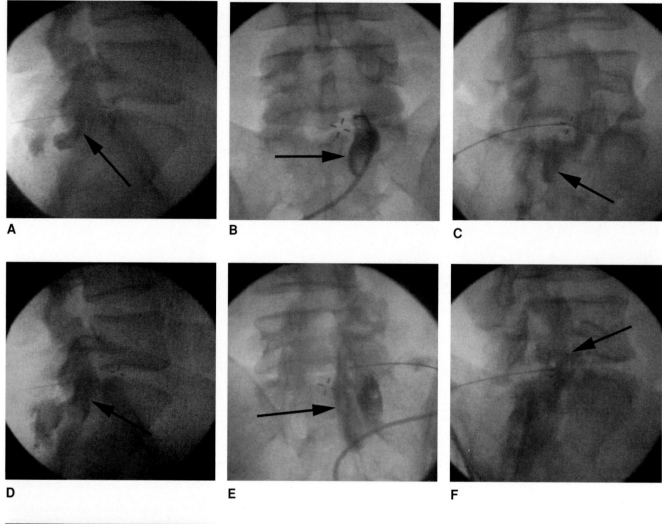

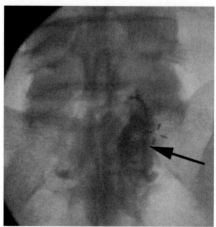

FIGURE 2–12

Epimembranous Injection versus Intra-Articular Injection, Converted to Epidural Injection. This 39-year-old man with low back pain and multilevel degenerative disc disease had received good pain relief in the past from epidural steroid injection. He returned for additional injection. *A,* Lateral fluoroscopic view obtained as contrast material appeared to flow freely into the spinal canal (arrow). Note the more posterior collection of contrast material from prior trial injection in the posterior perifascial tissues. *B,* Frontal view demonstrates that the needle tip is somewhat lateral to midline. Contrast dissects inferiorly from the point of injection (arrow). The contrast pattern in this view suggests possible intra-articular injection into the right L5-S1 facet joint. *C,* An oblique view, however, fails to demonstrate a convincing arthrogram, with no thin line of contrast into the superior margin of the joint. Furthermore, there is contrast material projecting well below what should be the inferior margin of the joint (arrow). *D,* Return to the lateral projection with advancement of the needle tip 1 to 2 mm resulted in flow of contrast material away from the needle tip inferiorly (arrow), in a configuration much more typical of a epidural injection. *E,* A left posterior oblique view demonstrates two distinct contrast collections, the first located lateral to the second (arrow). *F,* A right posterior oblique view also demonstrates the two contrast collections. Note the lack of any contrast material in the right L5-S1 facet joint, arguing against an intra-articular position of the needle tip on the original injection. *G,* Final frontal view demonstrates a typical epidurogram, with the initial injection of contrast material still collected inferolaterally on the right (arrow).

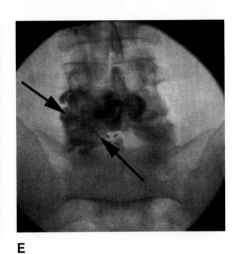

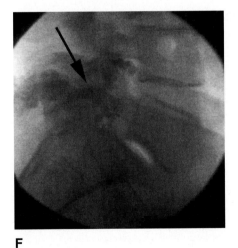

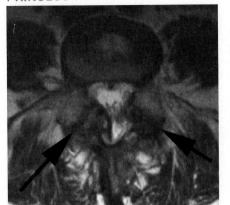

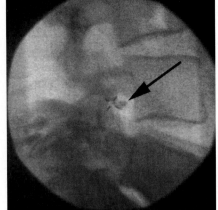

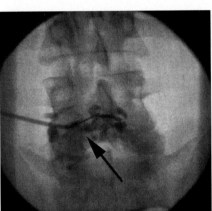

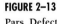

FIGURE 2–13

Pars Defects Injection via Interlaminar Injection. This 55-year-old man had known lytic spondylolisthesis with L5-S1 right foraminal stenosis and leg numbness and pain. *A*, Sagittal T2-weighted magnetic resonance imaging scan demonstrates a forward slip of L5 (arrow) on S1 along with degenerative loss of disc height and hydration at L5-S1 (and also at T11-12 and T12-L1). *B*, Axial T2-weighted magnetic resonance imaging scan demonstrates bilateral pars defects with fibroproliferative changes (arrows) as well as anteroposterior elongation of the vertebral canal. *C*, Lateral study performed after injection following loss of resistance to flow demonstrates ill-defined posterior contrast, as well as contrast projecting within the vertebral canal (arrow). *D*, Frontal view taken after injection of 2 to 3 mL of contrast material demonstrates flow along the left laminae (arrow) and laterally into the left L5 pars defect. *E*, Further contrast injection appears to collect predominantly in and around the left pars defect (arrows), without free flow into the epidural space. *F*, Final lateral view demonstrates contrast in the pars defect (arrow). Note the L5-S1 lytic spondylolisthesis.

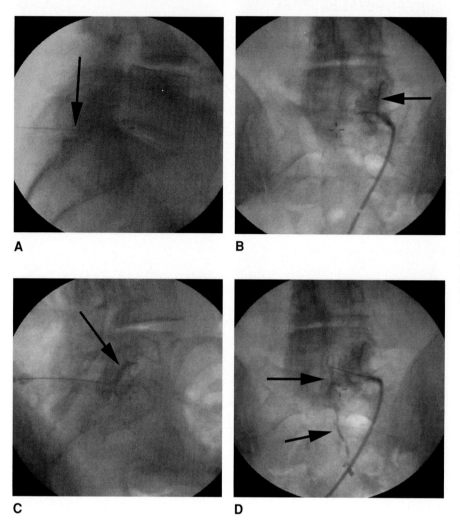

A

B

C

D

FIGURE 2–14

Facet Joint Injection During Interlaminar Lumbar Injection. This 82-year-old woman had multilevel spinal stenosis and low back and right leg pain. L2-3 through L4-5 had poor access, with degenerative spondylolisthesis at L4-5, so an L5-S1 interlaminar approach was taken. *A,* Initial lateral examination just after contrast material began to flow demonstrates the needle tip in the posterior spinal canal (arrow) with little evidence of contrast at this time. *B,* Frontal examination demonstrates a relatively central position of the needle tip and contrast flow away from the needle tip toward the right lateral aspect of the vertebral canal. In addition, there is a well-defined linear band of contrast material, suggesting an arthrogram on the right side (arrow). *C,* A right posterior oblique view demonstrates a definite right L5-S1 arthrogram (arrow). *D,* Frontal view following repositioning of the needle tip demonstrates epidural flow of contrast material, which appears to preferentially fill a middle to lower sacral circumneural sheath (arrows).

FACET JOINT INJECTION

On occasion, contrast material will spread from a relatively midline point of injection into an ipsilateral facet joint (Fig. 2–14). This may represent either communication of the facet joint with the posterior epimembranous space or inadvertent puncture of a distended facet joint capsule (or synovial cyst). This problem usually arises when the needle is relatively far from the midline.

PLICA MEDIANA DORSALIS

Occasionally, the epidural space is separated into right and left components by the plica mediana dorsalis (Luyendjik 1976). Injection between laminae on the right will result in spread within the right half of the epidural space, whereas injection on the left will result in spread within the left half of the epidural space (Fig. 2–15). Since prior to injection, there is no way to predict whether a given individual will

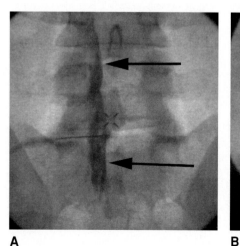

A

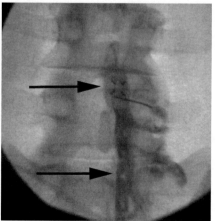

B

FIGURE 2–15

Complete Plica Mediana Dorsalis. This 44-year-old man had low back pain, occasionally worse on the right and occasionally worse on the left. *A,* Frontal view of L5-S1 interlaminar injection from slightly to the left of midline resulted in exclusively left-sided contrast material secondary to a complete and intact plica mediana dorsalis (arrows). *B,* Subsequent right L4-5 interlaminar injection done 1 week later again demonstrates a complete plica mediana dorsalis (arrows) and exclusively right-sided contrast material.

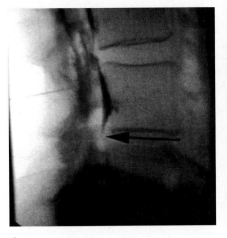

A

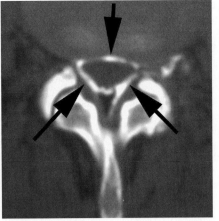

B

FIGURE 2–16

Poor Flow Past an Area of Stenosis. This 69-year-old woman had low back and bilateral leg pain and weakness with degenerative spondylolisthesis and vertebral canal stenosis at L4-5. *A,* Lateral study shows contrast above the L4-5 level with no flow inferior to this level. *B,* Axial computed tomographic scan at the L3-4 level subsequent to injection shows abundant contrast material in the epidural space (arrows). *C,* Axial computed tomographic scan at the L4-5 level subsequent to injection shows a paucity of contrast material in the epidural space (arrows). *D,* Axial computed tomographic scan at the L5-S1 level subsequent to injection shows no contrast material in the epidural space (arrows).

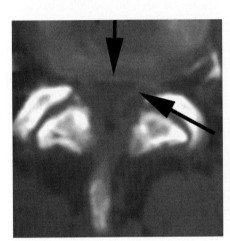

C

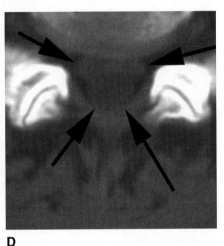

D

have a well-developed and intact plica mediana dorsalis, it makes sense to inject on the side of the culprit lesion when performing epidural steroid injections.

LACK OF FLOW PAST AN AREA OF STENOSIS

Injection above or below an area of spinal canal stenosis may lead to a lack of injectate reaching the side opposite the injection (Fig. 2–16). If the patient continues to have pain following injection on one side of a relatively complete block, subsequent injection on the other side of the block may provide better pain relief.

PECULIAR FLOW PATTERNS

Interlaminar injection into the epidural space may occasionally lead to preferential flow into the circumneural sheaths (Fig. 2–17). Such flow patterns may prevent the steroid from reaching a target lesion, and injection along a different route may prove beneficial.

FIGURE 2–17

Peculiar Flow Pattern Along Circumneural Sheath. This 83-year-old man had osteoporosis and multilevel degenerative disease with low back pain. *A,* Lateral examination after injection via a left interlaminar L3-4 approach shows a small amount of contrast material in the posterior spinal canal (arrow). *B,* Frontal view demonstrates contrast material flowing predominantly along the left L3 circumneural sheath (arrow). The patient had new left hip and groin pain, and no relief of back pain, following the injection.

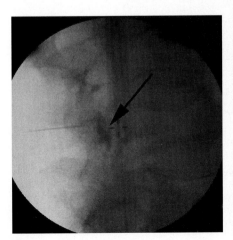

A

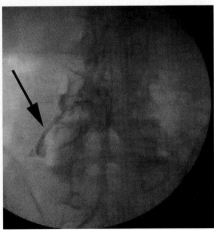

B

TABLE 2–5. Step-by-Step Description of L1–5 Transforaminal Lumbar Epidural Steroid Injection

1. Position C-arm to obtain a clear view of the appropriate pedicle. In the mid-lumbar spine, the angle is usually axial; in the upper lumbar spine, the angle may need to be adjusted in a more cranial direction, whereas in the lower lumbar spine, a more caudal angulation is often necessary.
2. Insert the needle along the course of the x-ray beam far enough so that it is anchored. Insertion should be through a skin site that has been prepped and draped in a sterile fashion.
3. Check position with the C-arm fluoroscope.
4. Adjust as necessary.
5. Advance the needle until the patient has radicular pain *or* the needle rests on bone. If the patient has radicular pain, inject 1.0 mL of an anesthetic agent.
6. Go to frontal position and confirm the needle tip position beneath the pedicle.
7. Inject 1.0 mL of nonionic contrast material and document circumneural sheath location. Make particular note of any suspected arterial flow toward the spinal canal, especially toward the conus (Houten 2002); avoid injecting when this happens.
8. Inject steroid and anesthetic agents and take frontal and oblique images.
9. Monitor for pain response and record percentage of pain relief at 30 minutes.
10. Release patient when stable. Provide patient with a telephone number to call if there is persistent or increased pain or numbness or if fever, swelling, or redness develops.

TRANSFORAMINAL LUMBAR EPIDURAL STEROID INJECTION

Transforaminal injections may better relieve radicular pain than the posterior interlaminar approach described earlier. In addition, transforaminal injections probably deliver more drug to the anterior spinal canal. Significant differences exist between injection in the lumbar spine (transforaminal injections done at levels L1 through L5) and injection at S1. Table 2–5 describes and Figures 2–18 through 2–22 illustrate lumbar transforaminal epidural steroid injection. Table 2–6 describes and Figures 2–23 through 2–25 illustrate S1 transforaminal epidural steroid injection. Reports for transforaminal injections are similar to those for interlaminar epidural steroid injections (see earlier discussion).

Text continued on page 39

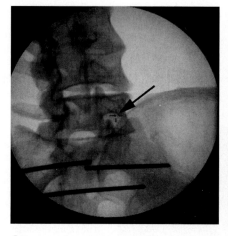 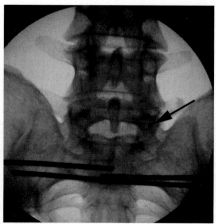

A   B

FIGURE 2–18

Skeletal Specimen Radiograph Demonstrating Target Position for Transforaminal L5 Lumbar Epidural Steroid Injection. *A*, Oblique specimen radiograph with a metallic bead (arrow) taped along the inferior, lateral aspect of the L5-S1 intervertebral nerve root canal (foramen). This is the correct angle for the C-arm at the start of the procedure. The cross-hairs of the laser aiming device target the bead. (The metallic bars through the pelvis hold the sacrum and pelvis together in this specimen.) *B*, Frontal view with the metallic bead (arrow) seen beneath the right L5 pedicle. Note that the target position projects slightly medial to the lateral margin of the vertebral body on a frontal view.

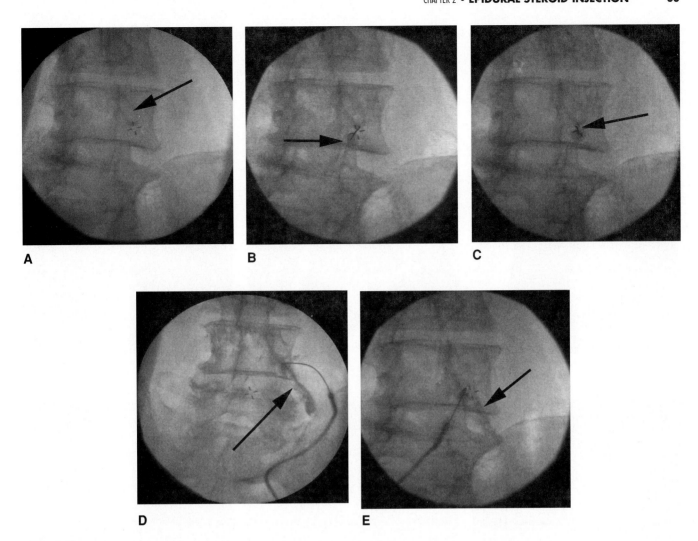

FIGURE 2–19

Step-by-Step L4 Transforaminal Epidural Steroid Injection. This 66-year-old man had right thigh pain suggesting an L4 distribution. Magnetic resonance imaging showed multilevel degenerative disc disease without foraminal disc herniation, stenosis, or synovial cyst formation. *A,* Right posterior oblique view demonstrates the L4 pedicle to good advantage (arrow). The cross-hairs of the laser aiming device are positioned directly beneath the L4 pedicle. *B,* A 22-gauge needle has been anchored in the skin. Fluoroscopic visualization shows the hub of the needle to have an associated faint radiopacity (arrow). Therefore, the tip of the needle is slightly superior and lateral to ideal position, since it is tracking up and anterior and if advanced will miss the target location immediately below the pedicle. The bevel should be turned superolateral as the needle is advanced. *C,* After the needle has been advanced, the tip angles slightly into a more ideal position beneath the pedicle (arrow). The patient did not experience any sharp radicular pain, and the needle eventually contacted bone. The fluoroscope was turned to the frontal position. *D,* Frontal view after injection of contrast material shows flow along the right L4 circumneural sheath (arrow), along with some flow into the spinal canal. *E,* Oblique view after injection of contrast material shows flow along the right L4 circumneural sheath (arrow).

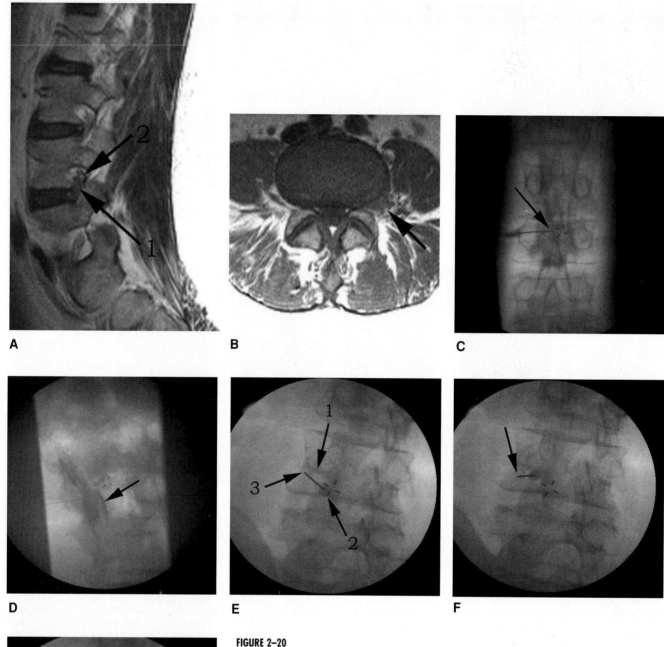

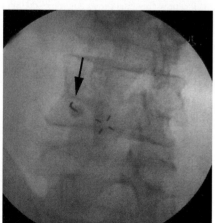

FIGURE 2–20

Interlaminar Injection Followed by Transforaminal Injection with Better Pain Relief. This 55-year-old woman had chronic low back pain and new-onset left thigh pain in a distribution consistent with L4. *A,* Left parasagittal T2-weighted magnetic resonance imaging scan demonstrates an L4-5 foraminal disc extrusion (arrow 1) displacing and compressing the L4 ganglion (arrow 2). *B,* Axial T1-weighted magnetic resonance imaging scan demonstrates the foraminal and far lateral extraforaminal disc extrusion (arrow). Compare the appearance with that of the opposite side. *C,* Frontal view taken during injection of an interlaminar L2-3 injection. The needle tip (arrow) is at the level of the L3 pedicles, with contrast material flowing both proximally and distally from the needle tip. *D,* Lateral view taken during the interlaminar injection demonstrates flow proximally and distally in the epidural space. Note that even with a limited volume of injectate (less than 3 mL total), contrast material reaches the ventral aspect of the epidural space (arrow) along the dorsal aspect of the L3 vertebral body. *E,* Oblique view after insertion of the needle far enough to anchor it in the skin during an L4 transforaminal injection. Target position is beneath the midpoint of the L4 pedicle (arrow 1). The needle hub (arrow 2) is inferior and medial to the target, while the tip (arrow 3) projects too far anterior. The bevel of the needle tip was turned anterior while the needle was advanced from this position. *F,* Oblique view after advancing the needle demonstrates a better position of the needle tip, slightly more posterior to the position in part E. *G,* Oblique view after further advancing of the needle demonstrates that the needle is in a nearly ideal position, close to the midpoint of the L4 pedicle (arrow). The patient described some leg pain at this time. A small amount of nonionic contrast material was injected at this point, which appeared to track along the course of the L4 circumneural sheath. However, injection of contrast material did not cause any significant radicular pain. The C-arm was switched from an oblique to a frontal projection.

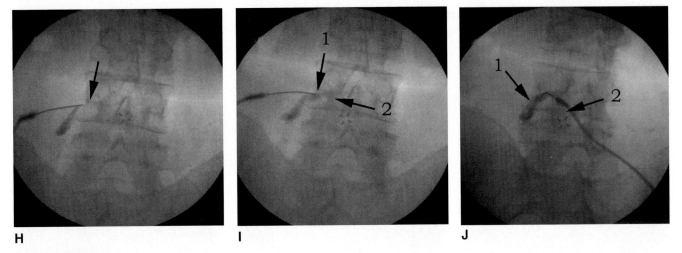

H   **I**   **J**

FIGURE 2–20 CONTINUED

H, Frontal view of injection of a small amount of contrast material. The contrast appears to flow in a course suggesting a circumneural sheath (arrow), but does not demonstrate the typical filling defect of the nerve. In addition, the needle tip is well lateral to the ideal position at or medial to the lateral edge of the pedicle (arrow 2). *I,* Frontal view after the needle tip was advanced 2 mm (which resulted in radicular pain). The tip is now at the lateral margin of the pedicle (arrow 1), and 0.2 mL of injected contrast material demonstrates flow in the circumneural sheath beneath the L4 pedicle and into the epidural space within the spinal canal (arrow 2). *J,* Oblique radiograph following injection of an additional 0.5 mL of contrast material demonstrates flow along the L4 circumneural sheath (arrow 1) and within the epidural space within the spinal canal (arrow 2). The patient had much better pain relief following the transforaminal injection than she had with the interlaminar injection.

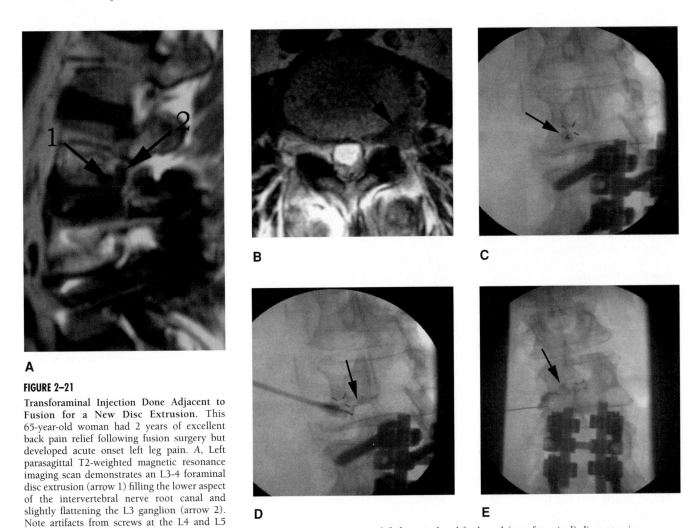

A

B   **C**

D   **E**

FIGURE 2–21

Transforaminal Injection Done Adjacent to Fusion for a New Disc Extrusion. This 65-year-old woman had 2 years of excellent back pain relief following fusion surgery but developed acute onset left leg pain. *A,* Left parasagittal T2-weighted magnetic resonance imaging scan demonstrates an L3-4 foraminal disc extrusion (arrow 1) filling the lower aspect of the intervertebral nerve root canal and slightly flattening the L3 ganglion (arrow 2). Note artifacts from screws at the L4 and L5 pedicles. *B,* Axial T2-weighted magnetic resonance imaging scan demonstrates a left foraminal and far lateral (extraforaminal) disc extrusion (arrow). *C,* Oblique view following needle placement. The faint opacity of the hub projects over the needle (arrow), which courses slightly from anterior to posterior. The cross-hairs of the laser aiming device target ideal position beneath the left L3 pedicle. Note pedicle screws and posterior interconnecting hardware at L4 and L5. The patient experienced her typical radicular pain with the needle in this position. *D,* Oblique view following injection of 0.3 mL of nonionic contrast material shows flow beneath the pedicle along the course of the L3 nerve (arrow). *E.* Frontal view following injection of an additional 0.3 mL of nonionic contrast material shows flow beneath the L3 pedicle into the epidural space within the spinal canal (arrow). Note that the needle tip is still at or slightly lateral to the lateral aspect of the L3 pedicle. Again seen is hardware beneath the injected level. The patient achieved excellent pain relief with the transforaminal injection.

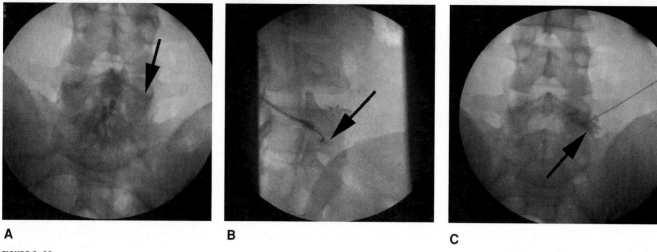

A   B   C

FIGURE 2–22

Transforaminal L5 Injection Providing Superior Pain Relief Compared with an Interlaminar Injection. This 29-year-old man had low back pain radiating into the right buttock and lateral thigh. An outside magnetic resonance imaging examination (not shown) demonstrated a small L5-S1 foraminal disc protrusion without accompanying neural compression. *A,* Frontal view following L5-S1 interlaminar epidural injection shows symmetric flow centered at the L5-S1 level. There is a paucity of flow past the right L5 pedicle (arrow). *B,* Oblique view following injection of 0.1 mL of contrast material during a right L5 transforaminal epidural steroid injection. Injection in this position reproduced the patient's typical back, buttock, and thigh pain. *C,* Frontal view shows the needle tip beneath the right L5 pedicle and contrast material flowing laterally past the edge of the pedicle along the L5 circumneural sheath (arrow). The patient received much better pain relief with this injection than with the interlaminar injection.

TABLE 2–6. Step-by-Step Description of S1 Transforaminal Lumbar Epidural Steroid Injection

1. Position C-arm to obtain a clear view through the S1 foramen. This usually requires considerable caudal angulation of the beam, as well as mild ipsilateral angulation. A relatively straight frontal view will demonstrate the arc of the anterior margin of the foramen, but passage of a needle toward the bottom of this arc will not succeed in reaching the foramen because the posterior opening is considerably higher (see Fig. 2–23). If it is not possible to see "down the barrel" of the S1 foramen, the bottom of the S1 pedicle may be used as a landmark. If this, too, cannot be accomplished, then starting superior to the anterior arch with the needle 2 to 3 cm from midline on the ipsilateral side is probably the best option.
2. Insert the needle along the course of the x-ray beam far enough so that it is anchored. Insertion should be through a skin site that has been prepped and draped in a sterile fashion.
3. Check position with the C-arm fluoroscope. The needle should be directed toward the superior, lateral aspect of the lucency formed by the S1 neural foramen.
4. Adjust as necessary.
5. If the patient has radicular pain, inject 1.0 mL of an anesthetic agent. Patients have radicular pain less frequently with S1 than with lumbar transforaminal injections.
6. When the needle is clearly along the course of the S1 foramen, go to lateral position and check for needle position projecting within the sacrum.
7. Inject 1.0 to 2.0 mL of nonionic contrast material and document circumneural sheath location. Make particular note of any suspected arterial flow toward the spinal canal, especially toward the conus (Houten 2002); avoid injecting when this happens.
8. Inject steroid and anesthetic agents and take frontal and oblique images.
9. Monitor for pain response and record percentage of pain relief at 30 minutes.
10. Release patient when stable. Provide patient with a telephone number to call if there is persistent or increased pain or numbness or if fever, swelling, or redness develops.

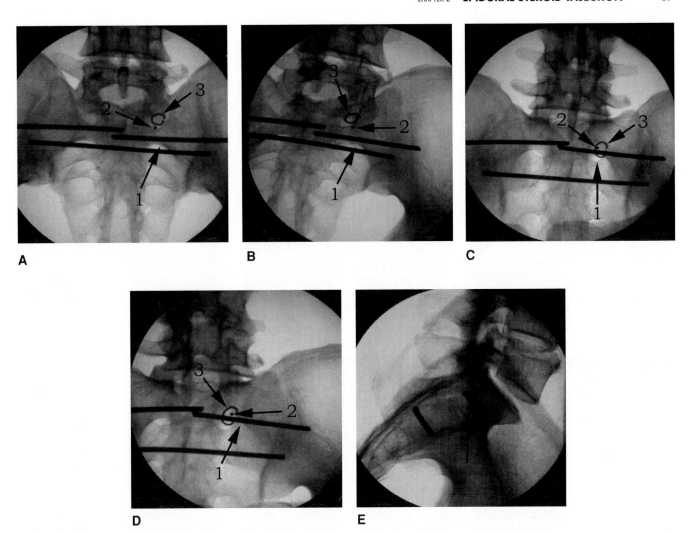

FIGURE 2–23

Skeletal Specimen Radiograph Demonstrating Target Position for Transforaminal S1 Lumbar Epidural Steroid Injection. *A,* Frontal view of a specimen radiograph. (The metallic bars through the pelvis hold the sacrum and pelvis together in this specimen and unfortunately somewhat obscure anatomy in the sacrum.) The anterior arch of the S1 foramen (arrow 1) is clearly visualized. However, any attempt to pass a needle directly toward this landmark would fail, because bone covers the posterior aspect of the foramen from this angle. A metallic marker has been placed in the target position within the middle of the S1 neural foramen (arrow 2). The posterior opening of the S1 neural foramen has been marked with an incomplete metal ring (arrow 3). Note that only passage through this opening will allow access to the S1 level. *B,* Oblique view of a specimen radiograph with ipsilateral angulation alone (and no caudal angulation). The S1 neural foramen (arrow 1) projects well below the metallic marker at the target position (arrow 2), which, in turn, projects below the posterior opening of the neural foramen (arrow 3). The posterior opening is at the inferior margin of the S1 pedicle, a difficult landmark to recognize (even on this specimen radiograph). Note that aiming toward the anterior neural arch with only ipsilateral angulation (and without associated caudal angulation) would not result in reaching the target position. *C,* Frontal view of the specimen radiograph with considerable (nearly 45 degrees) caudal angulation. The S1 neural arch is now seen as a marked lucency (arrow 1). Note, however, that placing the needle directly at the middle of this lucency might still not succeed in reaching the target (arrow 2), as the posterior opening (arrow 3) is above most of the lucency. *D,* Oblique view with caudal angulation of the beam. The S1 anterior neural arch (arrow 1) is somewhat obscured by the metallic pin in this image. The target position (arrow 2) is centered within the posterior opening (arrow 3), however, making the target most accessible from this route. *E,* Lateral examination demonstrates the metallic marker (arrow) in target position within the S1 neural foramen. Note that this position projects well within the body of the S1 vertebra.

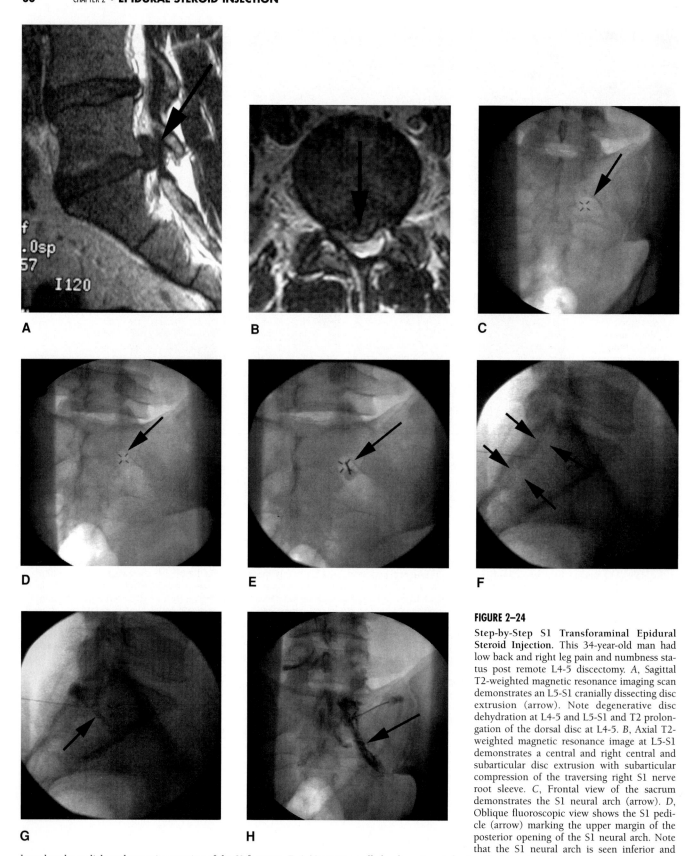

FIGURE 2–24

Step-by-Step S1 Transforaminal Epidural Steroid Injection. This 34-year-old man had low back and right leg pain and numbness status post remote L4-5 discectomy. *A*, Sagittal T2-weighted magnetic resonance imaging scan demonstrates an L5-S1 cranially dissecting disc extrusion (arrow). Note degenerative disc dehydration at L4-5 and L5-S1 and T2 prolongation of the dorsal disc at L4-5. *B*, Axial T2-weighted magnetic resonance image at L5-S1 demonstrates a central and right central and subarticular disc extrusion with subarticular compression of the traversing right S1 nerve root sleeve. *C*, Frontal view of the sacrum demonstrates the S1 neural arch (arrow). *D*, Oblique fluoroscopic view shows the S1 pedicle (arrow) marking the upper margin of the posterior opening of the S1 neural arch. Note that the S1 neural arch is seen inferior and lateral to the pedicle and posterior opening of the S1 foramen. *E*, A 22-gauge needle has been inserted using the laser aiming device. It is on track to pass beneath the S1 neural arch (arrow). *F*, Lateral view demonstrates that the needle tip projects within the sacral spinal canal (arrows). *G*, A small amount of contrast material has been injected, some of which flows along the right S1 circumneural sheath (arrow). Note that visualization of this contrast is difficult, but compare directly to part *F*. Dual monitor C-arm equipment, wherein a view can be stored on one screen while another screen is "live," will help visualization of such subtle collections of contrast material. *H*, A frontal view after further contrast injection shows that most of the contrast material flows along the right S1 circumneural sheath (arrow), although some has flowed superiorly and tracks within the vertebral canal and along the contralateral, left L5 circumneural sheath.

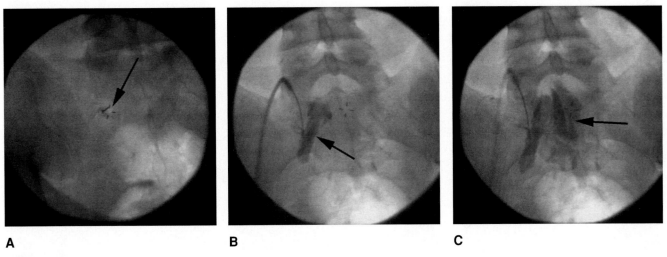

A   **B**   **C**

FIGURE 2–25

Transforaminal S1 Injection. This is the same patient illustrated in Figure 2–5, a 26-year-old man with low back and left leg pain. Although the interlaminar injections were providing good relief of back pain, the patient had ongoing left buttock and posterior thigh pain, so a transforaminal S1 injection was performed. *A,* Frontal radiograph during injection demonstrates the needle projecting within the lucency of the S1 neural foramen (arrow). There is caudal and ipsilateral angulation of the tube (note that the L5-S1 intervertebral disc is in-plane, indicating considerable caudal angulation of the x-ray beam). *B,* Frontal radiograph following injection of 0.5 mL of nonionic contrast material demonstrates flow along the S1 circumneural sheath (arrow). *C,* Frontal radiograph after injection of an additional 2.0 mL of nonionic contrast material demonstrates flow into the epidural space in the upper sacral spinal canal (arrow). The patient had excellent relief of leg pain following this injection.

As in lumbar interlaminar injections, there are occasional problems with transforaminal injections. Table 2–7 lists these. With regard to difficulties encountered during lumbar transforaminal injection, note the following:

Intrathecal injection. One of the benefits of transforaminal injection is that inadvertent intrathecal injection is distinctly unusual. Areas of extensive degenerative change or postoperative change are probably at higher risk (Fig. 2–26).

Venous injection. Venous injection (Fig. 2–27) occurs 10% to 20% of the time (Furman 2000, Sullivan 2000), particularly at S1 (Furman 2000). Slight

adjustment of needle tip position usually results in exclusive epidural flow.

Facet joint injection. Inadvertent injection into the facet joint at the level of the injection results from redundancy of the capsule of the facet, synovial cyst formation, or a lower than ideal needle position (Fig. 2–28).

Discography. Inadvertent discography often occurs when a patient has a large foraminal disc extrusion (Fig. 2–29) or spondylolisthesis with a redundant annulus (Fig. 2–30). Given enough caudal dissection with the disc extrusion, it is even possible (although very unusual) to perform discography at the superior adjacent level (Fig. 2–31). When this complication occurs, it is probably prudent to inject a small amount (0.5–1.0 mL) of 100 mg/mL cefazolin to help prevent the dreaded complication of discitis, although these degenerated discs are usually relatively well vascularized and thus at least theoretically at somewhat less risk of infection.

TABLE 2–7. Problems Encountered During Lumbar Transforaminal Epidural Steroid Injection

Intrathecal injection (see Fig. 2–26)
Venous injection (see Fig. 2–27)
Facet joint injection (see Fig. 2–28)
Intradiscal injection (see Figs. 2–29, 2–30, and 2–31)

Text continued on page 43

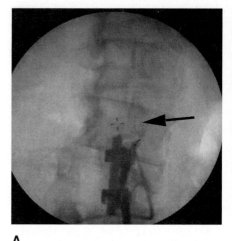
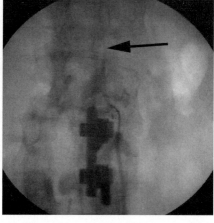

A   B

FIGURE 2–26

L2 Transforaminal Epidural Steroid Injection with Intrathecal Injection. This 74-year-old man was status post L3 through sacral spine fusion with adjacent segment L2-3 degenerative disc disease and right groin pain. *A,* Right posterior oblique examination demonstrates a 22-gauge needle beneath the right L2 pedicle (arrow). *B,* Repeat right posterior oblique examination following contrast injection demonstrates contrast flow around the undersurface of the right L2 pedicle as well as into the vertebral canal. A thin narrow strip of contrast material tracks superiorly along the right side of the vertebral canal that is probably intrathecal (arrow). Shortly after the injection, the patient lost urinary continence and experienced transient paraplegia for the duration of the local anesthetic.

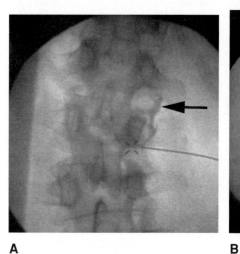
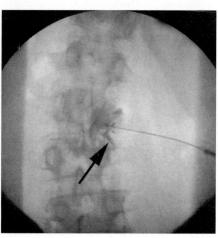

A   B

FIGURE 2–27

Transforaminal with Vascular Injection. This 67-year-old man had middle back pain radiating into the right side and groin region. *A,* Frontal view with the needle beneath the L2 pedicle demonstrates a combination of epidural and venous (arrow) flow. *B,* Frontal view following needle tip adjustment shows better epidural flow, including flow along the right L2 circumneural sheath (arrow).

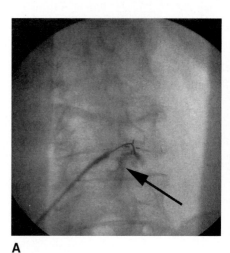
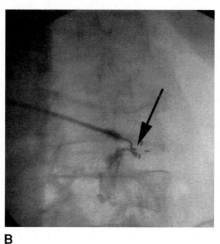
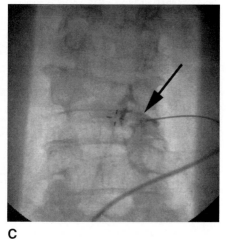

A   B   C

FIGURE 2–28

Transforaminal with Facet Joint Injection. This 75-year-old woman had right medial thigh and leg pain. *A,* Right posterior oblique view demonstrates that the needle has taken a curved course en route to beneath the right L3 pedicle. It deflected off the transverse process when inserted. There is contrast material in the right L3-4 facet joint (arrow). *B,* The needle was withdrawn slightly and the needle bevel directed inferiorly so that the needle tip would track superiorly (arrow). The needle is still somewhat inferior to ideal position. *C,* Frontal examination after additional contrast injection shows contrast flow into the vertebral canal and along the right L3 circumneural sheath. Again, the needle is inferior to ideal position, but contrast is tracking along the target L3 level.

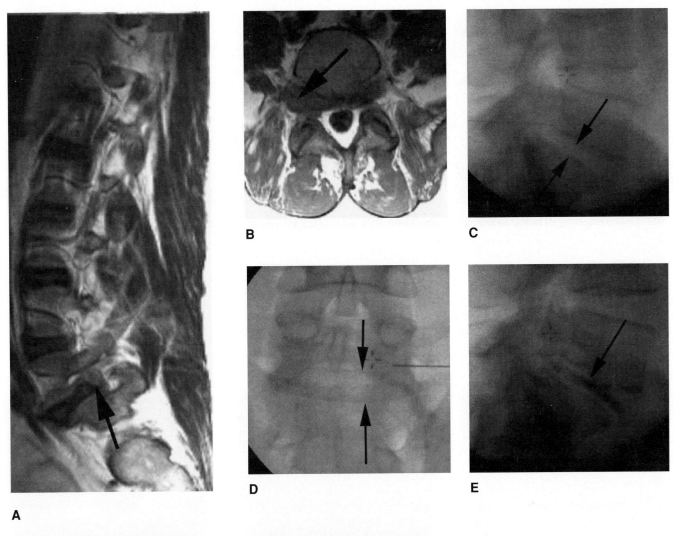

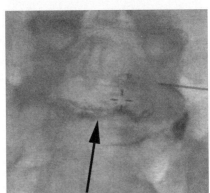

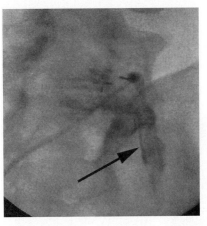

FIGURE 2–29

Transforaminal with Discography from a Foraminal Disc Herniation. This 35-year-old truck driver had chronic bilateral sciatica and two recent injuries with severe right lower extremity pain in an L5 distribution. *A*, Right parasagittal T2-weighted magnetic resonance imaging scan demonstrates spondylolisthesis of L5 on S1 secondary to spondylolysis along with a large foraminal disc extrusion (arrow). *B*, Axial T1-weighted magnetic resonance imaging scan just above the level of the L5-S1 intervertebral disc demonstrates a large right foraminal disc extrusion (arrow). The needle was positioned in the usual oblique manner and frontal and lateral films were obtained. *C*, Lateral film demonstrates the needle superior to the L5-S1 intervertebral disc (arrows). *D*, Frontal film demonstrates that the needle is superior to the disc (arrows), which is oblique to the plane of imaging on this study. *E*, Lateral examination made after contrast injection demonstrates an L5-S1 discogram (arrow). *F*, Frontal view after contrast injection also demonstrates an L5-S1 discogram (arrow). *G*, Oblique view following repositioning of the needle and injection of additional contrast material demonstrates flow along the right L5 circumneural sheath (arrow).

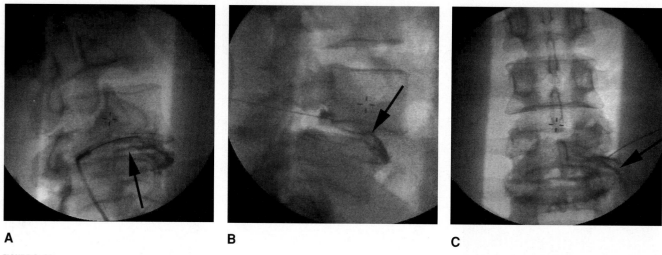

A　　　　　**B**　　　　　**C**

FIGURE 2–30

Transforaminal Injection with Discography from Spondylolisthesis and Annular Redundancy. This 28-year-old man had right anterior thigh pain and L4-5 lytic spondylolisthesis. *A,* Right posterior oblique view demonstrates the needle tip beneath the right L4 pedicle, with contrast tracking not only anterior, but also beneath the needle in a linear fashion (arrow). At first glance, the contrast anterior to the needle appears to be along the right L4 circumneural sheath. *B,* Lateral examination demonstrates lytic spondylolisthesis of L4 on L5, the needle tip superior to the disc level, and an L4-5 discogram (arrow). *C,* Frontal view obtained after adjustment of the needle tip and additional contrast injection demonstrates contrast material in the right L4 circumneural sheath.

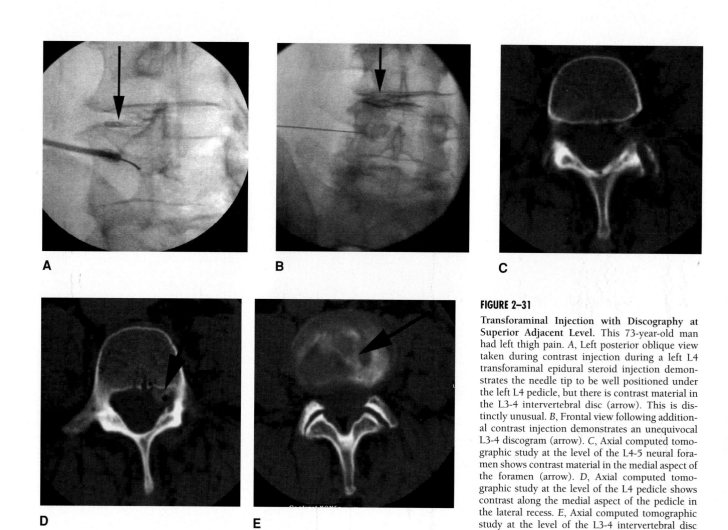

A　　　　　**B**　　　　　**C**

D　　　　　**E**

FIGURE 2–31

Transforaminal Injection with Discography at Superior Adjacent Level. This 73-year-old man had left thigh pain. *A,* Left posterior oblique view taken during contrast injection during a left L4 transforaminal epidural steroid injection demonstrates the needle tip to be well positioned under the left L4 pedicle, but there is contrast material in the L3-4 intervertebral disc (arrow). This is distinctly unusual. *B,* Frontal view following additional contrast injection demonstrates an unequivocal L3-4 discogram (arrow). *C,* Axial computed tomographic study at the level of the L4-5 neural foramen shows contrast material in the medial aspect of the foramen (arrow). *D,* Axial computed tomographic study at the level of the L4 pedicle shows contrast along the medial aspect of the pedicle in the lateral recess. *E,* Axial computed tomographic study at the level of the L3-4 intervertebral disc shows contrast tracking back into the nucleus of this disc (arrow), along with a small foraminal and subarticular disc contour abnormality. The patient appears to have a caudally dissecting disc extrusion extending from the disc margin to the L4-5 neural foramen.

TABLE 2–8. Step-by-Step Description of Caudal Epidural Steroid Injection

1. Position the C-arm fluoroscope so that a clear view of the sacrum is possible.
2. Palpate the sacral hiatus and anesthetize the overlying skin. Insertion should be through a skin site that has been prepped and draped in a sterile fashion.
3. Place the injection needle into the sacral canal.
4. Check the position of the needle with the C-arm fluoroscope.
5. Adjust as necessary.
6. Go to frontal position and confirm the position of the needle tip between the sacral pedicles.
7. Inject 2.0 mL of nonionic contrast material and document the epidural location of the injected material.
8. Inject steroid and 10 mL of a dilute anesthetic agent.
9. Monitor for pain response and record percentage of pain relief at 30 minutes.
10. Release patient when stable. Provide patient with a telephone number to call if there is persistent or increased pain or numbness or if fever, swelling, or redness develops.

Caudal Epidural Steroid Injection

Table 2–8 describes and Figures 2–32 and 2–33 illustrate caudal epidural steroid injection. Although most patients find caudal injections more painful than interlaminar injections, caudal injections have the advantage of relatively fewer complications. Intrathecal injection is distinctly uncommon, and the only frequently encountered problems are venous injection, which occurs about 10% of the time (Renfrew 1991) (Fig. 2–34) and incorrect needle placement (Fig. 2–35), both of which are relatively easy to remedy at the time of the procedure.

Text continued on page 46

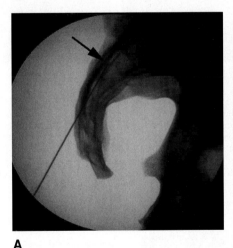
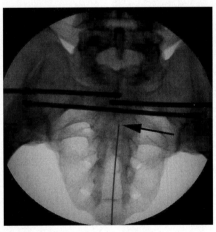

A   B

FIGURE 2–32

Skeletal Specimen Radiograph with a Needle in Position, Demonstrating Ideal Needle Placement for a Caudal Epidural Steroid Injection. *A,* Lateral view of a specimen radiograph. The needle tip projects within the sacral spinal canal at the S3 level (arrow). *B,* Frontal view of the specimen radiograph demonstrates the needle tip located centrally within the sacral spinal canal (arrow). (The metallic bars through the pelvis hold the sacrum and pelvis together in this specimen.)

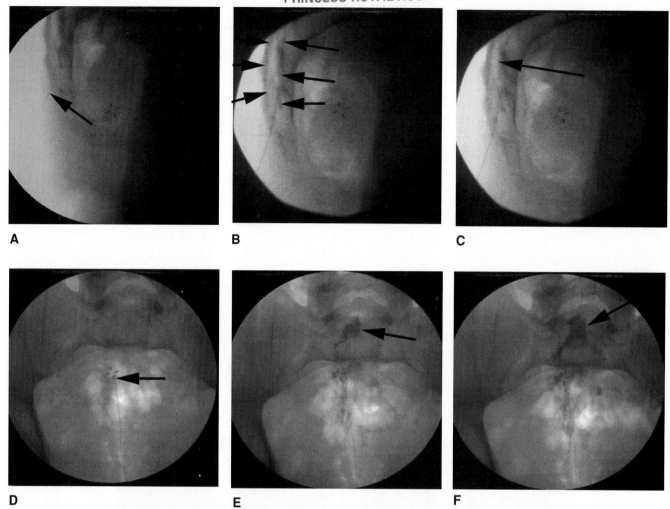

FIGURE 2–33

Step-by-Step Caudal Epidural Steroid Injection. This 22-year-old patient had coccydynia and low back pain following trauma. *A*, A lateral view of the sacrum obtained with a 25-gauge anesthetization needle (arrow) in place demonstrates that the needle is in the inferior sacral canal (this patient was very slender). *B*, Lateral view of the sacrum with a 25-gauge spinal needle in the anterior sacral spinal canal (arrows). *C*, The needle has been further advanced so that the tip is more superior in the sacral spinal canal (arrow). *D*, Frontal view demonstrates the needle with its tip (arrow) located slightly to the left of midline. *E*, Frontal view following injection of 2.0 mL of contrast material demonstrates flow proximally into the spinal canal, which reaches the level of the L5-S1 intervertebral disc (arrow). *F*, Injection of steroid and anesthetic has propelled the contrast material further superior within the sacral spinal canal (arrow).

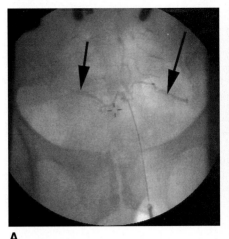

A

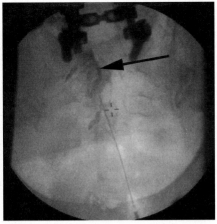

B

FIGURE 2–34

Venous Injection from Caudal Route. This 85-year-old woman had good relief of low back pain and leg symptoms for several years, following multilevel fusion surgery with subsequent return of low back pain. *A,* Initial injection with the needle somewhat low in the sacral spinal canal demonstrates the typical tubular, evanescent filling of veins (arrows). There is hardware from prior fusion surgery. *B,* After adjustment of the needle, the epidural space is opacified (arrow).

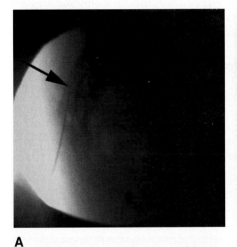

A

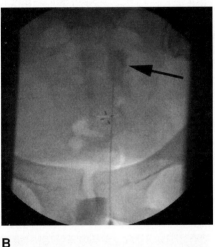

B

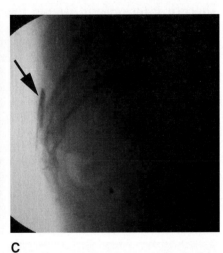

C

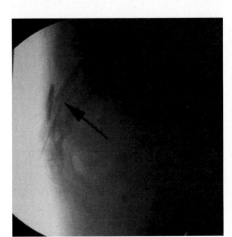

D

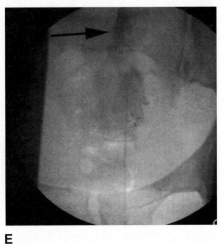

E

FIGURE 2–35

Initial Posterior Injection Followed by Correction of Needle Placement. This 46-year-old woman was status post L5-S1 discectomy with left leg pain radiating from the buttocks to the posterior heel, suggesting S1 radicular pain. Imaging demonstrated no disc extrusion or neural compression. *A,* Lateral examination demonstrates the needle tip at the level of the lower sacrum. The tip appears to project along the posterior spinal canal. *B,* Frontal examination following injection of 1.0 mL of contrast material. The needle tip is to the right of midline. Contrast pools around the needle tip with "feathered" edges, suggesting a location other than the epidural space. No filling of circumneural sheaths is identified. *C,* Lateral examination demonstrates contrast that is definitely posterior to the spinal canal. The needle tip is located too far posterior. *D,* Without complete needle withdrawal from the skin, the needle was drawn back and reinserted. A repeat lateral view now shows the needle tip to project anterior to the contrast collection, in a position consistent with the sacral spinal canal. *E,* Frontal view following contrast injection with the needle in the revised position. Contrast flows away from the needle tip into the upper sacral spinal canal epidural space (arrow).

TABLE 2–9. Step-by-Step Description of Thoracic Interlaminar Epidural Steroid Injection

1. Position the C-arm fluoroscopy so that a clear view of the chosen interlaminar space is possible. Extreme angulation may be necessary. It may not be possible to visualize an interlaminar space. In these cases, placing the needle along the dorsal aspect of a lamina and "walking off" the lamina by successive superior placement of the needle tip may be necessary.
2. Insert the needle along the course of the x-ray beam far enough so that it is anchored. Insertion should be through a skin site that has been prepped and draped in a sterile fashion. Check position with the C-arm fluoroscope.
3. Adjust as necessary.
4. Move to the lateral position and check position with the C-arm fluoroscope.
5. When needle is just behind the spinal canal, inject 0.1 to 0.2 mL of nonionic contrast material and confirm position in the posterior soft tissues.
6. Advance the needle *very slowly* with one hand while pressurizing the syringe with the other. When a thin line of nonionic contrast spreads along the posterior epidural space, *immediately stop advancing the needle!*
7. Inject 2.0 to 3.0 mL of nonionic contrast material under fluoroscopic control. Confirm that the contrast injection pattern is typical for the epidural space.
8. Inject steroid and anesthetic agents and take frontal and lateral images.
9. Monitor for pain response and record percentage of pain relief at 30 minutes.
10. Release patient when stable. Provide patient with a telephone number to call if there is persistent or increased pain or numbness or if fever, swelling, or redness develops.

Thoracic Interlaminar Steroid Injection

Table 2–9 describes and Figures 2–36 through 2–38 illustrate thoracic interlaminar epidural steroid injection. The interlaminar lumbar and interlaminar thoracic injections differ in that relatively steep craniocaudd angulation of the C-arm may be necessary in the thoracic spine because of the broad, angulated laminae. In addition, a 25-gauge needle is usually used in the thoracic spine, and this will make the "meniscus quiver" test for entry into the epidural space described earlier for lumbar injections unreliable. A "loss of resistance" method can be used instead. Complications are similar to those reviewed for lumbar interlaminar epidural steroid injection, including intrathecal injection.

Thoracic Transforaminal Steroid Injection

Thoracic transforaminal epidural steroid injection is similar to lumbar transforaminal epidural steroid injection (see earlier), with the exception that it is more difficult to obtain ideal needle placement because the ribs may block the best access route to the circumneural sheath.

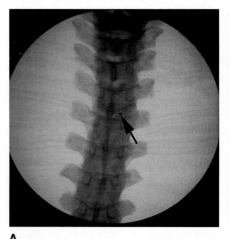 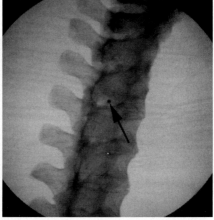 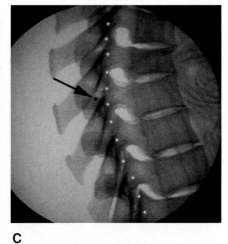

A   B   C

FIGURE 2–36

Skeletal Specimen Radiograph with a Metallic Marker Along the Inferior Aspect of the T6 Lamina. *A,* Frontal view of the mid-thoracic spine. A metallic marker (arrow) has been taped along the inferior aspect of the T6 lamina. Note that the laminar margins are difficult to identify with confidence, even in this specimen radiograph (without the overlapping soft tissues present in patients). *B,* Oblique, magnified view demonstrates the marker (arrow) along the inferior aspect of the T6 lamina. *C,* Lateral view demonstrates the metallic marker (arrow) along the undersurface of the T6 lamina. Note that the posterior margin of the epidural space (marked by white dots) is slightly anterior to the lamina. The specimen has a T6 compression fracture.

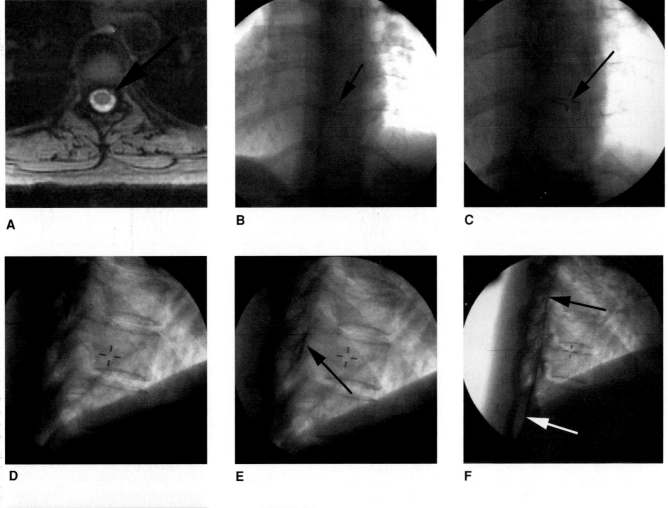

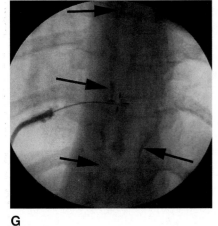

FIGURE 2–37

Step-by-step Thoracic Interlaminar Epidural Injection. This 41-year-old woman had pain in the lower thoracic spine. *A,* Axial magnetic resonance imaging scan demonstrates a T9-10 disc protrusion (arrow). *B,* Slightly oblique view demonstrates the cross-hairs of the laser aiming device between the T9 (arrow) and T10 laminae. *C,* Slightly oblique view following needle insertion demonstrates the needle on course toward the interlaminar space. *D,* Lateral examination demonstrates the needle tip (arrow) approaching the posterior aspect of the thoracic vertebral canal. Note that the ribs superimpose perfectly posteriorly. This is a key to good positioning in the thoracic spine. In this position, the contrast within the connecting tube is pressurized by the practitioner putting pressure on the syringe while very slowly advancing the needle under fluoroscopic guidance. *E,* Lateral examination performed just after loss of resistance on the syringe. Contrast material tracks along the posterior thoracic vertebral canal (arrow). *F,* With further injection, contrast material tracks superiorly and inferiorly within the thoracic epidural space (arrows). *G,* Frontal view also demonstrates widespread distribution of contrast material within the epidural space (arrows).

TABLE 2–10. *Step-by-Step Description of Cervical Epidural Steroid Injection*

1. Position the C-arm fluoroscope so that a clear view of the chosen interlaminar space between the C7 and T1 vertebrae is visualized. Moderate angulation may be necessary.
2. Insert the needle along the course of the x-ray beam far enough so that it is anchored. Insertion should be through a skin site that has been prepped and draped in a sterile fashion.
3. Check position with the C-arm fluoroscope.
4. Adjust as necessary.
5. Move to the oblique position and check position with the C-arm fluoroscope.
6. When the needle is just behind the spinal canal, inject 0.2 to 0.3 mL of nonionic contrast material and confirm position in the posterior soft tissues.
7. Advance the needle very slowly with one hand while pressurizing the syringe with the other. When a thin line of contrast spreads along the posterior epidural space, *immediately stop advancing the needle!*
8. Inject 2.0 to 3.0 mL of nonionic contrast material under fluoroscopic control.
9. Inject a steroid agent and take frontal and lateral images.
10. Monitor for pain response and record percentage of pain relief at 30 minutes.
11. Release patient when stable. Provide patient with a telephone number to call if there is persistent or increased pain or numbness or if fever, swelling, or redness develops.

Cervical Epidural Steroid Injection

Table 2–10 and Figures 2–39 through 2–43 illustrate cervical epidural steroid injection. Table 2–11 lists difficulties encountered with cervical epidural steroid injection. With regard to these problems, note the following:

Intrathecal and spinal cord injection. If the needle is advanced slowly under pressurization and using an oblique, magnified view, it will appear to be far more anterior than it actually is within the spinal canal. This is a good thing, because it reinforces how *extremely dangerous* these injections may be if the needle is in an inappropriate location (Hodges 1998). If the needle is advanced under direct fluoroscopic visualization with advancement stopped when contrast material exits along the needle tip, it should never be in the thecal sac (and never, *ever*, in the spinal cord).

Venous injection. Venous injection within the cervical spinal canal is unusual (Fig. 2–44). It has the same characteristics as venous flow elsewhere: evanescent tubular filling followed by quick dispersal as the injection is terminated.

Facet joint injection. On rare occasion, the contrast pattern will demonstrate flow to one (Fig. 2–45) or both facet joints (Fig. 2–46). Presumably, the cause of this injection pattern is some variation of the epimembranous space and/or degenerative changes of the facet joints with capsular expansion (see earlier discussion under Lumbar Interlaminar Epidural Steroid Injection) (Okada 1981).

Injecting above C7-T1 via the interlaminar approach is riskier because the epidural space diminishes in size above this level.

As stated above in the Patient Selection section, I do not perform transforaminal cervical epidural steroid injections because of the risk of catastrophic complications.

TABLE 2–11. *Problems Encountered During Cervical Interlaminar Epidural Steroid Injections*

Intrathecal injection
Cord injection
Venous injection (see Fig. 2–44)
Facet joint injection (see Figs. 2–45 and 2–46)

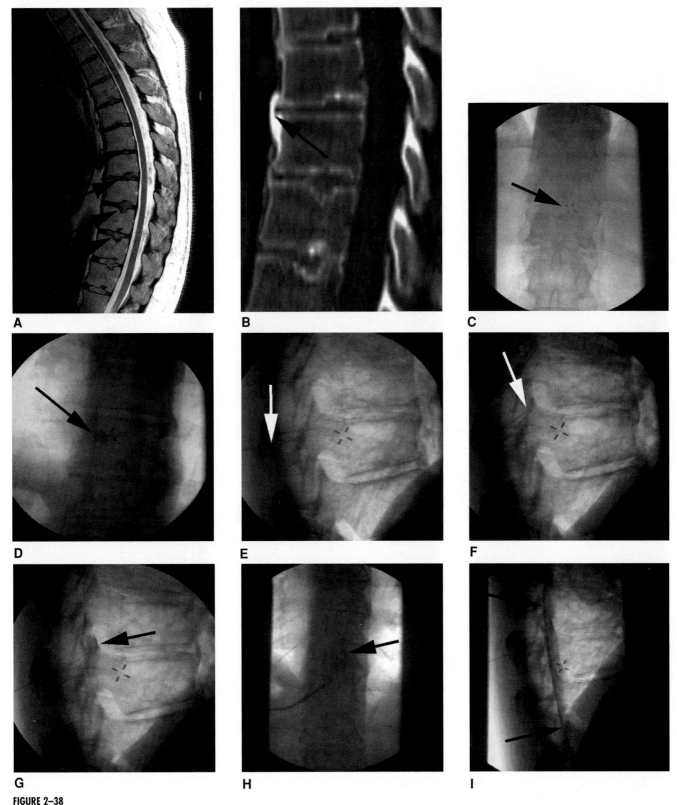

A   B   C

D   E   F

G   H   I

FIGURE 2–38

Thoracic Epidural Steroid Injection. This 45-year-old man had increasingly severe central back pain. *A*, Sagittal T2-weighted magnetic resonance imaging scan demonstrates multilevel intervertebral disc dehydration and Schmorl's node formation (arrows) as well as slight accentuation of thoracic kyphosis. The findings are those of Scheuermann's disease, although the patient does not meet the strict criteria of having 5 degrees of thoracic wedging at three adjacent levels. *B*, Sagittal computed tomographic reconstruction demonstrates multilevel Schmorl's nodes as well as anterior osteophytic spurring (arrow). *C*, Frontal view of the thoracic spine. The patient's skin was marked at the level of maximum tenderness, and the laser aiming device placed at this level, which appears to be at the T10-11 level (arrow). *D*, Oblique view following needle placement. The needle hub (arrow) is located medial to the tip of the needle, so the needle bevel needs to be directed laterally as the needle is advanced. Note that it is very difficult to identify the interlaminar space. The orientation of the C-arm was switched to lateral at this time. *E*, Lateral view demonstrates the needle tip (arrow) posterior to the thoracic spinal canal. The needle was resting on bone at this time. It was withdrawn and advanced more superiorly in 1 to 2 mm increments. *F*, Lateral view demonstrates the needle tip (arrow) deflected superiorly as it "rides up" the T10 lamina. *G*, Lateral view following injection of 0.3 mL of nonionic contrast material demonstrates flow in the epidural space (arrow). *H*, Frontal view demonstrates contrast material tracking superiorly and inferiorly within the thoracic epidural space (arrow). *I*, Additional lateral view demonstrates widespread flow of contrast material in the thoracic epidural space (arrows).

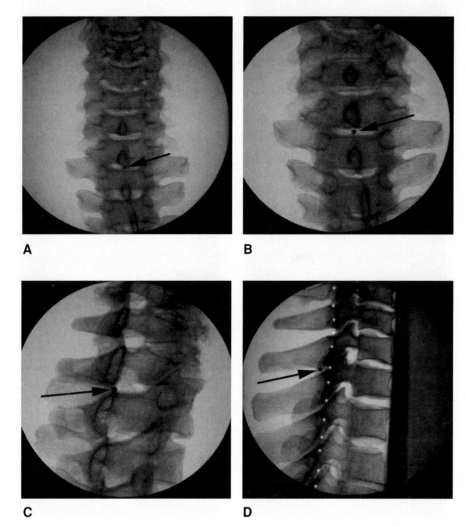

A

B

C

D

FIGURE 2–39

Skeletal Specimen Radiograph with a Metallic Marker Along the Inferior Aspect of the C7 Lamina. *A*, Frontal view of the mid-thoracic spine. A metallic marker (arrow) has been placed at the junction of the right and left laminae at the midline. Note that on the frontal projection, the C7 spinous process projects over the marker and prevents direct access to the spinal canal (and epidural space). *B*, Frontal view after cranial angulation and magnification. The metallic bead (marker) now projects in the interlaminar space at the C7-T1 level. *C*, Oblique magnified view shows the metallic marker (arrow) between the C7 and T1 spinous processes. The bead is actually at least 3 to 4 mm posterior to the spinal canal at this location. The arrow shows the path of the needle for cervical interlaminar epidural steroid injection. *D*, Lateral view with the metallic bead (arrow) as above. The posterior margin of the epidural space is marked by a series of white dots. The arrow shows the path of the needle for cervical interlaminar epidural steroid injection.

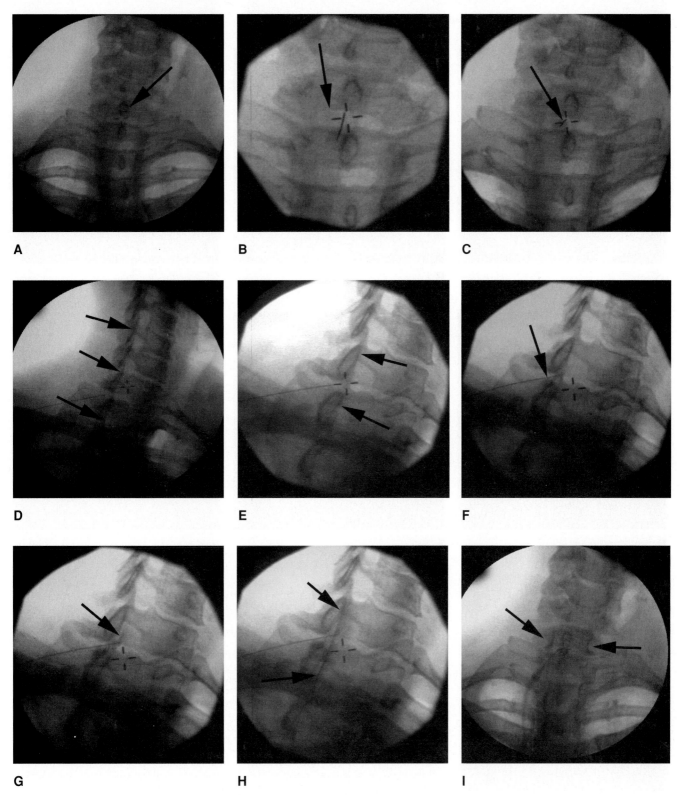

FIGURE 2–40

Step-by-Step Cervical Epidural Steroid Injection. This 47-year-old woman had neck pain and degenerative disc disease from C3-4 through C5-6. *A*, Frontal view shows the cross-hairs of the laser aiming device pointed between the C7 (arrow) and T1 spinous processes. *B*, Frontal view following placement of a needle at the location of the laser aiming device, near the midline and inferior to the inferior margin of the C7 lamina (arrow). *C*, The needle (arrow) has been carefully advanced with the bevel pointing up, bringing it into a more nearly horizontal plane with respect to the C7 spinous process. *D*, An oblique view demonstrates the needle tip posterior to the equivalent of the spinolaminar line (arrows) on the oblique view. Note degenerative disc disease at C3-4, C4-5, and C5-6. From this position, the image intensifier is put on a "magnification" setting and the needle very slowly advanced under direct fluoroscopic guidance. *E*, The needle is still well behind the equivalent of the spinolaminar line (arrows). At this time, the contrast within the connecting tube is pressurized by the practitioner's placing pressure on the syringe plunger. The needle tip is advanced very slowly under direct fluoroscopic guidance, with observation of contrast flow pattern. *F*, A small amount of contrast material has flowed back along the needle track, outside of the cervical vertebral canal (and epidural space). Needle advance is continued very slowly from this position. *G*, Contrast has begun to flow superiorly within the cervical spinal canal (arrow). *H*, Contrast continues to flow in a thin, even line within the epidural space (arrows). *I*, Frontal view demonstrates relatively widespread, predominantly caudal flow of contrast material within the epidural space (arrows). Placing the patient in a head-down position may move injected material to a more cranial location.

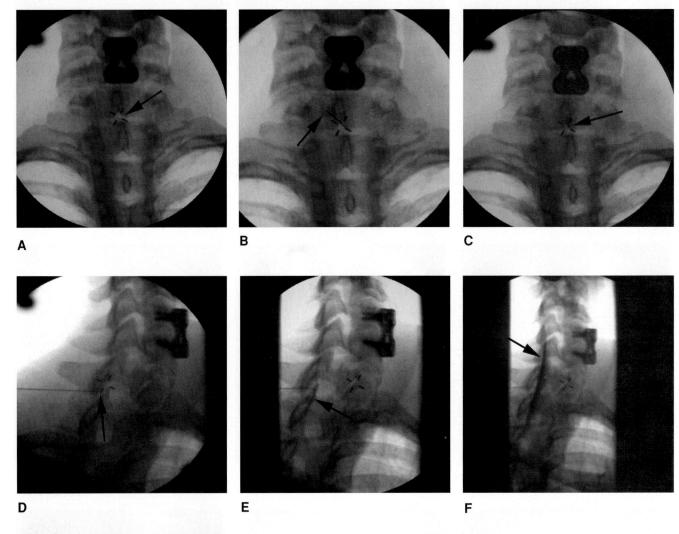

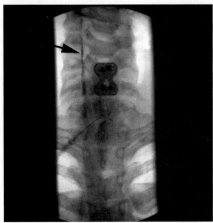

FIGURE 2–41

Cervical Interlaminar Epidural Steroid Injection in a Postoperative Patient. This 34-year-old woman had surgery 2 years prior to this cervical epidural steroid injection. Fusion was performed at C6-7, with excellent relief of arm pain, and with a decrease in neck pain. The patient's ongoing neck pain had been treated with periodic (every 6 months) cervical interlaminar epidural steroid injections with good benefit. *A,* Frontal view of the lower cervical spine with cranial angulation and magnification demonstrates the C7-T1 interlaminar space targeted by the cross-hairs of the laser aiming device (arrow). *B,* Frontal view following initial needle placement demonstrates the needle to be markedly oblique to the correct path. The needle hub (arrow) is superior and lateral. The needle was withdrawn and readvanced with the bevel directed inferiorly and to the left. Great care was taken to ensure that the needle was not advanced to the level of the spinal canal. *C,* Repeat frontal view after needle repositioning demonstrates the needle as a single dot (arrow), indicating that the needle is precisely aligned with the central ray of the x-ray beam. *D,* Oblique view taken after viewing the needle with oblique fluoroscopy and advancing it until the tip (arrow) was at or posterior to the most posterior aspect of the epidural space. *E,* Oblique view following injection of 0.2 mL of nonionic contrast material demonstrates flow within the epidural space along the posterior aspect of the upper thoracic spinal canal (arrow). *F,* Oblique view following injection of an additional 1.5 mL of nonionic contrast material demonstrates additional inferior flow, as well as flow into the more superior cervical spinal canal (arrow). *G,* Frontal view after injection of a total of 2.0 mL of nonionic contrast material shows flow well superior in the epidural space of the cervical spinal canal (arrow). This is predominantly left-sided. The patient had approximately 5 months of good pain relief following this injection.

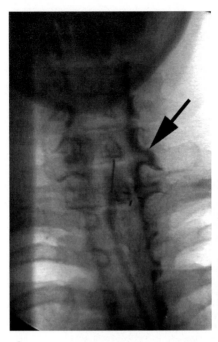
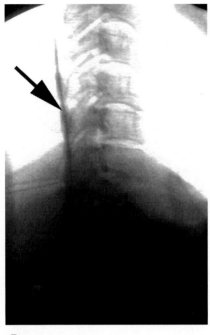

A   **B**

FIGURE 2–42

Cervical Interlaminar Epidural Steroid Injection with Extensive Flow. This 43-year-old woman had neck and bilateral arm pain. Magnetic resonance imaging examination (not shown) demonstrated degenerative disc disease at C5-6 and C6-7, including disc narrowing and bulging. No soft tissue disc extrusion or severe cord compression or spinal stenosis was present. A, Frontal view of the cervical spine with contrast in the epidural space. There is extensive flow of 3 mL of contrast material, including along several cervical circumneural sheaths (arrow). B, Lateral view demonstrates contrast most obvious in the posterior epidural space (arrow). Note that this view, taken at the same time as the frontal view (part A) does not demonstrate the contrast located anteriorly along the circumneural sheaths.

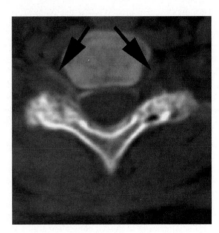

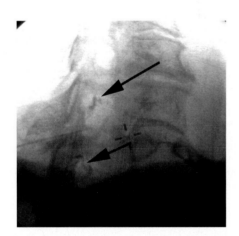

FIGURE 2–43

Cervical Computed Tomographic Scan Obtained After Epidural Injection. This 62-year-old woman had pain in the lower neck and right shoulder. Axial computed tomographic scan performed after epidural contrast (and steroid) injection. Both the injection and this image were at the C7-T1 level. There is extensive degenerative facet arthropathy. Contrast surrounds the spinal canal and extends along the C8 circumneural sheaths (arrows).

FIGURE 2–44

Cervical Epidural Steroid Injection with Venous Flow. This 48-year-old woman had neck and bilateral arm pain with multilevel degenerative disc disease. Right posterior oblique view taken during interlaminar epidural steroid injection demonstrates evanescent contrast material in small cervical epidural veins (arrows).

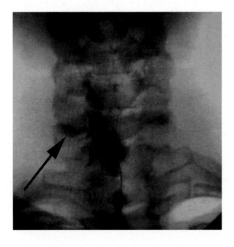

FIGURE 2–45

Cervical Epidural Steroid Injection with Unilateral Facet Joint Filling. This 43-year-old woman had neck and bilateral arm pain. Frontal examination with contrast material injected demonstrates epidural contrast but also contrast within the left C6-7 facet joint (arrow).

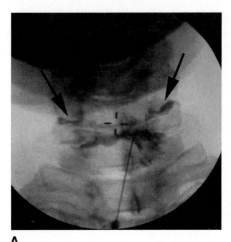

A

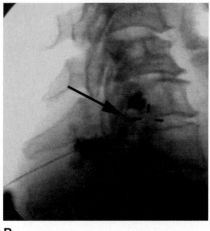

B

FIGURE 2–46

Cervical Epidural Steroid Injection with Bilateral Facet Joint Filling. This 66-year-old woman had neck pain. *A*, Frontal examination made during injection demonstrates bilateral C6-7 facet joint filling with contrast (arrows). Note that the needle tip is significantly to the right of midline. *B*, Lateral examination confirms intra-articular injection of contrast material (arrow).

References

Benzon HT. Epidural steroid injections for low back pain and lumbosacral radiculopathy. Pain 1986; 24:277–295.

Berman AT, Garbarino JL, Fisher SM, Bosacco SJ. The effects of epidural steroid injection of local anesthetics and corticosteroids on patients with lumbosciatic pain. Clin Orthop Rel Res 1984; 188:144–151.

Boden SD, Wiesel SW, Spengler DM. Lumbar spine algorithm. In Wiesel SW et al (eds): The Lumbar Spine, 2nd ed. Philadelphia, W.B. Saunders, 1996.

Botwin KP, Gruber RD, Bouchlas CG, Torres-Ramos FM, Freeman TL, Slaten WK. Complications of fluoroscopically guided transforaminal lumbar epidural injections. Arch Phys Med Rehabil 2000; 81:1045–1050.

Brouwers PJ, Kottink EJ, Simon MA, Prevo RL. A cervical anterior spinal artery syndrome after diagnostic blockade of the right C6-nerve root. Pain 2001; 91:397–399.

Burn JMB, Langdon L. Lumbar epidural injection for the treatment of chronic sciatica. Rheum Phys Med 1970; 10:368–374.

Bush K, Hillier S. A controlled study of caudal epidural injections of triamcinolone plus procaine for the management of intractable sciatica. Spine 1991; 16:572–575.

Chiba K, Toyama Y, Matsumoto M, Maruiwa H, Watanabe M, Nishizawa T. Intraspinal cyst communicating with the intervertebral disc in the lumbar spine: discal cyst. Spine 2001; 26:2112–2118.

Coomes EN. A comparison between epidural anaesthesia and bed rest in sciatica. Br Med J 1961; 1:20–24.

Cuckler JM, Bernini PA, Wiesel SW, Booth RE, Rothman RH, Pickens GT. The use of epidural steroids in the treatment of lumbar radicular pain. J Bone Joint Surg Am 1985; 67:63–66.

Daly P. Caudal epidural anesthesia in lumbosciatic pain. Anaesthesia 1970; 25:346–348.

Davidson JT, Robin GC. Epidural injections in the lumbosciatic syndrome. Br J Anesth 1961; 33:595–598.

Debi R, Halperin N, Mirovsky Y. Local application of steroids following lumbar discectomy. J Spinal Disord Techniques 2002; 15:273–276.

Dilke TFW, Burry HC, Grahame R. Extradural corticosteroid injection in management of lumbar nerve root compression. Br Med J 1973; 2:635–637.

Evans W. Intrasacral epidural injection in the treatment of sciatica. Lancet 1930; 2:1225–1229.

Fredman B, Nun MB, Zohar E, Iraqi G, Shapiro M, Gepstein R, Jedeikin R. Epidural steroids for treating "failed back surgery syndrome": is fluoroscopy really necessary? Anesth Analg 1999; 88:367–372.

Furman MB, O'Brien EM, Zgleszewski TM. Incidence of intravascular penetration in transforaminal lumbosacral epidural steroid injections. Spine 2000; 25:2628–2632.

Goldie I, Peterhoff V. Epidural anaesthesia in low-back pain and sciatica. Acta Orthop Scand 1968; 39:261–269.

Gundry CR, Heithoff KB. Epidural hematoma of the lumbar spine: 18 surgically confirmed cases. Radiology 1993; 187:427–431.

Guyer DW, Wiltse LL, Eskay ML, Guyer BH. The long-range prognosis of arachnoiditis. Spine 1989; 14:1332–1341.

Hayashi N, Weinstein JN, Meller ST, Lee HM, Spratt KF, Gebhart GF. The effect of epidural injection of betamethasone or bupivacaine in a rat model of lumbar radiculopathy. Spine 1998; 23:877–885.

Heithoff KB, Gundry CR, Burton CV, Winter RB. Juvenile discogenic disease. Spine 1994; 19:335–340.

Heyse-Moore GH. A rational approach to the use of epidural medication in the treatment of sciatic pain. Acta Orthop Scand 1978; 49:366–370.

Hodges SD, Castleberg RL, Miller T, Ward R, Thornburg C. Cervical epidural steroid injection with intrinsic spinal cord damage: two case reports. Spine 1998; 23:2137–2142.

Hogan QH. Lumbar epidural anatomy: a new look by cryomicrotome section. Anesthesiology 1991; 75:767–775.

Hogan QH. Epidural catheter tip position, distribution of injectate evaluated by computed tomography. Anesthesiology 1999; 90:964–970.

Houten JK, Errico TJ. Paraplegia after lumbosacral nerve root block: report of three cases. Spine J 2002; 2:70–75.

Johnson BA, Schellhas KP, Pollei SR. Epidurography and therapeutic epidural injections: technical considerations and experience with 5334 cases. Am J Neuroradiol 1999; 20:697–705.

Karppinen J, Malmivaara A, Kurunlahti M, Kyllonen E, Pienimaki T, Nieminen P, Ohinmaa A, Tervonen O, Vanharanta H. Periradicular infiltration for sciatica: a randomized controlled trial. Spine 2001a; 26:1059–1067.

Karppinen J, Ohinmaa A, Malmivaara A, Kurunlahti M, Kyllonen E, Pienimaki T, Nieminen P, Tervonen O, Vanharanta H. Cost effectiveness of periradicular infiltration for sciatica: subgroup analysis of a randomized controlled trial. Spine 2001b; 23:2587–2595.

Kelman H. Epidural injection therapy for sciatic pain. Am J Surg 1944; 64:183–190.

Knight JW, Cordingly JJ, Palazzo MGA. Epidural abscess following epidural steroid and local anesthetic injection. Anaesthesia 1997; 52:576–585.

Koes BW, Scholter RJ, Mens JM, Bouter JM. Efficacy of epidural steroid injections for low-back pain and sciatica: a systematic review of randomized clinical trials. Pain 1995; 63:279–288.

Lee HM, Weinstein JN, Meller ST, Hayashi N, Spratt KF, Gebhart GF. The role of steroids and their effects on phospholipase A2: an animal model of radiculopathy. Spine 1998; 23:1191–1196.

Link SC, El-Khoury GY, Guilford WB. Percutaneous epidural and nerve root block and percutaneous lumbar sympatholysis. Radiol Clin North Am 1998; 36:509–521.

Lutz GE, Vad VB, Wisneski RJ. Fluoroscopic transforaminal lumbar epidural steroids: an outcome study. Arch Phys Med Rehabil 1998; 79:1363–1366.

Luyendjik W. The plica mediana dorsalis of the dura mater and its relation to lumbar periradiculopathy (canalography). Neuroradiology 1976; 11:147–149.

Mamourian AC, Dickman CA, Drayer BP, Sonntag VKH. Spinal epidural abscess: three cases following spinal epidural injection demonstrated with magnetic resonance injection. Anesthesiology 1993; 70:204–207.

McCormick CC, Taylor JR, Twomey LT. Facet joint arthrography in lumbar spondylolysis: anatomic basis for spread of contrast material. Radiology 1989; 171:193–196.

McLain RF, Fry M, Hecht S. Transient paralysis associated with epidural steroid injection. J Spinal Disord 1997; 10:441–444.

McNeill TW, Andersson GBJ, Schell B, Sinkora G, Nelson J, Lavender SA. Epidural administration of methylprednisolone and morphine for pain after a spinal operation. J Bone Joint Surg Am 1995; 77:1814–1817.

Nelson DA, Vates TS, Thomas RB. Complications from intrathecal steroid therapy in patients with multiple sclerosis. Acta Neurol Scand 1973; 49:176–188.

Okada K. Studies on the cervical facet joints using arthrography of the cervical facet joints. Nippon Seikeigeka Gakkai Zasshi 1981; 55:563–580.

Raskin NH. Lumbar puncture headache: a review. Headache 1990; 30:197–200.

Renfrew DL, Moore TE, Kathol MH, El-Khoury GY, Lemke JH, Walker CW. Correct placement of epidural steroid injections: fluoroscopic guidance and contrast administration. Am J Neuroradiol 1991; 12:1003–1007.

Ridley MG, Kingsley GH, Gibson T, Grahame R. Outpatient lumbar epidural corticosteroid injection in the management of sciatica. Br J Rheum 1988; 27:295–299.

Riegelman RK, Hirsch RP. Studying a Study and Testing a Test: How to Read the Medical Literature, 2nd ed. Boston, Little, Brown, 1989.

Riew KD, Yin Y, Gilula L, Bridwell KH, Lenke LF, Lauryssen C, Goette K. The effect of nerve-root injections on the need for operative treatment of lumbar radicular pain. J Bone Joint Surg Am 2000; 82:1589–1593.

Rivest C, Katz JN, Ferrante FM, Jamison RN. Effects of epidural steroid injection on pain due to lumbar spinal stenosis or herniated disks: a prospective study. Arthritis Care Res 1998; 11:291–297.

Roy-Camille R, Mazel CH, Husson JL, Saillant G. Symptomatic spinal epidural lipomatosis induced by a long-term steroid treatment: review of the literature and report of two additional cases. Spine 1991; 16:1365–1371.

Schellinger D. Patterns of anterior spinal canal involvement by neoplasms and infections. Am J Neuroradiol 1996; 17:953–959.

Snoek W, Weber H, Jorgensen B. Double blind evaluation of extradural methylprednisolone for herniated lumbar discs. Acta Orthop Scand 1977; 48:635–641.

Stambough JL, Booth RE, Rothman RH. Transient hypercorticism after epidural steroid injection. J Bone Joint Surg Am 1984; 66:1115–1116.

Stojanovic MP, Vu TN, Caneris O, Slezak J, Cohen SP, Sang CN. The role of fluoroscopy in cervical epidural steroid injections: an analysis of contrast dispersal patterns. Spine 2002; 27:509–514.

Sullivan WJ, Willick SE, Chira-Adisai W, Zuhosky J, Tyburski M, Dreyfuss P, Prather H, Press JM. Incidence of intravascular uptake in lumbar spinal injection procedures. Spine 2000; 25:481–486.

Swerdlow M, Sayle-Creer W. A study of extradural medication in the relief of the lumbosciatic syndrome. Anaesthesia 1970; 25:341–345.

Vad VB, Bhat AL, Lutz GE, Cammisa F. Transforaminal epidural steroid injections in lumbosacral radiculopathy. Spine 2002; 27:11–16.

Victory RA, Hassett P, Morrison G. Transient blindness following epidural analgesia. Anaesthesia 1991; 46:940–941.

Waldman SD. Complications of cervical epidural nerve blocks with steroids: a prospective study of 790 consecutive blocks. Reg Anesth 1989; 14:149–151.

Wang JC, Lin E, Brodke DS, Youssef JA. Epidural injections for the treatment of symptomatic herniated discs. J Spinal Disord Techniques 2002; 15:269–272.

Warr AC, Wilkinson JA, Burn JMB, Langdon L. Chronic lumbosciatic syndrome treated by epidural injection and manipulation. Practitioner 1972; 209:53–59.

White AH, Derby R, Wynne G. Epidural injections for the diagnosis and treatment of low-back pain. Spine 1980; 5:78–86.

Williams KN, Jackowski A, Evans PJ. Epidural haematoma requiring surgical decompression following repeated cervical epidural steroid injections for chronic pain. Pain 1990; 42:197–199.

Wiltse LL, Fonseca AS, Amster J, Dimartino P, Ravessoud FA. Relationship of the dura, Hofmann's ligaments, Batson's plexus, and a fibrovascular membrane lying on the posterior surface of the vertebral bodies and attaching to the deep layer of the posterior longitudinal ligament: an anatomical, radiologic, and clinical study. Spine 1993; 18:1030–1043.

3 Nerve Root Block

DONALD L. RENFREW

Definition

Transforaminal epidural steroid injection (Botwin 2000, Johnson 1999, Link 1998, Lutz 1998, Vad 2002) uses injection of steroid within the circumneural sheath, usually along with anesthetic, for therapeutic purposes. A *nerve root block* (Dooley 1988, Haueisen 1985, Krempen 1974, MacNab 1971, North 1996, Schutz 1973, Stanley 1990, Tajima 1980) uses the same injection route, with the injection of a small amount of an anesthetic agent, sometimes along with a steroid drug, for diagnostic purposes. In a nerve root block, the volume of injectate is reduced to minimize reflux into the spinal canal (and hence maximize the specificity of the injection).

Literature Review

The nerve root block procedure has been in use for more than 50 years, with, for example, a detailed description of the anatomy and methods of performing blocks using anatomic landmarks published in an anesthesia textbook by Pitkin in 1953 (Pitkin 1953). MacNab (1971) described a technique using fluoroscopy and injection of an oil-based contrast medium for studying patients who had undergone negative disc exploration. MacNab's paper focused on the causes of "negative disc exploration" in patients with severe sciatic pain, and his final categories of diagnoses were as follows: "migration of a disc fragment into the intervertebral foramen, nerve-root kinking by the pedicle, articular process impingement on the nerve root, spinal stenosis, and extraforaminal lateral disc herniation." For his injections, MacNab described fluoroscopic visualization of needle tip position, reproduction of patient pain upon needle placement, visualization of the circumneural sheath by injection of oil-based contrast material, and anesthetization of the nerve using 1 mL of 2% lidocaine.

Multiple subsequent studies found similar results. Schutz and colleagues (Schutz 1973) also described image-guided needle localization, reproduction of typical pain upon injection, injection of an oil-based contrast material, and anesthetization of the nerve (with 1 mL of procaine). The authors used this technique in 15 patients who later went to surgery, and 13 of these demonstrated corresponding lesions. The authors also state, "The test was helpful in the management of 7 of 8 patients in whom no operation

was performed." Krempen and Smith (Krempen 1974) used the same technique to evaluate 22 patients with "complicated back problems who were seen with sciatica as the major problem" and found that "evaluation by this method permitted precise diagnosis of the level and side of the lesion in 18 patients, and appropriate surgical treatment in 16." Tajima and colleagues (Tajima 1980) described evaluation of an additional 106 patients with a similar technique; however, Tajima and colleagues used water-soluble ionic contrast material and also injected "water-soluble corticosteroid." They found the technique useful for "disorders featuring nerve root entrapment in the lateral foraminal recess, in which accurate localization cannot be determined by other auxiliary diagnostic measures." Haueisen and colleagues (Haueisen 1985) reported on an additional 105 patients and found that of 55 undergoing subsequent surgery, nerve blocks provided an accurate diagnosis in 43 (93%), whereas myelography was accurate in only 13 (24%). Dooley and colleagues (Dooley 1988) described an additional 62 similar injections, wherein they classify patients into three categories: patients with both reproduction of typical pain upon needle placement and relief of typical pain upon injection of anesthetic; patients with reproduction of typical pain but no relief; and patients with neither reproduction nor relief of pain. Patients with the reproduction/relief pattern typically underwent surgical exploration, with herniated discs, bony stenosis, and/or scarring found in nearly all cases. Stanley and colleagues (Stanley 1990) similarly classified responses into those with reproduction of symptoms and pain relief and those without; patients with the former pattern they considered candidates for surgery, and patients with the latter pattern they did not.

Contradicting these encouraging results, North and colleagues (North 1996) published a controlled, randomized study of 33 patients with sciatica who underwent (in random order) (1) selective nerve blocks, (2) sciatic nerve blocks, (3) medial branch posterior primary ramus blocks, and (4) subcutaneous lidocaine injections. They concluded (based on the good pain relief for many patients undergoing medial branch blocks or sciatic nerve blocks) that there is a "limited role for uncontrolled local anesthetic blocks in the diagnostic evaluation of sciatica." Although the nerve blocks provided better pain relief than the sciatic blocks and medial branch blocks, the differences were not statistically significant; more important than the differences between groups is the fact that, in a given patient with sciatica, good pain relief may follow from medial branch blocks or a sciatic

57

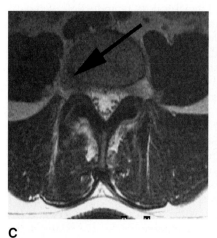

A

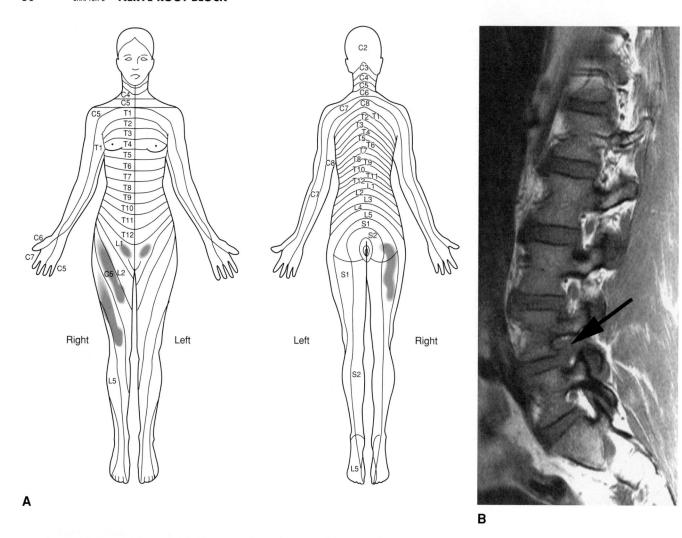

B

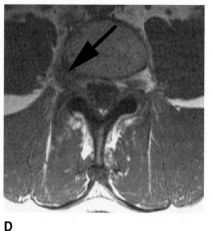

C   **D**

FIGURE 3–1

Patient with a Far Lateral Disc Extrusion Who Would Have Been a Candidate for a Diagnostic Nerve Block in an Earlier Era. This 49-year-old man had right groin and thigh pain and low back pain. *A,* Pain diagram. The patient indicated predominantly right anterior thigh pain. *B,* Right parasagittal T1-weighted magnetic resonance imaging (MRI) examination demonstrates a right foraminal disc extrusion (arrow). Compare the soft tissue fullness of the L4-5 neural foramen with the normal appearance of the L3-4 and L5-S1 neural foramina, which demonstrate fat surrounding the nerve in both instances. *C,* Axial T2-weighted MRI study at the level of the L4-5 disc demonstrates a right extraforaminal disc extrusion (arrow). Compare to the contralateral (normal) side, where the relatively brighter signal intensity of fat fills the lateral foramen and extraforaminal paravertebral space. *D,* Axial T1-weighted MRI study at the level of the L4-5 disc demonstrates to better advantage the right extraforaminal disc extrusion (arrow). Note the improved differentiation of the left ganglion and foraminal and extraforaminal paravertebral fat on the contralateral side. Two points deserve mention. First, this lesion would be impossible to see with plain films or oil myelography and difficult to see with water-soluble myelography and computed tomography. Second, even with high-quality MRI, this lesion is subtle (it is particularly hard to see on the T2-weighted images, where most viewers spend much of their effort). Nonetheless, given the patient's pain pattern and clinical history, the lesion is unequivocally the cause of the patient's symptoms, and diagnostic nerve blocks are not needed to make the diagnosis or plan therapy.

nerve block, indicating that the response to injection is not specific. Schwarzer and colleagues (Schwarzer 1994) have published similar findings regarding medial branch blocks. A recent pair of editorials in the journal *Spine* (Slosar 1998) reviewed the issue of whether selective nerve root blocks were diagnostic, therapeutic, or a placebo.

Rationale for Procedure

As noted earlier (see Table 1–1), we assume that needle placement close to the site of a symptomatic structure will stimulate nociceptors and thus reproduce the patient's typical pain, and that anesthetic agents placed through the needle will (at least temporarily) decrease activity within nociceptors and thus relieve the patient's pain. This rationale is reiterated in the language of many of the articles reviewed in Literature Review (Dooley 1988, Haueisen 1985, Krempen 1974, MacNab 1971, Schutz 1973, Stanley 1990, Tajima 1980). For many of the patients in these reported series, surgeons based their operative planning on the patient's response to diagnostic needle studies. In these situations, nerve blocks can be used in the evaluation of patients with radicular pain in two circumstances: when imaging studies demonstrate no definite anatomically corresponding abnormality, and when imaging studies demonstrate multilevel disease and it is not clear which level is responsible for the patient's radicular pain.

Diagnostic nerve root blocks originated in an era when oil-based myelography was the most sophisticated means available to evaluate the spine. For this reason, many of the patients undergoing diagnostic nerve blocks had diagnoses such as foraminal or far lateral (extraforaminal) disc herniation and subarticular and foraminal stenosis. With water-soluble contrast myelography, computed tomography, and magnetic resonance imaging (MRI) (the current imaging method of choice), these causes of radicular pain are readily diagnosed. Modern imaging would thus have eliminated many of the patients in the published studies on diagnostic nerve blocks (Fig. 3–1). If a patient demonstrates unequivocal single-level radiculopathy in the absence of any causative pathologic condition (and such pathologic findings may be subtle) along the course of the suspected nerve roots and nerve within the spine, surgeons are unlikely to operate regardless of the results of a nerve block (whether controlled or not). It is probably more prudent to search further proximally (with brain, cervical, or thoracic MRI) or distally (with pelvic or extremity MRI) for sources of lower extremity radicular pain (Bickels 1999) than to perform a nerve block hoping that it provides "definitive" results. The fact that a block at a given location along the pathway from peripheral

TABLE 3–1. Equipment and Supplies for Nerve Root Block

C-arm fluoroscope
Surgical scrub solution
Needles
Syringes
Connecting tube
Nonionic contrast material
Anesthetic agent
Steroid (optional)

nociceptors to the brain brings pain relief does not indicate that operating at the site of the block will eradicate that pain, particularly if the pain's origin is not at the site of the block. So, in the case of radicular pain, if there is a corresponding pathologic lesion at an anatomically appropriate location, diagnostic nerve blocks are usually redundant, whereas if no corresponding pathologic lesion is seen in the examined area, it is usually more appropriate to search elsewhere than to perform a diagnostic nerve block.

In those cases with multilevel disease, imaging will demonstrate that several adjacent levels all show possible causes of radicular pain, and injections are undertaken to differentiate which lesion is responsible for most or all of the patient's symptoms. However, probably because of factors such as the overlap of dermatomes and reflux of even small amounts of anesthetic drug into the spinal canal (with associated cross-anesthetization of proximal and distal nerves), such injections often add little to surgical planning. This is not to say that such injections, particularly when combined with steroid, may not be beneficial in providing pain relief; however, when performed in this manner, the injection is properly called a *transforaminal epidural steroid injection* rather than a nerve block.

Additional imaging technology may provide the solution to the conundrum of patients with radicular pain and negative or equivocal imaging study findings. In a study evaluating a device for loading the lumbar spine during MRI, Willen and Danielson (Willen 2001) found significant additional information in 14% of patients with sciatica when comparing unloaded (usual) and loaded MRI scans. In the cervical spine, performing studies with the patient in flexion and in extension may demonstrate pathologic lesions not evident when the spine is in a neutral position (Muhle 1999).

Equipment and Supplies[1]

Table 3–1 lists equipment required for nerve root blocks.

A standard fluoroscope can be used for nerve block injections, but it is generally much more difficult to obtain ideal positioning (particularly at the S1 level) than when using a C-arm device. A laser aiming device (an attachment that shows a cross-hair on the fluoroscopic screen corresponding in position to a red dot on the skin surface) is extremely helpful for proper needle placement. Selection of needle type varies with the operator; a 22-gauge spinal needle for most lumbar injections and a 25-gauge spinal needle for thoracic injections work well. These needles are inexpensive, are readily available, and can usually be inserted without prior local anesthetic. Everything injected into the patient must be as safe as possible and preferably safe for intrathecal use, since there will be occasions when, despite the utmost diligence on the part of the operator, some of the injected materials will reach the thecal sac. For this reason, nonionic contrast material approved for intrathecal injection, an anesthetic agent approved for intrathecal injection (consult the package insert), and the most benign steroid obtainable should be used. In addition, if the contrast

---

[1]This section is virtually identical to the Equipment and Supplies section in Chapter 2 and can be skipped if the reader is already familiar with this material.

injection pattern suggests that the injection is intrathecal, it is usually best to stop injecting, abandon the procedure, and reschedule the procedure for another day.

In addition to the equipment listed in Table 3–1, a crash cart should be readily available to handle medical emergencies (e.g., contrast media and drug reactions).

Informed Consent Issues[2]

Informed consent issues can be divided into three topics: description of the procedure, warning the patient about possible drug side effects, and delineation of material risks. Informed consent also implies that alternatives to the proposed treatment have been described; for a general description of such alternatives, see Chapter 1.

Either the performing physician or a trained subordinate should completely explain the entire procedure in detail to the patient prior to performance of the procedure. Patients who know what to expect are much less anxious than those who do not. A step-by-step description, including reassurance that the procedure takes only a few minutes, that many patients undergo similar procedures every day, and that the amount of pain caused by needle insertion is similar to that caused by drawing blood or starting an intravenous access line, provides a considerable calming effect in most patients.

The performing physician or a trained subordinate should also explain that local anesthetic may cause numbness and weakness of the leg. Patients should be warned that the injection may recreate or exacerbate their pain. While this side effect typically relents within moments of injection of local anesthetic, occasionally it will persist. In those cases in which a steroid is injected, review of steroid side effects should be undertaken. These side effects include changes in mood (usually mild euphoria but occasionally anxiety), appetite (usually increased), insomnia, sweating, hot flashes, facial flushing, rash, and gastrointestinal upset. Some patients benefit from medications to relieve anxiety or insomnia.

Complications can be subdivided into two categories: occasional (but inevitable) and rare but reported in the literature. Vasovagal reactions (treated with time, intravenous fluids, and atropine as necessary) and inadvertent thecal puncture constitute the first category. Any recognized thecal puncture should result in immediate removal of the needle and rescheduling of the procedure. Inadvertent injection of local anesthetic into the lumbar thecal sac usually results in a spinal block, urinary incontinence, and inability to move the lower extremities for the duration of the block. Inadvertent injection of steroid into the thecal sac will probably not result in such obvious immediate problems but carries the risk of arachnoiditis (Benzon 1986, Nelson 1973). Some patients who have had an inadvertent thecal puncture, as well as some who undergo myelography or diagnostic lumbar puncture, may develop a "post-tap headache." Treatment of such headaches includes bedrest, caffeine, pain killers, and an epidural "blood

patch" (or saline injection) (Raskin 1990). The epidural blood patch is performed as indicated in Chapter 2 for an interlaminar epidural steroid injection, with injection of 10 to 15 mL of freshly drawn venous blood from the patient injected into the epidural space.

Less frequent but either reported or theoretical complications of nerve blocks are similar to those for epidural steroid injection (minus the steroid-specific complications if no steroid is injected) and are listed in Table 3–2. Patients should cease taking all anticoagulants and other agents that might increase the risk of epidural hematoma formation prior to performance of the epidural injection. With respect to anaphylactic reaction, patients should be screened for sensitivity to contrast media. If a patient has had a prior minor reaction to an intravenous contrast agent, either reassurance or oral prednisone prior to the procedure is advised. For prior major reactions, the best option is probably to perform the procedure with fluoroscopic guidance and to forego steroid injection, since intrathecal injection of steroids may result in adhesive arachnoiditis, which is essentially incurable (Guyer 1989). Nonlatex gloves and surgical scrub solution without iodine may be used as appropriate.

After hearing of possible complications (however rare), patients may wish to reconsider or decline nerve blocks. In the interests of balancing these infrequent complications with the usual course of events, the performing physician or a trained subordinate may wish to review with the patient the experience reviewed by Botwin and colleagues (2000). This group reported on 322 transforaminal injections (comparable to nerve blocks) with one vasovagal reaction, one case of intraoperative hypertension, and one case of transient elevation of blood sugar in an insulin-dependent diabetic patient, without any serious or permanent ill effects. The blood sugar elevation would not have occurred without steroid injection.

Patient Selection

As indicated in the Rationale for Procedure section, modern imaging has eliminated the need for diagnostic nerve blocks

TABLE 3–2. Reported or Theoretical Complications of Nerve Root Blocks

Reported in epidural steroid injection procedures, no steroid injected
 Transient paralysis (McLain 1997)
 Epidural abscess (Knight 1997, Mamourian 1993)
 Epidural hematoma (Williams 1990)
 Paraplegia following transforaminal lumbar injection (Houten 2002)
Reported in epidural steroid injection procedures, steroid injected
 Transient hypercorticism (Stambough 1984)
 Epidural lipomatosis (Roy-Camille 1991)
 Retinal hemorrhage with transient blindness (Victory 1991)
Theoretical (but reported for other procedures)
 Anaphylactic reaction to contrast material
 Anaphylactic reaction to anesthetic agent
 Anaphylactic reaction to steroid drug
 Anaphylactic reaction to latex, surgical scrub solution, etc.

---

[2]This section is very similar to the Informed Consent Issues section of Chapter 2 and can be skipped if the reader is already familiar with this material.

TABLE 3–3. Step-by-Step Description of L1-5 Transforaminal Lumbar Nerve Root Blocks

1. Position the C-arm fluoroscope to obtain a clear view of the appropriate pedicle. In the midlumbar spine, the angle is usually axial; in the upper lumbar spine, the angle may need to be adjusted in a more cranial direction, whereas in the lower lumbar spine, a more caudal angulation is often necessary.
2. Insert needle along the course of the x-ray beam far enough so that it is anchored. Insertion should be through a skin site that has been prepped and draped in a sterile fashion.
3. Check position with C-arm fluoroscope.
4. Adjust as necessary.
5. Advance needle until the patient has radicular pain *or* the needle rests on bone.
6. Go to frontal position and confirm needle tip position beneath the pedicle.
7. Inject 0.5 mL of nonionic contrast material and document circumneural sheath location. Make particular note of any suspected arterial flow toward the spinal canal, especially toward the conus (Houten 2002); avoid injecting if this happens.
8. Inject 0.5 to 1.0 mL of local anesthetic while monitoring displacement of the nonionic contrast material. If there is extensive flow into the spinal canal, stop injecting.
9. Take frontal and oblique images.
10. Monitor patient for pain relief. If the patient does not achieve pain relief, consider blocking more proximal or distal levels.
11. Release patient when stable. Provide patient with a telephone number to call if there is persistent increased pain or numbness or if fever, swelling, or redness develops.

in many patients. In the absence of any imaging evidence of causative pathologic conditions, the utility of nerve blocks is limited. There may be cases of unequivocal radicular pain but equivocal pathologic findings wherein the nerve block is used. Some authors prefer to use the injection for its negative prognostic value given this scenario: if the patient fails to respond to a block at this level, then no surgery will be performed, whereas if the patient does get pain relief upon injection, no conclusion regarding surgical benefits can be made (Slosar 1998).

Procedure Description

The procedure is very similar to that of transforaminal epidural steroid injection (see Chapter 2). Table 3–3 describes and Figures 3–2 and 3–3 illustrate the lumbar nerve root block procedure. Table 3–4 describes and Figure

3–4 illustrates the S1 nerve root block procedure. See also Chapter 2, particularly the illustrations concerning transforaminal epidural steroid injection. One problem with nerve root blocks is that although large volumes (2.0–3.0 mL) of injected material will sometimes flow exclusively distally within the circumneural sheath (Figs. 3–4 and 3–5), on other occasions even tiny volumes (0.1–0.2 mL) of injected material may show passage into the spinal canal (Fig. 3–6), regardless of the exact needle position with respect to the pedicle. Therefore, when performing nerve blocks, it is essential to document with hard copy (and indicate in the report) whether reflux has occurred and thus whether the block can be considered specific. The record should also indicate, of course, whether the patient had reproduction of typical symptoms and the degree and duration of pain relief. Since negative control blocks either above, below, or both above and below the suspected level lend credibility to the results, it is worthwhile to consider

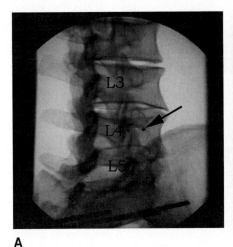
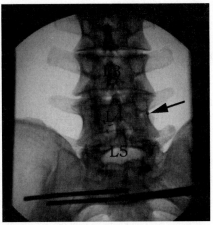

A   **B**

FIGURE 3–2

Skeletal Radiograph Demonstrating Target Position for an L4 Nerve Block. Compare with Figure 2–18, a skeletal radiograph depicting the anatomy for an L5 transforaminal epidural steroid injection. *A,* Oblique specimen radiograph with a metallic bead (arrow) taped along the inferior lateral aspect of the L4-5 intervertebral nerve root canal (foramen). This is the correct angle for the C-arm at the start of the procedure. The cross-hairs of the laser aiming device project posterior to the target point, so either the C-arm needs to be lowered or the table needs to be elevated for ideal positioning. (The metallic bars through the pelvis hold the sacrum and pelvis together in this specimen.) *B,* Frontal view with the metallic bead (arrow) seen beneath the right L4 pedicle.

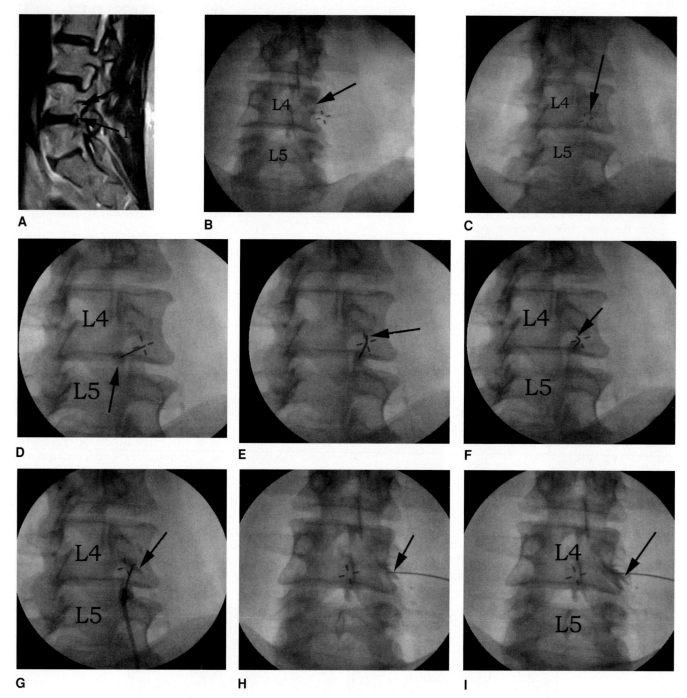

FIGURE 3–3

Step-by-Step Right L4 Nerve Block. This 55-year-old woman had low back and right lateral and anterior thigh pain. *A,* Right parasagittal T2-weighted magnetic resonance imaging examination shows a right foraminal disc protrusion with relative T2 prolongation (arrow 1). There is no significant flattening of the exiting right L4 ganglion, however (arrow 2). Interlaminar therapeutic injections provided minimal benefit. *B,* Frontal view demonstrates the cross-hairs of the laser aiming device just beneath the right L4 pedicle (arrow). From this position, the C-arm needs to be rotated toward the patient's right side. *C,* Oblique view following rotation of the C-arm. The cross-hairs of the laser aiming device (arrow) are positioned under the anterior aspect of the right L4 pedicle, in appropriate position for needle placement. Positioning the needle too high may result in the inability to advance the needle to an appropriate position under the pedicle because the transverse process may block the needle path. *D,* Oblique magnified view following needle placement demonstrates that the needle tip is centered in the cross-hairs of the laser aiming device. The needle hub (arrow) projects more posteriorly and inferiorly. Although the needle tip is currently projecting in the correct location, if advanced it will pass superior and lateral to the target position. Placing the bevel so that it faces superiorly and to the right will help prevent this from happening. *E,* Oblique magnified view following advancement of the needle tip with the bevel facing anteriorly and superiorly. The needle tip (arrow) is now directed more posteriorly but is still somewhat superior and may be blocked by the transverse process. *F,* Oblique magnified view following further advancement of the needle tip with the bevel directed superiorly. The tip (arrow) is now located in good position beneath the right L4 pedicle. The patient had reproduction of typical right anterior thigh pain at this time. *G,* Oblique magnified view following injection of 0.1 mL of nonionic contrast material demonstrates flow along the right L4 circumneural sheath distally. Note that there is no reflux of contrast or flow into the epidural space within the spinal canal. *H,* Frontal magnified view following injection of 0.1 mL of nonionic contrast material again demonstrates flow along the right L4 circumneural sheath distally. As on the oblique view, there is no reflux of contrast or flow into the epidural space within the spinal canal. *I,* Frontal magnified view following injection of a total of 0.3 mL of nonionic contrast material demonstrates additional flow distally along the right L4 circumneural sheath. Although a small amount of contrast also tracks proximally along the sheath, no reflux into the epidural space of the spinal canal is identified. Following injection of 0.5 mL of 2% lidocaine, the patient had complete pain relief for the duration of the local anesthetic, consistent with right L4 ganglionic irritation as the source of the patient's symptoms.

TABLE 3–4. Step-by-Step Description of S1 Nerve Root Block

1. Position the C-arm fluoroscope to obtain a clear view through the S1 foramen. This usually requires considerable caudal angulation of the beam, as well as mild ipsilateral angulation. A relatively straight frontal view will demonstrate the arc of the anterior margin of the foramen, but passage of a needle toward the bottom of the arc will not succeed in reaching the foramen because the posterior opening is considerably higher. If it is not possible to see "down the barrel" of the S1 foramen, the bottom of the S1 pedicle may be used as a landmark. If this, too, cannot be accomplished, then starting superior to the anterior arch with the needle 2 to 3 cm from midline on the ipsilateral side is probably the best option.
2. Insert needle along the course of the x-ray beam far enough so that it is anchored. Insertion should be through a skin site that has been prepped and draped in sterile fashion.
3. Check position with the C-arm fluoroscope. The needle should be directed toward the superior, lateral aspect of the lucency formed by the S2 neural foramen.
4. Adjust as necessary.
5. When the patient has radicular pain, or when the needle is clearly along the course of the S1 foramen, go to lateral position and check needle position. Ideal position is in approximately the middle of the sacrum in the anterior-posterior direction.
6. Inject 0.5 mL of nonionic contrast material and document circumneural sheath location. Make particular note of any suspected arterial flow toward the spinal canal, especially toward the conus (Houten 2002); avoid injecting if this happens.
7. Inject 0.5 to 1.0 mL of local anesthetic while monitoring displacement of the nonionic contrast material. If there is extensive flow into the spinal canal, stop injecting.
8. Take frontal and lateral images.
9. Monitor patient for pain relief. If the patient does not achieve pain relief, consider blocking more proximal or distal levels.
10. Release patient when stable. Provide patient with a telephone number to call if there is persistent increased pain or numbness or if fever, swelling, or redness develops.

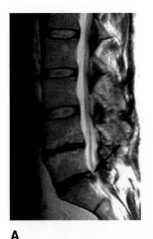 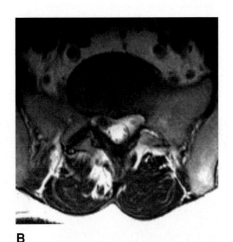 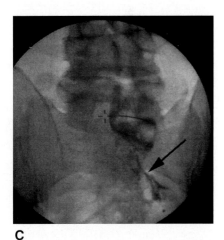

A B C

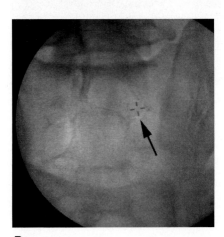 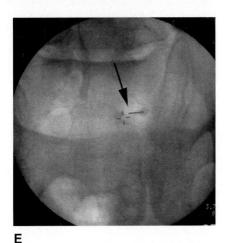

D E

FIGURE 3–4

S1 Nerve Root Block. This 44-year-old man had low back pain radiating to the right posterior thigh for 5 weeks. He had a history of remote prior L4-5 discectomy with relief of contralateral lower extremity symptoms. *A,* Right parasagittal T2-weighted magnetic resonance imaging examination demonstrates L4-5 and L5-S1 loss of disc height and hydration with subchondral changes at L4-5. At the L5-S1 level, there is a caudally dissecting disc extrusion (arrow). Note the smooth disc margin at the postoperative L4-5 level. *B,* Axial T2-weighted magnetic resonance imaging scan at the L5-S1 disc level demonstrates the right subarticular disc extrusion (arrow). The disc extrusion and the traversing right S1 nerve root are difficult to differentiate.

C, Frontal view from an interlaminar lumbar epidural steroid injection demonstrates that the needle is in place via a right-sided L5-S1 approach. There is contrast at, above, and below the level of the needle, with contrast along the right S1 circumneural sheath (arrow). The patient achieved minimal if any pain relief following this injection. An S1 nerve root block was planned to see whether significant pain relief could be achieved by anesthetization of the S1 nerve. *D,* Frontal view of the sacrum prior to placing the needle for an S1 nerve root block. The cross-hairs of the laser imaging device is just superior to the foramen for the S1 nerve (arrow). Caudal angulation has been used to visualize the neural foramen as a lucency. *E,* Frontal view following introduction of a needle. The needle tip is on line to pass into or through the right S1 neural foramen (arrow). *(Figure continues on following page)*

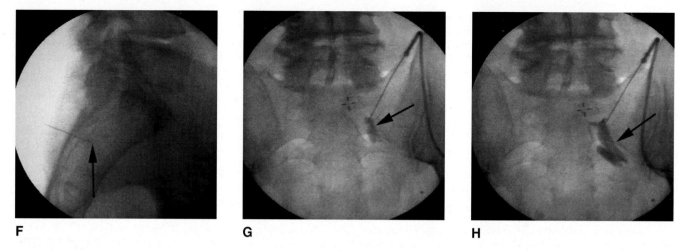

F   G   H

FIGURE 3–4 CONTINUED

F, Lateral view following needle insertion. The needle tip (arrow) projects over the posterior aspect of S1, in a position consistent with the dorsal aspect of the S1 neural foramen. *G*, Frontal view after injection of 0.3 mL of nonionic contrast material, which flows distally along the right S1 circumneural sheath (arrow). Note the oblique course of the needle now that the C-arm has been returned to neutral position. *H*, Frontal view after injection of 0.5 mL of local anesthetic and an additional 1.0 mL of contrast material demonstrates exclusively distal flow along the S1 circumneural sheath (arrow), without reflux of contrast material into the spinal canal. The patient had approximately 50% pain relief. This result, while better than the pain relief offered by the interlaminar injection done at L5-S1, implies that the S1 nerve root irritation may not be the sole source of lower extremity symptoms, given incomplete pain relief despite placement of an adequate amount of local anesthetic along the right S1 nerve root.

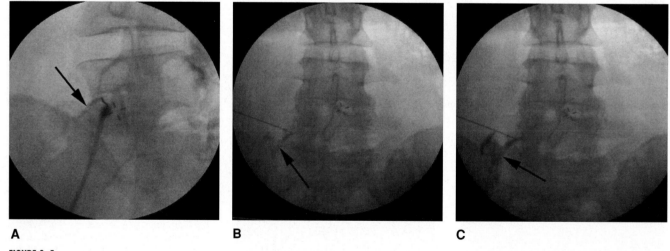

A   B   C

FIGURE 3–5

Injected Material Flowing Distally Along the Circumneural Sheath. This 55-year-old woman had left leg pain in an L5 distribution. *A*, Oblique view obtained following injection of 0.3 mL of contrast material. The needle is laterally located beneath the L5 pedicle. Contrast flows peripherally along the left L5 circumneural sheath (arrow). *B*, Frontal view obtained after injection of an addition 0.5 mL of contrast material. Note that the material is flowing preferentially distally along the circumneural sheath (arrow), with no reflux into the epidural space within the spinal canal. *C*, Frontal view after an additional 1.0 mL of contrast material has been injected. Again, the material flows exclusively distally, without reflux into the epidural space within the spinal canal. Such exclusive, distal flow guarantees that the injection will be "specific" in the sense that the attendant pain relief may be attributed to anesthetization of the selected nerve and not secondary to reflux within the spinal canal and anesthetization of adjacent segment nerves. Of course, a positive response could also be secondary to the placebo effect, which may be (at least partially) controlled for by additional injections done at other levels.

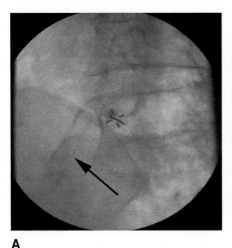
A

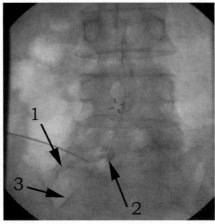
B

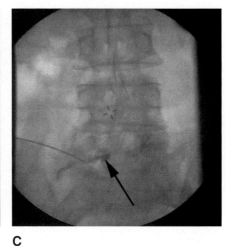
C

FIGURE 3–6

Injected Material Flowing Proximally into the Epidural Space of the Spinal Canal. This 70-year-old woman had left leg pain in an L5 distribution. *A*, Oblique view obtained prior to injection of contrast material. Note that the needle tip is located somewhat more medial in relation to the L5 pedicle than in Figure 3–5B. No contrast material has been injected, but there is somewhat confusing calcification of the left common iliac artery (arrow). *B*, Frontal view obtained after injection of 0.2 mL of contrast material. Note that the material is flowing freely not only distally along the L5 circumneural sheath (arrow 1) but also proximally into the epidural space within the spinal canal (arrow 2). Calcification along the iliac artery (arrow 3) mimics contrast along a lower circumneural sheath. *C*, Frontal view after an additional 1.0 mL of contrast material has been injected. Much of the injected material is flowing into the epidural space within the spinal canal. Flow of anesthetic in this manner would compromise the specificity of a nerve block, because the material may reach more proximal and distal nerve roots.

including a "control" block as part of the procedure. The following is a report of the case illustrated in Figure 3–3:

INTRODUCTION

The patient has low back and right thigh pain in what appears to be an L4 distribution. The patient has foraminal narrowing at L4-5 with some possible contact of the exiting right L4 nerve root on MRI examination.

TECHNICAL INFORMATION

Informed consent was obtained. Using sterile technique and fluoroscopic guidance, a 22-gauge spinal needle was placed into the right L4 circumneural sheath. Confirmation of needle tip position was established via fluoroscopic visualization of contrast material in the right L4 circumneural sheath. A total of 0.3 mL of iohexol (Omnipaque) 240 mg/mL contrast material was injected, and 0.5 mL of 2.0% lidocaine was injected.

INTERPRETATION

Frontal and lateral films demonstrate contrast distribution exclusively along the L4 circumneural sheath without significant reflux into the spinal canal. The patient experienced reproduction of typical symptoms upon injection, followed by 100% pain relief for the duration of the local anesthetic.

CONCLUSION

1. Technically successful lumbar L4 nerve block with injection of nonionic contrast material and local anesthetic.
2. The patient achieved complete pain relief for the duration of the local anesthetic, although she did not have similar pain relief with prior interlaminar

lumbar epidural steroid injections. This set of circumstances indicates that foraminal narrowing and associated right L4 ganglionic irritation is probably a significant source of the patient's right leg pain.

References

Benzon HT. Epidural steroid injections for low back pain and lumbosacral radiculopathy. Pain 1986; 24:277–295.

Bickels J, Kahanovitz N, Rubert CK, Henshaw RM, Moss DP, Meller I, Malawer MM. Extraspinal bone and soft-tissue tumors as a cause of sciatica: clinical diagnosis and recommendations—analysis of 32 cases. Spine 1999; 24:1611–1616.

Botwin KP, Gruber RD, Bouchlas CG, et al. Complications of fluoroscopically guided transforaminal lumbar epidural injections. Arch Phys Med Rehabil 2000; 81:1045–1050.

Dooley JF, McBroom RJ, Taguchi T, MacNab I. Nerve root infiltration in the diagnosis of radicular pain. Spine 1988; 13:79–83.

Guyer DW, Wiltse LL, Eskay ML, Guyer BH. The long-range prognosis of arachnoiditis. Spine 1989; 14:1332–1341.

Haueisen DC, Smith BS, Myers SR, Pryce ML. The diagnostic accuracy of spinal nerve injection studies: their role in the evaluation of recurrent sciatica. Clin Orthop Rel Res 1985; 198:179–183.

Houten JK, Errico TJ. Paraplegia after lumbosacral nerve root block: report of three cases. Spine J 2002; 2:70–75.

Johnson BA, Schellhas KP, Pollei SR. Epidurography and therapeutic epidural injections: technical considerations and experience with 5334 cases. Am J Neuroradiol 1999; 20:697–705.

Knight JW, Cordingly JJ, Palazzo MGA. Epidural abscess following epidural steroid and local anesthesic injection. Anaesthesia 1997; 52:576–585.

Krempen JF, Smith BS. Nerve-root injection: a method for evaluating the etiology of sciatica. J Bone Joint Surg Am 1974; 56:1435–1444.

Link SC, El-Khoury GY, Guilford WB. Percutaneous epidural and nerve root block and percutaneous lumbar sympatholysis. Radiol Clin North Am 1998; 36:509–521.

Lutz GE, Vad VB, Wisneski RJ. Fluoroscopic transforaminal lumbar epidural steroids: an outcome study. Arch Phys Med Rehabil 1998; 79:18-1363–1366.

MacNab I. Negative disc exploration: an analysis of the causes of nerve-root involvement in sixty-eight patients. J Bone Joint Surg Am 1971; 53:891–903.

Mamourian AC, Dickman CA, Drayer BP, Sonntag VKH. Spinal epidural abscess: three cases following spinal epidural injection demonstrated with magnetic resonance injection. Anesthesiology 1993; 70:204–207.

McLain RF, Fry M, Hecht S. Transient paralysis associated with epidural steroid injection. J Spinal Disord 1997; 10:441–444.

Muhle C, Metzner J, Weinert D, et al. Kinematic MR imaging in surgical management of cervical disc disease, spondylosis, and spondylolytic myelopathy. Acta Radiol 1999; 40:146–153.

Nelson DA, Vates TS, Thomas RB. Complications from intrathecal steroid therapy in patients with multiple sclerosis. Acta Neurol Scand 1973; 49:176–188.

North RB, Kidd DH, Zahurak M, Piantadosi S. Specificity of diagnostic nerve blocks: a prospective, randomized study of sciatica due to lumbosacral spine disease. Pain 1996; 65:77–85.

Pitkin GP. Conduction Anesthesia, 2nd ed. Philadelphia, J.B. Lippincott, 1953.

Raskin NH. Lumbar puncture headache: a review. Headache 1990; 30:197–200.

Roy-Camille R, Mazel CH, Husson JL, Saillant G. Symptomatic spinal epidural lipomatosis induced by a long-term steroid treatment: review of the literature and report of two additional cases. Spine 1991; 16:1365–1371.

Schutz H, Lougheed WM, Wortzman G, Awerbuck BG. Intervertebral nerve-root in the investigation of chronic lumbar disc disease. J Can Surg 1973; 16:217–221.

Schwarzer AC, Aprill CN, Derby R, Fortin J, Kine G, Bogduk N. The false-positive rate of uncontrolled diagnostic blocks of the lumbar zygapophysial joints. Pain 1994; 58:195–200.

Slosar PJ, White AH, Wetzel FD. The use of selective nerve root blocks: diagnostic, therapeutic, or placebo? Spine 1998; 23:2253–2256.

Stambough JL, Booth RE, Rothman RH. Transient hypercorticism after epidural steroid injection. J Bone Joint Surg Am 1984; 66:1115–1116.

Stanley D, McLaren MI, Euinton HA, Getty CJM. A prospective study of nerve root infiltration in the diagnosis of sciatica: a comparison with radiculography, computed tomography, and operative findings. Spine 1990; 15:540–543.

Tajima T, Furukawa K, Kuramochi E. Selective lumbosacral radiculography and block. Spine 1980; 5:68–77.

Vad VB, Bhat AL, Lutz GE, Cammisa F. Transforaminal epidural steroid injections in lumbosacral radiculopathy. Spine 2002; 27:11–16.

Victory RA, Hassett P, Morrison G. Transient blindness following epidural analgesia. Anaesthesia 1991; 46:940–941.

Willen J, Danielson B. The diagnostic effect from axial loading of the lumbar spine during computed tomography and magnetic resonance imaging in patients with degenerative disorders. Spine 2001; 26:2607–2614.

Williams KN, Jackowski A, Evans PJ. Epidural haematoma requiring surgical decompression following repeated cervical epidural steroid injections for chronic pain. Pain 1990; 42:197–199.

4 Sacroiliac Joint Injection

DONALD L. RENFREW

Definition

Sacroiliac joint injection is just that: injection into the sacroiliac joint. Sacroiliac joint injection is predominantly a diagnostic tool, with evaluation of whether typical symptoms are elicited upon injection and are then relieved with local anesthetic. Steroid can be injected into the sacroiliac joint for therapeutic purposes.

Literature Review

There is far less literature regarding sacroiliac joint injection than there is regarding epidural steroid injection or even nerve blocks. A century ago, the sacroiliac joint was thought to be the cause of low back pain in a high proportion of back pain sufferers (Fortin 1995, Goldthwait 1911), but that view changed starting with Mixter and Barr's 1934 article (Mixter 1934) introducing the concept of a herniated disc.

Although earlier authors had suggested the possibility of blind sacroiliac joint injection (Haldeman 1938), Miskew and colleagues (Miskew 1979) first described fluoroscopically directed insertion (for aspiration purposes in cases of infection rather than diagnosis or treatment by injection). In 1982, Hendrix and colleagues (Hendrix 1982) published an injection technique they described as "quick, simple, and reliable." A 1995 paper by Bollow and colleagues (Bollow 1995) illustrates an example of computed tomographically directed needle placement into the sacroiliac joint of a patient with spondyloarthropathy, and a 2000 paper by Pereira (Pereira 2000) describes a magnetic resonance imaging directed injection technique.

Many signs and symptoms have been proposed as indicative of pain originating in the sacroiliac joint (Fortin 1995, Simon 2001). By and large, these have not been found predictive of relief of pain provided by intra-articular injection of lidocaine (Dreyfuss 1996, Maigne 1996, Schwarzer 1995), although, in general terms, if pain is maximal above the L5 level, it is unlikely to be relieved by sacroiliac joint injection. Unlike the situation with the facet joints that have discrete innervation (see Chapter 5), the sacroiliac joints are diffusely innervated and thus cannot be "blocked" by anesthetic placed at the location of supplying nerves (Dreyfuss 2002).

Intra-articular injection of steroid has been evaluated in cases of spondyloarthropathy (Bollow 1996, Braun 1996, Maugars 1992, Maugars 1996) with mixed, mostly positive results, but little or nothing has been published regarding evaluation of pain relief from intra-articular injection of steroids in those patients whose pain is presumed to be secondary to degenerative change or whose pain is relieved by intra-articular injection of an anesthetic agent (Dreyfuss 2002).

Rationale for Procedure

As stated by Schwarzer and colleagues (Schwarzer 1995), "Needles can be precisely placed in the joint to inject radiographic contrast medium and local anesthetic. In this way, pain may be provoked and relieved.... Infiltration of the joint with local anesthetic should anesthetize all nociceptors within the joint and thereby relieve any pain stemming from it" (see Table 1–1). Similarly, a steroid may be introduced on the theory that this may provide long-term benefit (although literature support is lacking, at least in patients without spondyloarthropathy).

Equipment and Supplies[1]

Table 4–1 lists equipment required for sacroiliac joint injection.

A standard fluoroscope can be used for sacroiliac joint injections, but it is generally much more difficult to obtain

TABLE 4–1. Equipment and Supplies for Sacroiliac Joint Injection

C-arm fluoroscope
Surgical scrub solution
Needles
Syringes
Connecting tube
Nonionic contrast material
Anesthetic agent
Steroid (optional)

---

[1]This section is virtually identical to the Equipment and Supplies section in Chapter 2 and can be skipped if the reader is already familiar with this material.

TABLE 4–2. Step-by-Step Description of Sacroiliac Joint Injection

1. Position the C-arm fluoroscope so that a clear view of the inferior aspect of the sacroiliac joint is obtained. *Caudal angulation* will better visualize the posterior (target) portion of the joint. Angulation *away from* the side to be injected may better visualize the inferior (target) portion of the joint, although this varies considerably from patient to patient and it is usually best to check several medial-to-lateral angulation options while visualizing the inferior aspect of the joint.
2. Insert the needle along the course of the x-ray beam far enough so that it is anchored.
3. Check the position of the needle with a C-arm fluoroscope.
4. Adjust needle position as necessary while advancing in 3 to 5 mm increments.
5. Advance the needle until the needle tip encounters bone, feels as if it has entered the joint, or demonstrates a curve in its distal aspect. If on bone, adjust until the needle is within the joint.
6. Inject 0.1 to 0.2 mL of contrast material and document an intra-articular position of the injected material. Reposition if not intra-articular.
7. Inject 1.0 to 1.5 mL of anesthetic for a diagnostic block. Inject steroid if desired.
8. Monitor patient for significant pain relief.
9. Release patient when stable. Provide patient with a telephone number to call if there is persistent or increased pain or numbness or if fever, swelling, or redness develop.

ideal positioning than with a C-arm device. A laser aiming device (an attachment that shows a cross-hair on the fluoroscopic screen corresponding in position to a red dot on the skin surface) is extremely helpful for proper needle placement. Selection of needle type varies with the operator; 22-gauge spinal needles work well. These needles are inexpensive, are readily available, and can usually be inserted without prior local anesthetic. Everything injected into the patient must be as safe as possible.

In addition to the equipment listed in Table 4–1, a crash cart should be readily available to handle medical emergencies (e.g., contrast media and drug reactions).

Informed Consent Issues[2]

Informed consent issues can be divided into three topics: description of the procedure, warning the patient about possible drug side effects, and delineation of material risks. Informed consent also implies that alternatives to the proposed treatment have been described; for a general description of such alternatives, see Chapter 1.

Either the performing physician or a trained subordinate should completely explain the entire procedure in detail to the patient prior to performance of the procedure. Patients who know what to expect are much less anxious than those who do not. A step-by-step description, including reassurance that the procedure takes only a few minutes, that many patients undergo similar procedures every day, and that the amount of pain caused by needle insertion is similar to that caused by drawing blood or starting an intravenous access line, provides a considerable calming effect in most patients.

The performing physician or a trained subordinate should also explain that local anesthetic injected during a sacroiliac joint injection may, by flowing out of the anterior aspect of the joint capsule, cause anesthetization of the sacral plexus and thus numbness and weakness of the leg (Fortin 1995). Patients should be warned that the injection may recreate or exacerbate their pain. While this side effect typically relents within moments of injection of local anesthetic, occasionally it will persist. In those cases in which a

steroid is injected, review of steroid side effects should be undertaken. These side effects include changes in mood (usually mild euphoria but occasionally anxiety), appetite (usually increased), insomnia, sweating, hot flashes, facial flushing, rash, and gastrointestinal upset. Some patients benefit from medications to relieve anxiety or insomnia.

Complications can be subdivided into two categories: occasional (but inevitable) and rare but reported or theoretical. In the occasional but inevitable category, vasovagal reactions are usually best treated with time, intravenous fluids, and atropine as necessary.

Rare but potential complications of sacroiliac joint injections with steroids include local hemorrhage and infection, transient hypercorticism, and retinal hemorrhage with transient blindness. Patients should cease taking all anticoagulants prior to performance of sacroiliac joint injection. With respect to anaphylactic reaction, patients should be screened for sensitivity to contrast media. If a patient has had a prior minor reaction to an intravenous contrast agent, either reassurance or oral prednisone prior to the procedure is advised. For prior major contrast reactions, the best option is probably to perform the procedure with fluoroscopic guidance but without contrast injection. Nonlatex gloves and surgical scrub solution without iodine can be used as appropriate.

Patient Selection

Since signs and symptoms are not particularly predictive of response to sacroiliac joint injection (Dreyfuss 1996, Schwarzer 1995), selection of appropriate patients is difficult. On the other hand, since neither intra-articular steroids nor any other method of treatment of sacroiliac pain has been demonstrated to be efficacious in controlled trials, making the diagnoses might be considered unnecessary. Surgeons rarely fuse the sacroiliac joint. Dreyfuss (Dreyfuss 2002) suggests that the injections not be performed if pain is maximal above the L5 level, if another cause of pain is apparent and more likely, if pain responds to other, more conservative measures, or if there is no need to establish the diagnosis. One rationale for securing the diagnosis is that it prevents further search for other causes of pain (Dreyfuss 2002), but this rationale makes sense only if the patient is content to stop seeking diagnosis and treatment if the injection is "positive."

---

[2]This section is very similar to the Informed Consent Issues section of Chapter 2 and can be skipped if the reader is already familiar with this material.

Procedure Description

The literature provides several descriptions of injection techniques (Dreyfuss 2002, Dussault 2000, Hendrix 1982). None of these are uniformly successful, and on occasion multiple attempts, even repeatedly using the same technique or trying different techniques, all fail. Difficulty in injection follows from the complex anatomy of the joint, which has complex interdigitating surfaces on both a macro- and a microlevel (Vleeming 1990). A single frontal projection of the joint, for example, will frequently demonstrate at least two "joint cavities" at its inferior aspect; the more medial of these spaces usually represents the posterior aspect of the joint.

Table 4–2 describes and Figure 4–1 illustrates the technique described by Dussault and colleagues (Dussault 2000) for sacroiliac joint injection. The following is the report associated with the case illustrated in Figure 4–1:

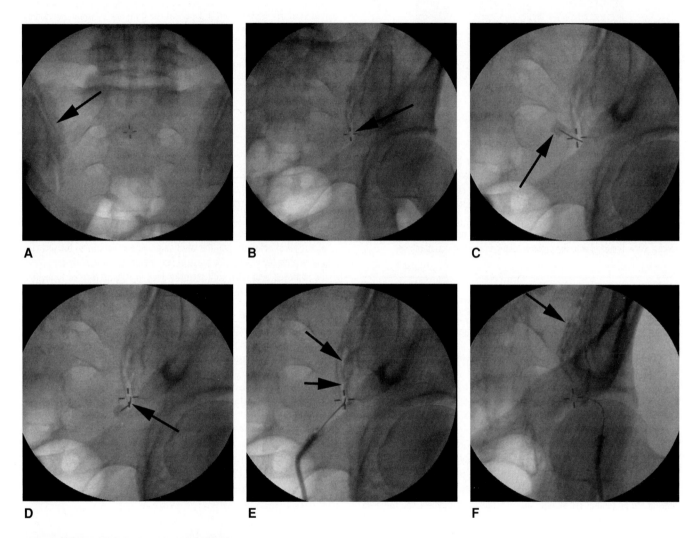

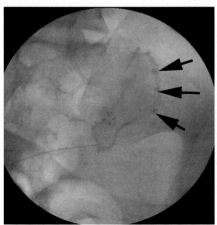

FIGURE 4–1

Step-by-Step Illustration of Sacroiliac Joint Injection. *A,* Frontal view of the pelvis with the central beam directed at the midline. Note that whereas the superior aspect of the sacroiliac joint demonstrates the "two cavity" appearance with multiple lines (arrow), the inferior aspect of the joint in this particular patient is more purely sagittal in orientation. *B,* The C-arm has been moved to the right and angulated in the caudal direction until the inferior-most aspect of the sacroiliac joint projects just above the superior pubic ramus (arrow). The cross-hairs of the laser aiming device are on the target position at the inferior aspect of the joint. *C,* A 25-gauge needle has been inserted. Note that the needle hub (arrow) is superomedial, so the needle is directed inferolaterally. The needle bevel should be directed inferiorly and laterally (in the 5 o'clock position) when the needle is being advanced to bring the point of the needle into a more superior and lateral position. *D,* The needle has been advanced into the joint. Note the curve at the distal aspect of the needle (arrow), where it has entered the joint. *E,* After injection of 0.5 mL of contrast material, there is tracking of contrast into the more superior aspect of the joint (arrows). *F,* An ipsilateral, right posterior oblique view demonstrates contrast in the more superior portion of the joint, along with a diverticulum along the joint margin (arrow). *G,* The contralateral, left posterior oblique view demonstrates the typical "auricular" (ear-shaped) appearance of the sacroiliac joint when viewed from this angle. Note multiple small diverticula along the joint margin (arrows). For further details of this injection, see the sample report in the text.

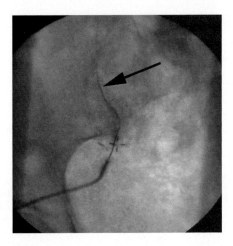

FIGURE 4–2

Intra-articular Sacroiliac Joint Injection. Frontal view with needle in place and contrast tracking into the sacroiliac joint. Note that there are two "lines" of contrast, the more medial and denser (arrow) in a position consistent with the more posterior aspect of the joint and a fainter, lateral collection of contrast in a position consistent with the anterior portion of the joint. These two meet at the inferior aspect of the joint, where the needle is inserted. The patient had excellent pain relief for the duration of the local anesthetic procedure, with return of pain followed by a repeat sacroiliac joint injection with, again, complete but transient pain relief.

INTRODUCTION

The patient describes persistent right leg and hip and to a lesser extent back pain. Prior transforaminal epidural steroid injections, facet joint injections, and interlaminar epidural steroid injections as well as hip injections have been incompletely successful at pain relief. Lumbar magnetic resonance imaging examination demonstrates facet arthropathy.

The procedure and possible complications as well as alternatives to the procedure were discussed with the patient. Informed consent was obtained.

TECHNICAL INFORMATION

Using sterile technique and fluoroscopic guidance, a 25-gauge needle was used to puncture the right sacroiliac joint along its inferior aspect. A total of 1.0 mL of iohexol (Omnipaque) 240 mg/mL was injected. A total of 2.0 mL of 0.5% bupivacaine-epinephrine (Sensorcaine) and 1.0 mL of methylprednisolone acetate (Depo-Medrol) 40 mg/mL was injected.

INTERPRETATION

Frontal and oblique films demonstrate contrast distribution within the right sacroiliac joint. No contrast extravasation or capsular tear was identified, although there are several diverticula of the joint. The patient experienced reproduction of typical symptoms upon injection. There were no immediate complications of the procedure. For at least the next 2 hours, the patient had complete

pain relief, which was much more dramatic and complete than responses to earlier injections.

CONCLUSION

1. Technically successful right sacroiliac joint injection.
2. The patient's response of having typical pain provoked during the injection with relief of pain following the injection provide evidence that the sacroiliac joint is probably at least one cause of her symptoms, particularly considering the improved pain relief with sacroiliac joint injection compared to multiple alternative injections that the patient has had.

Ventral capsule rupture is a weak predictor of response to intra-articular injection of lidocaine (Schwarzer 1995), but in general the relationship of imaging to symptoms is under ongoing investigation (Fortin 1995). The morphologic features of the joint may be reported, but their significance is mostly speculative at this time. Reports of diagnostic sacroiliac joint injections must include specific mention of the degree and duration of pain relief. Complete relief of pain, or complete relief of at least some component of the patient's pain, when combined with a negative control block (or a second intra-articular injection of lidocaine with repeated pain relief) constitutes evidence that the patient's sacroiliac joint is the pain-producing structure.

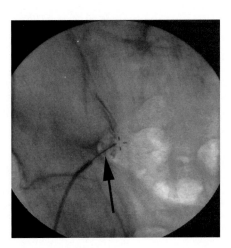

FIGURE 4–3

Intra-articular Sacroiliac Joint Injection. Contrast is seen within the joint, with a small amount of contrast pooling along the inferior aspect of the joint (arrow) oblique to the plane of the x-ray beam and thus not as linear and sharp as the more superior collection. The patient had complete, transient pain relief.

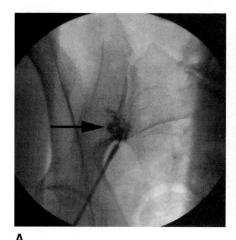

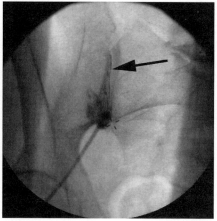

A   **B**

FIGURE 4–4

Extra-articular, Followed by Intra-articular, Sacroiliac Joint Injection. *A,* Frontal view taken during needle placement for sacroiliac joint injection demonstrates a pool of contrast material around the needle tip, documenting an extra-articular position of the needle tip. The needle tip was adjusted multiple times with additional small aliquots of contrast material all pooling around the needle tip. *B,* After final manipulation, injection resulted in intra-articular flow of contrast (arrow). Unlike this case, repeated manipulation is not always successful at intra-articular positioning. This patient had a small foraminal disc protrusion at L3-4, and a transforaminal epidural steroid injection done at the L3 level provided no benefit. The sacroiliac joint injection provided complete pain relief.

Figures 4–2 and 4–3 offer additional examples of intra-articular injection of contrast material, whereas Figure 4–4 shows an initially extra-articular injection followed by an intra-articular injection.

References

Bollow M, Braun J, Hamm B, Eggens U, Schilling A, Konig H, Wolf KJ. Early sacroiliitis in patients with spondyloarthropathy: evaluation with dynamic gadolinium-enhanced MR imaging. Radiology 1995; 194:529–536.

Bollow M, Braun J, Taupitz M, et al. CT-guided intra-articular corticosteroid injection into the sacroiliac joints in patients with spondyloarthropathy: indication and follow-up with contrast-enhanced MRI. J Comput Assist Tomogr 1996; 20:512–521.

Braun J, Bollow M, Seyrekbasan F, Haberle HJ, Eggens U, Mertz A, Distler A, Sieper J. Computed tomography–guided corticosteroid injection of the sacroiliac joint in patients with spondyloarthropathy with sacroiliitis: clinical outcome and follow-up by dynamic magnetic resonance imaging. J Rheumatol 1996; 23:659–664.

Dreyfuss P. Practice guidelines and protocols: sacroiliac joint blocks. In the International Spinal Injection Society Syllabus for the 9th Annual Scientific Meeting, Orlando, Florida, February, 2002. San Francisco, ISIS, 2002.

Dreyfuss P, Michaelsen M, Pauza K, McLarty J, Bogduk N. The value of history and physical examination in diagnosing sacroiliac joint pain. Spine 1996; 21:2594–2602.

Dussault RG, Kaplan PA, Anderson MW. Fluoroscopy-guided sacroiliac joint injections. Radiology 2000; 214:273–277.

Fortin JD. Sacroiliac joint injection and arthrography with imaging correlation. In Lennard TA (ed). Physiatric Procedures in Clinical Practice. Philadelphia, Hanley & Belfus, 1995.

Goldthwait JE. The lumbo-sacral articulation: an explanation of many cases of "lumbago," "sciatica" and paraplegia. Boston Med Surg J 1911; 164:365–372.

Haldeman KO, Soto-Hall R. The diagnosis and treatment of sacroiliac condition by the injection of procaine. J Bone Joint Surg Am 1938; 20:675–685.

Hendrix RW, Lin PJP, Kane WJ. Simplified aspiration or injection technique for the sacro-iliac joint. J Bone Joint Surg Am 1982; 64:1249–1252.

Maigne JY, Aivalikis A, Pfefer F. Results of sacroiliac joint double block and value of sacroiliac pain provocation tests in 54 patients with low back pain. Spine 1996; 21:1889–1892.

Maugars Y, Mathis C, Vilon P, Prost A. Corticosteroid injection of the sacroiliac joint in patients with seronegative spondyloarthropathy. Arthritis Rheum 1992; 35:564–568.

Maugars Y, Mathis C, Berthelot J. Assessment of the efficacy of sacroiliac corticosteroid injections in spondyloarthropathies: a double-blind study. Br J Rheum 1996; 35:767–770.

Miskew DB, Block RA, Witt PF. Aspiration of infected sacro-iliac joints. J Bone Joint Surg Am 1979; 61:1071–1072.

Mixter WJ, Barr JS. Rupture of the intervertebral disc with involvement of the spinal canal. N Engl J Med 1934; 211:210–215.

Pereira PL, Gunaydin I, Trubenbach J, Dammann F, Remy CT, Kotter I, Schick F, Koenig CW, Claussen CD. Interventional MR imaging for injection of the sacroiliac joints in patients with sacroiliitis. AJR 2000; 175:265–266.

Schwarzer AC, Aprill CN, Bogduk N. The sacroiliac joint in chronic low back pain. Spine 1995; 20:31–37.

Simon S. Sacroiliac joint injection and low back pain. In Waldman SD (ed). Interventional Pain Management, 2nd ed. Philadelphia, W.B. Saunders, 2001.

Vleeming A, Stoeckart R, Volkers ACW, Snijders CJ. Relation between form and function in the sacroiliac joint. Part I: clinical anatomical aspects. Spine 1990; 15:130–132.

5 Facet Joint Procedures

DONALD L. RENFREW

Definition

This chapter reviews four different procedures regarding the facet joints:

Facet joint injection: Injection of contrast, anesthetic, and/or steroid agent into the facet or zygapophyseal joint. The injection may be used as a diagnostic tool, to elicit typical symptoms upon injection of joint and elimination of symptoms with placement of local anesthetic. The injection may also be used as a therapeutic tool, with instillation of local anesthetic steroids into the joint to provide long-lasting pain relief.

Facet joint block: Anesthetization of the facet joint by application of local anesthetic to its nerve supply. Innervation of the facet joints is relatively simple with, in most cases, two well-defined nerves located in constant relation to bony targets providing sensation for the joint. Anesthetization of these small branches blocks sensation from the joint and is used as a diagnostic test to ascertain whether the patient's pain is coming from the facet joints.

Facet joint rhizotomy: Thermal ablation of the facet joint nerve supply. The nerve supply may be destroyed by cauterization using percutaneously placed needles and radiofrequency-induced tissue heating.

Synovial cyst injection/rupture: Injection into the facet joint with the goal of rupturing a synovial cyst. Degenerative changes of the facet joints may lead to the development of synovial cysts. When these cysts compress nerve roots or ganglia, radiculopathy and radicular pain may result. These lesions can be treated with intra-articular injection.

Because of the close anatomic relationship between pars defects (spondylolysis lesions) and the facet joints, a discussion of *pars injections* is also included in this chapter.

Literature Review

Hundreds of articles address the clinical significance of the facet joints. The following discussion highlights a few of the more historically and clinically pertinent articles with the goal of providing background information for the described procedures. Note that while this chapter describes five different procedures, the earlier literature grounds the discussion of all of these procedures.

Background Information

Goldthwait ascribed low back pain to the facet joints in 1911 (Goldthwait 1911), Ghormley coined the term *facet syndrome* in 1933 (Ghormley 1933), and Hirsch and colleagues induced pain in the low back by injection of hypertonic saline in the region of the facet joints in 1963 (Hirsch 1963). Mooney and Robertson published a single study with two parts in 1976 (Mooney 1976). For the first part of the study, 20 patients (5 healthy volunteers and 15 patients with "chronic back pain and sciatica") underwent fluoroscopically guided facet joint injections of 1 to 3 mL of hypertonic saline. The patients perceived "an uncomfortable sensation which was located in the low back region, greater trochanter, and then radiated down the posterior lateral portion of the thigh" (Fig. 5–1). Injection of 2 to 5 mL of 1% xylocaine obliterated the patient's pain. The authors found that patients with symptoms had worse pain

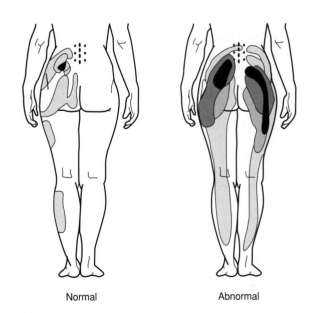

Normal   Abnormal

FIGURE 5–1

Pain Referral Patterns from Lumbar L4-5 and L5-S1 Facet Joint Injections. On the left are areas of pain drawn by asymptomatic subjects following injection of hypertonic saline into the facet joints, and on the right are areas of pain drawn by patients with chronic back and leg pain who had similar injections. The different methods of shading indicate different patients. (From Mooney V, Robertson J. The facet syndrome. Clin Orthop Rel Res 1976; 115:149–156.)

than the volunteers, that pain increased with injectate volume, and that patterns of pain were similar upon injection of the L4-5 or L5-S1 joints. The authors also found reversible abnormalities on electromyelography studies, improved straight-leg raising, and improved reflex abnormalities. For the second portion of the study, the authors studied 100 consecutive patients with back pain and no neurologic signs who underwent bilateral, fluoroscopically guided intra-articular injection of 1 mL methylprednisolone acetate (Depo-Medrol) and 2 to 5 mL of local anesthetic. Sixty-two of these patients had initial pain relief; follow-up of these patients revealed that 20 reported complete relief at 6 months, 32 partial relief at 6 months, and 10 no relief at 6 months.

In 1980, Carrera (Carrera 1980a) described fluoroscopically directed facet joint injection using 0.5 to 1.0 mL of (ionic) contrast material, 2.0 to 3.0 mL of 1% lidocaine, and 10 mg of methylprednisolone acetate. In a companion article (Carrera 1980b), he reported complete immediate pain relief in 13 of the 20 patients; 6 of these remained pain free at 6 months. In 1981, Dory also described arthrography of the facet joints, and stated, "The articular capsule nearly always bursts during or after arthrography, and the path followed by the leaking contrast medium provides an explanation of how injected anesthetics and steroids act in relieving low back pain" (Dory 1981). Dory noted that leakage could occur laterally (at the site of joint innervation) or medially (into the epidural space) and that anesthetic and steroid at these locations could account for pain relief. Raymond and Dumas (Raymond 1984) also emphasized the effects of joint rupture. In their study of 25 patients wherein they strictly controlled maximum injection volume to 1 mL to avoid capsular rupture, only 4 patients achieved pain relief. Similarly, Moran and colleagues (Moran 1988) limited injection volume and found that only 9 of 54 patients (16.7%) with pain suspected on clinical grounds to be arising from the facet joints had their pain provoked and relieved.

While not addressing the issue of intra- versus extracapsular spread of intra-articular injectate, three studies published between 1986 and 1991 provided a control group. Lynch and colleagues (Lynch 1986), in 1986, studied 50 patients with pain of more than 6 months' duration that worsened on hyperextension and that was accompanied by paraspinal tenderness. They attempted unilateral, two-level intra-articular injection in all patients, using 0.5 mL of contrast material and 50 mg of methylprednisolone (with an unstated volume). Intra-articular injection frequently failed, providing three groups of patients: those with two intra-articular injections, those with one intra- and one extra-articular injection, and those with two extra-articular injections. At 2 weeks, 25 of 33 patients (75%) with two intra-articular injections had pain relief, which was graded as total (in 9, or 33%) or partial (in 16, or 48%). In the same 2-week time period, six of eight patients (75%) with one intra- and one extra-articular injection had pain relief, which was total in two (25%) and partial in four (50%). In 15 patients in whom both injections were extra-articular, 8 (53%) achieved partial pain relief and none total pain relief. Differences between groups achieved statistical significance. Lilius and colleagues (Lilius 1989) randomly injected 109 patients who had had more than 3 months of unilateral back pain with three different methods: with cor-

tisone and local anesthetic into two facet joints, with the same mixture around two facet joints, and with physiologic saline into two facet joints. Patients in all groups had significant improvements in work attendance, pain, and disability scores regardless of the method of injection, with no significant difference between groups. The volume of injectate in this group was 8 mL for all groups. Carette and colleagues (Carette 1991) randomized patients who had at least 50% pain relief with intra-articular anesthetic into two groups, those who received 2 mL of isotonic saline and those who received 20 mg of methylprednisolone in 2 mL of saline. At 1 month, 20 of 48 patients (42%) undergoing steroid injection had "marked" or "very marked" pain relief by self-report, with 16 of 48 (33%) of the saline injection patients having "marked" or "very marked" pain relief. At 6 months, 22 of the 48 (46%) steroid injection patients reported "marked" or "very marked" pain relief, versus 7 of the 48 (15%) saline injection patients. Although the 6-month results difference was statistically significant (note the threefold difference in percentage of patients achieving "marked" or "very marked" pain relief), the authors dismissed this difference; they noted that they could think of "no plausible pharmacologic or biologic basis" for improvement between 1 and 6 months following injection (note two additional patients had "marked" or "very marked" pain reduction at 6 months versus 1 month in this group), that concurrent interventions were more frequent in the steroid group, and that other outcome measures differed. For these reasons, they concluded that "injections of methylprednisolone into facet joints have very little efficacy in patients with chronic low back pain." The authors thus make the unusual argument that we should reject the null hypothesis (that groups treated with steroid and saline do not differ in pain relief) not on the basis of the data from the study (which supports this rejection, and perforce adoption of the alternative hypothesis that the groups *do* differ), but rather because of the poor quality of the study. This is an exceptionally peculiar argument, and one that perhaps reveals more about the biases of the authors than it does about the efficacy of facet joint injection.

While studies regarding the facet joints generally use signs and symptoms, and occasionally radiographic criteria, for patient inclusion, two studies specifically addressed the role of signs and symptoms and one the role of radiographic findings in patients with suspected facet joint origin for their pain. In 1988, Jackson and colleagues (Jackson 1988) studied 127 variables by assessing 454 patients with facet joint injections. While several variables (including older age, prior history of low back pain, normal gait, maximum pain on extension following forward flexion, absence of leg pain, muscle spasms, and aggravation of pain on Valsalva) demonstrated significant ($P < .05$) correlation with post-injection pain relief, the authors concluded, "We were not able to identify clinical facet joint syndromes or predict patients responding better to this procedure." Similarly, Schwarzer and colleagues (Schwarzer 1994b) stated, "The zygapophyseal joint is an important source of pain, but the existence of a 'facet syndrome' must be questioned." They based this conclusion on the lack of predictive value of clinical features with respect to response of back pain to injections and noted, "In particular, rotation of the lumbar spine and rotation combined with extension were poor discriminators of

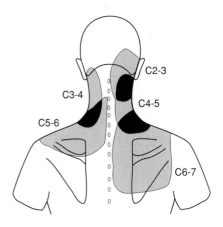

FIGURE 5–2

Pain Referral Patterns from Cervical C2-3 through C6-7 Facet Joint Injections. Shaded areas indicate areas of pain experienced by asymptomatic volunteers after injection of facet joints C2-3 through C6-7. (From Dwyer AB, Aprill C, Bogduk N. Cervical zygapophyseal joint pain patterns. I: A study in normal volunteers. Spine 1990; 15:453–457.)

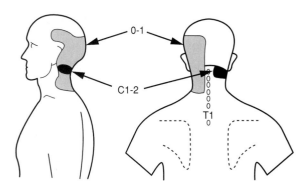

FIGURE 5–3

Pain Referral Patterns from the Atlanto-occipital (O-C1) and Lateral Atlantoaxial (C1-2) Joints. The larger, lightly shaded area is the location of pain induced by injection of the atlanto-occipital (O-C1) joints of asymptomatic volunteers, and the more darkly shaded areas are from similar injections of the lateral atlantoaxial joints (C1-2). (From Dreyfuss P, Michaelsen M, Fletcher D. Atlanto-occipital and lateral atlanto-axial joint pain patterns. Spine 1994; 19:1125–1131.)

zygapophyseal joint pain; referral of pain below the knee was not any more common or less common" in patients responding to injection. In another study, Schwarzer and colleagues (Schwarzer 1995) showed that facet degenerative changes demonstrated by computed tomography were also not predictive of patient response to injection.

A separate study by Schwarzer and colleagues (Schwarzer 1994a) questioned the reliability of single blocks to demonstrate facet joint pain. The authors found that while 83 of 176 (47%) of back pain patients had pain relief with injection of lignocaine, only 26 (15%) of the same patients had relief 2 weeks later with 0.5% bupivacaine, and concluded that "uncontrolled diagnostic blocks will always be associated with an unacceptably low positive predictive value." Whether because of a large number of false-positive results associated with single blocks or for other reasons, a study by Esses and colleagues (Esses 1993) found no correlation between facet block results and the outcome of either operative arthrodesis or nonoperative treatment.

Kaplan and colleagues in 1998 published a study investigating the basic premises of facet injection, namely, whether pain may arise from the joint, and whether such

pain may be blocked by anesthetization of the joint's innervating nerves (Kaplan 1998). They subjected 18 volunteers to articular distension (without extravasation) until pain was provoked, demonstrating that intra-articular injection could be painful. One week later, these subjects returned for either saline ($n = 5$) or lidocaine ($n = 9$) injection at the source of innervation. Thirty minutes later, the subjects had repeat intra-articular injections performed; all five in the saline group had reproduction of pain whereas eight of the nine "blocked" group had no pain. The authors concluded that "lumbar medial branch blocks successfully inhibit pain associated with capsular distention of the lumbar zygapophysial joints at a rate of 89%." Dwyer and colleagues (Dwyer 1990) had earlier documented pain patterns (Fig. 5–2) elicited in healthy volunteers upon cervical facet joint injection. An associated study by the same authors (Aprill 1990) vindicated the use of these pain patterns in patients. Dreyfuss and colleagues (Dreyfuss 1994) later elucidated pain patterns for the atlanto-occipital and lateral atlantoaxial joints in the same manner (Fig. 5–3).

Table 5–1 summarizes the literature of facet joint "blocks." The following sections review the more specific

TABLE 5–1. Summary of Literature Review on Facet Joint Injection

The facet joints appear to be a significant cause of pain in at least some patients with low back pain. The percentage of all patients with low back pain who have a significant proportion of their pain attributable to the facet joints varies from 15% to 50% in published series, and many patients with facet joint pain probably have pain coming from other structures in the back as well.

Pain from L4-5 and L5-S1 demonstrates considerable overlap in terms of perceived location within the back and lower extremity (Mooney 1976) (see Fig. 5–1). Pain from cervical levels also demonstrates overlap, although helpful generalizations are available (see Figs. 5–2 and 5–3).

"Facet joint syndrome" in the sense of an identifiable constellation of signs and symptoms predictive of response to facet joint injection does not exist (Jackson 1988, Schwarzer 1994b).

Imaging findings are also not predictive of response to facet joint injections (Schwarzer 1995).

The facet joints have a small capacity, and injection of more than approximately 1.0 mL will lead to rupture (Dory 1981, Raymond 1984). Material extravasated from the joint will reach the source of joint innervation and/or the epidural space.

False-positive results of a single injection cloud the issue and either a repeat injection or a negative "control" injection of another structure (or with saline) is necessary to implicate the facet joint as the cause of pain in most cases (Schwarzer 1994a).

but related issues of rhizotomy, synovial cyst injection, and pars injection.

Rhizotomy

Shealy (1975) first described percutaneous radiofrequency denervation of the facet joints in 1975. Gallagher and colleagues (Gallagher 1994) published a controlled, randomized study comparing radiofrequency facet joint denervation with a placebo procedure (identical to the experimental group except for the heat treatment). Patients who had good relief of pain with a single block showed statistically significant improvements of mean visual analogue scores (by a factor of approximately 2) at 1 and 6 months after the procedure when compared with similar patients treated with placebo. In 1999, van Kleef and colleagues (van Kleef 1999) published a second randomized trial of 31 patients with a similar study design, in which they found decreased pain and also a decrease in the intake of analgesics and improvement of disability status. Dreyfuss and colleagues (Dreyfuss 2000) published a prospective audit in 15 carefully selected patients (responding to two sets of blocks), and found that 9 (60%) had at least 90% pain relief, and 13 (87%) had at least 60% pain relief, at 6 months. Leclaire and colleagues (Leclaire 2001) published a third randomized, controlled study of 70 patients, in which they failed to show any statistically significant differences in pain or disability between a group undergoing radiofrequency denervation and another group undergoing a sham control procedure. The patients in this study were chosen on the basis of "relief of their low back pain for at least 24 hours during the week after intra-articular facet injections" using lidocaine and triamcinolone. This inclusion criterion can be faulted on three grounds: (1) the 24-hour pain relief period is inconsistent with the duration of action of lidocaine or steroid; (2) there may have been a significant number of false-positive blocks given the single injection (Schwarzer 1994a); and (3) both the experimental and the control group would have been given an intra-articular steroid, a proven treatment for the disease under consideration (see earlier discussion regarding Carette 1991).

Cervical rhizotomy has been described for cervicogenic headaches (van Suijlekom 1998). Haldeman and Dagenais provide a critical review of cervicogenic headaches (Haldeman 2001); as they note, definition of this entity is undergoing evolution, despite relatively explicit criteria offered by Sjaastad and colleagues in 1990 and revised in 1998 (Sjaastad 1998). In general, cervicogenic headaches are headaches that "start in the neck or occipital region and are associated with tenderness of cervical paraspinal tissues" (Haldeman 2001). According to Sjaastad and colleagues (Sjaastad 1998), anesthetic blocks of "the major or minor occipital nerves, the C2 root, the third occipital nerve, facet joints, or of the lower cervical roots and branches on the symptomatic side—or a combination of them—should virtually abolish the pain." Although Lord and colleagues published a double-blind, sham controlled study demonstrating the efficacy of rhizotomy for treatment of lower cervical facet joints, they also specifically cautioned against lesioning of the C2-3 joint and third occipital nerve (C3 dorsal ramus) on the grounds of a high technical failure rate (Lord 1995).

Synovial Cyst Injections

Hemminghytt and colleagues (Hemminghytt 1982) originally described the computed tomographic (CT) appearance of a symptomatic synovial cyst in 1982. In a 1985 article describing surgical treatment of such cysts, Kurz and colleagues noted that "if a connection with a facet joint could be demonstrated, then aspiration of the cyst or aspiration and injection with steroid could be performed, perhaps avoiding an operation" (Kurz 1985). Bjorkengren and colleagues (Bjorkengren 1987) described such treatment in three patients. Jackson and colleagues (Jackson 1989) subsequently reported the magnetic resonance imaging (MRI) appearance of synovial cysts, with multiple subsequent reports detailing the usual (and not so usual) imaging appearance of synovial cysts (Apostolaki 2000, Awwad 1990, Davis 1990, Liu 1990, Silbergleit 1990, Yuh 1991). Parlier-Cuau and colleagues (Parlier-Cuau 1999) reported on 30 patients undergoing injection therapy for synovial cyst treatment, with 20 patients (67%) having good or excellent results at 1 month and 10 (33%) at 6 months (with these 10 continuing to have good results on follow-up 9 to 50 months later). Bureau and colleagues (Bureau 2001) reported on an additional 12 patients so treated; in their cases, they made a specific effort to rupture (rather than just inject) the cyst and to follow cases both clinically and with imaging. They reported excellent pain relief in nine patients (75%), with symptom relief usually (but not universally) accompanied by decreased cyst size on follow-up imaging; two patients with ongoing pain and one patient with recurrent symptoms demonstrated persistence of the cysts. Although synovial cysts are often referred to as "rare" or "uncommon," this assertion is somewhat undermined by reports of large series (60 by Sabo and colleagues in 1996 and 194 by Lyons in 2000), as well as the fact that in an imaging study of 25 patients with acute radiculopathy, 2 patients (8%) demonstrated synovial cysts as the causative lesion versus 18 (72%) demonstrating herniated discs as the causative lesion (Modic 1995).

Pars Interarticularis Injections

Ghelman and Doherty (Ghelman 1978) described a case wherein facet joint injection at L4-5 resulted in contrast opacification of a pars interarticularis defect; injection of local anesthetic resulted "only in minimal pain relief which lasted a few days." Maldague and colleagues (Maldague 1981) subsequently performed arthrography on 11 patients with spondylolysis, and in 9 showed a communication with the pars defect. In one of their cases, contrast flowed across the midline and connected the left and right pars defects. Five of the 11 patients injected with local anesthetic and steroids had significant pain relief "for periods lasting from 2 to 10 months." Suh and colleagues (Suh 1991) found that pars injections predicted surgical success in a small group of 10 patients: pain, dysfunction, disability, and return to work were all improved in patients achieving at least 80% pain relief for at least 60 minutes compared with subjects who had less pain relief following injection. Duprez and colleagues (Duprez 1999) reported two cases wherein the posterior channel described by Maldague and colleagues (Maldague 1981) expanded with fluid and caused symptomatic narrowing of the spinal canal.

Rationale for Procedure

As noted in Chapter 1 (see Table 1–1), we assume, when performing diagnostic and therapeutic injection, that pain may be secondary to inflammation in proximity to nociceptors, and that such inflammation (and therefore associated pain) may respond to steroid injection. Most authors do not, however, use provocation of pain by injection either within or adjacent to facet joints for diagnostic purposes. Pain relief response to a single injection, as reviewed earlier, may result in frequent false-positive study results (Schwarzer 1994a), and a single injection will not therefore necessarily secure the diagnosis of facet joint pain. Either intra-articular or nerve block injections may be used, as both are apparently equally diagnostic (Dreyfuss 1995).

In addition to the assumptions listed in Table 1–1, rhizotomy makes the additional assumption that ablation of the nerve supply to a symptomatic structure will provide long-term pain relief, whereas synovial cyst injection makes the additional assumption that treatment of a compressive lesion may relieve radicular pain.

Equipment and Supplies[1]

Table 5–2 lists the equipment required for facet joint procedures.

A C-arm device or dual-plane fluoroscope is necessary to perform facet joint injections. A laser aiming device (an attachment that shows a cross-hair on the fluoroscopic screen corresponding in position to a red dot on the skin surface) is extremely helpful for proper needle placement. Selection of needle type varies with the operator; a 22-gauge spinal needle for most lumbar injections and a 25-gauge spinal needle for thoracic and cervical injections work well. These needles are inexpensive, are readily available, and can usually be inserted without prior local anesthetic. Everything injected into the patient must be as safe as possible and preferably safe for intrathecal use, at least for intra-articular injections, since some of the injected materials (particularly in the procedures of intra-articular facet injection and pars injection) may reach the epidural space or even the thecal sac. For this reason, nonionic contrast material approved for intrathecal injection, anesthetic approved for intrathecal injection (consult the package insert), and the most benign steroid obtainable should be used. In addition, if the contrast injection pattern suggests that the injection is intrathecal, it is usually best to stop

TABLE 5–2. Equipment and Supplies for Facet Joint Procedures

C-arm fluoroscope
Surgical scrub solution
Needles
Syringes
Connecting tube
Nonionic contrast material
Anesthetic agent
Steroid (optional)
Radiofrequency needles and device (for rhizotomies)

injecting, since injection of an anesthetic agent may result in a spinal block and injection of a steroid may result in arachnoiditis.

In addition to the equipment listed in Table 5–2, a crash cart should be readily available to handle medical emergencies (e.g., contrast media and drug reactions).

Chemical rhizotomies have been described (Silvers 1990) but are not as widely used because of the potential for inadvertent spread of injectate (Gray 2001).

Informed Consent Issues[2]

Informed consent issues may be divided into three topics: description of the procedure, warning the patient about possible drug side effects, and delineation of material risks. Informed consent also implies that a description of alternatives to the proposed treatment has been given; for a general description of such alternatives, see Chapter 1.

Either the performing physician or a trained subordinate should completely explain the entire procedure in detail to the patient prior to performance of the procedure. Patients who know what to expect are much less anxious than those who do not. A step-by-step description, including reassurance that the procedure takes only a few minutes (although rhizotomy may take considerably longer), that many patients undergo similar procedures every day, and that the amount of pain caused by needle insertion is similar to that caused by drawing blood or starting an intravenous access line, provides a considerable calming effect in most patients.

The performing physician or a trained subordinate should also explain that local anesthetic may cause numbness and weakness of the leg in lumbar injections or arm in cervical injections. Cervical injection of local anesthetic may also result in dizziness. Patients should be warned that the injection may recreate or exacerbate their pain. While this side effect typically relents within moments of injection of local anesthetic, occasionally it will persist. In those cases in which steroid is injected, review of steroid side effects should be undertaken. These side effects include changes in mood (usually mild euphoria but occasionally anxiety), appetite (usually increased), insomnia, sweating, hot flashes, facial flushing, rash, and gastrointestinal upset.

---

[1]This section is virtually identical to the Equipment and Supplies section in Chapter 2 and can be skipped if the reader is already familiar with this material.

[2]This section is very similar to the Informed Consent Issues section of Chapter 2 and can be skipped if the reader is already familiar with this material.

Some patients benefit from medications to relieve anxiety or insomnia.

Complications may be subdivided into two categories: occasional (but inevitable) and rare but either reported in the literature or at least theoretical. Vasovagal reactions (treated with time, intravenous fluids, and atropine as necessary) and inadvertent thecal puncture constitute the first category. Inadvertent thecal sac puncture should virtually never occur with medial branch blocks, but it is possible to inadvertently enter the thecal sac when performing an intra-articular facet joint injection or pars injection, particularly if the needle is advanced through the joint or defect. Any recognized thecal puncture should result in immediate removal of the needle and rescheduling of the procedure. Inadvertent injection of local anesthetic into the lumbar thecal sac usually results in a spinal block, urinary incontinence, and inability to move the lower extremities for the duration of the block. Inadvertent injection of steroid into the thecal sac will probably not result in such obvious immediate problems, but carries the risk of arachnoiditis (Benzon 1986, Nelson 1973). Some patients who have had an inadvertent thecal puncture, as well as some who undergo myelography or diagnostic lumbar puncture, may develop a "post-tap headache." Treatment of such headaches includes bedrest, caffeine, pain killers, and an epidural "blood patch" (or saline injection) (Raskin 1990). The epidural blood patch is performed as indicated in Chapter 2 for an interlaminar epidural steroid injection, with injection of 10 to 15 mL of freshly drawn venous blood from the patient injected into the epidural space.

Less frequent but either reported or theoretical complications of facet joint procedures are listed in Table 5–3. Patients should cease taking all anticoagulants and other agents that might increase the risk of hematoma formation. With respect to anaphylactic reaction, patients should be screened for sensitivity to contrast media. If a patient has had a prior minor reaction to intravenous contrast material, either reassurance or oral prednisone prior to the procedure is advised. For prior major contrast reactions, the best option is probably to perform the procedure with fluoroscopic guidance only, and without contrast. The main purpose of using contrast in case of medial branch block is to document a nonvascular location of the needle tip (Kaplan 1998), and in intra-articular injections to document an intra-articular location of the needle tip. This information, while important, is not worth the risk of a major contrast reaction in those patients with a prior history of such reactions. If there is any doubt as to whether injected materials might reach the thecal sac when a procedure is performed without contrast, it is best to forego steroid injection, since intrathecal injection of steroids may result in adhesive arachnoiditis, which is essentially incurable (Guyer 1989). Nonlatex gloves and surgical scrub solution without iodine can be used as appropriate.

Patient and Procedure Selection

In facet joint injection procedures, two related issues must be addressed: first, the choice of procedure for a given patient, and second, at what levels to perform the procedure. For intra-articular facet joint injections and medial branch blocks, as noted in the Literature Review section, clinical and imaging features of patients who respond to injection vary. One paper (Schwarzer 1994b) suggests that lumbar injections are unlikely to benefit patients with predominantly central (nonlateralizing) pain. In general, patients undergoing diagnostic injections have severe, persistent pain not relieved by other measures. Obviously, if a

TABLE 5–3. Reported or Theoretical Complications of Facet Joint Procedures

Procedure	Complication
Medial branch blocks	Soft tissue abscess
	Soft tissue hematoma
Rhizotomy	As medial branch blocks, plus:
	Exacerbation of existing pain
	Inadvertent segmental nerve ablation
	(with numbness/paralysis in the affected distribution)
Intra-articular injection (without steroid)	Infectious arthritis
	Epidural abscess
	Soft tissue abscess
	Epidural hematoma
	Soft tissue hematoma
Intra-articular injection (with steroid)	As above, plus:
	Transient hypercorticism (reported in epidural steroid injection) (Stambough 1984)
	Epidural lipomatosis (reported in epidural steroid injection) (Roy-Camille 1991)
	Retinal hemorrhage with transient blindness (reported in epidural steroid injection) (Victory 1991)
Theoretical (reported for other procedures)	Anaphylactic reaction to contrast material
	Anaphylactic reaction to anesthetic agent
	Anaphylactic reaction to steroid drug
	Anaphylactic reaction to latex, surgical scrub solution, etc.
	Arterial injury with or without neural damage (particularly in the cervical spine)

patient does not have or cannot reproduce his or her typical pain at the time of the injection, there is no point in undertaking diagnostic intra-articular injections or medial branch blocks. Occasionally, patients will need to be sent away from clinic with instructions to call in for an injection when their pain returns.

Selection of injection level in the lumbar spine is difficult, given the overlap of the two common locations (L4-5 and L5-S1) of symptoms (see Fig. 5–1). In the cervical spine, either comparing the patient's pain diagram with Figures 5–2 and 5–3, or having the patient indicate which area most matches his pain from Figures 5–2 and 5–3, forms a helpful starting point. Since a negative control injection may be used as part of the evaluation of the patient, if the first set of injections provides incomplete or no relief but the patient is suspected of having a higher or lower level of origination of pain, having the patient return in 1 week for injections at these levels will provide enough information for management (either excluding the diagnosis of facet joint pain at any level or proceeding with rhizotomy; see later). Either intra-articular or medial branch/dorsal ramus injections can be used for diagnostic purposes (Dreyfuss 1995). In patients undergoing evaluation for possible rhizotomy, it probably makes more sense to perform blocks, because the studies demonstrating benefit from rhizotomy choose the patients on the basis of response to blocks (Gallagher 1994, van Kleef 1999). The two uppermost cervical levels (the atlanto-occipital and lateral atlanoaxial joints) are limited to diagnostic and therapeutic injection (no associated rhizotomy exists), and C2-3 facet joint rhizotomy has a high technical failure rate (Lord 1995).

For rhizotomy, patients should receive at least 50% (preferably 75%) pain relief on two different occasions with medial branch blocks of the level (Gray 2001, Schellhas 2000), or achieve such pain relief on one occasion with a negative control injection (which may be a negative block at another level or another type of injection). Cervical rhizotomy has been described for cervicogenic headaches (van Suijlekom 1998); such patients should undergo diagnostic testing in the same manner as patients with neck and back pain.

For synovial cyst injection, patients should have radicular pain in an anatomically appropriate location with a corresponding imaging abnormality.

For pars injection, response to injected anesthetic may be predictive of surgical results (Suh 1991), whereas injection of steroids may provide long-term pain relief in some patients (Maldague 1981).

Procedure Description

Description of medial branch blocks, intra-articular injection, and rhizotomy for lumbar and cervical levels follows. This section also describes synovial cyst injection and pars injection of the lumbar spine. For the thoracic spine, there is no currently accepted medial branch block technique (Dreyfuss 1995). Although synovial cysts occur in the thoracic and cervical spine (Howington 1999) (where they are genuinely, rather than just nominally, rare), injection of these lesions is not recommended because pressurization of the cyst could result in cord compression.

Anatomy

A few words regarding the anatomy of the medial branches are in order. Cervical facets C3-4 through C7-T1 are innervated by medial branches of the dorsal rami of the segmental nerves above and below the level of the joint, and these medial branches lie in the groove along the lateral mass near its midpoint. Therefore, to anesthetize or denervate the left C4-5 facet joint, the targets would be the midpoints of the rhomboids formed by the lateral masses of the C4 and C5 lateral masses. At the C2-3 level, the dorsal ramus of C3, also known as the third occipital nerve, should be blocked; this structure lies along the lateral aspect of the C2-3 joint (Dreyfuss 1995, Schellhas 2000). In the lumbar spine, the facet joints are innervated by the medial branch of the dorsal ramus of the nerve exiting under the pedicle at the same level and *from the nerve exiting one level above* (Dreyfuss 1995, Gray 2001, Silbergleit 2001) (Fig. 5–4). Therefore, the L3-4 facet joint is innervated by the L2 and L3 medial branches, which on first blush is quite confusing. However, note that the medial branches pass over the transverse processes one level below where they exit the spine, and therefore the L2 medial branch passes over the L3 transverse process, and the L3 medial branch passes over the L4 transverse processes. Therefore, to anesthetize the L3-4 facet joint, medial branch blocks performed at the level of the L3 and L4 transverse processes are appropriate, and so the confusion evaporates. In addition, note that the target for the L5 "medial branch" is actually at the location of the dorsal ramus of the L5 nerve, which lies in the notch of the ala of the sacrum, and that further block of the L5-S1 level can be obtained by injecting at the site of a communicating branch (or branches) from the dorsal ramus of S1 along the inferior aspect of the L5-S1 facet joint (Derby 1993).

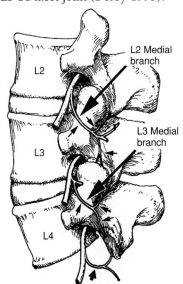

FIGURE 5–4

Anatomy of Medial Branches in the Midlumbar Spine. Innervation of the left L3-4 facet joint is from the medial branch from the L2 nerve, which crosses the L3 transverse process at the base of the superior articular process, and the medial branch from the L3 level, which crosses the L4 transverse process at the base of the superior articular process. Although the nomenclature is confusing, the end result is simple enough: anesthetization of the left L3-4 facet joint requires needle placement along the L3 and L4 transverse processes. (Modified from Schellinger D, Wener L, Ragsdale BD, Patronas NJ. Facet joint disorders and their role in the production of back pain and sciatica. Radiographics 1987; 7:923–944.)

TABLE 5–4. Step-by-Step Description of Lumbar Facet Joint Nerve Blocks

1. Identify the angle between the superior articular process and the transverse process (for lumbar medial branches), the sacral notch (for the dorsal ramus of L5), or the inferior aspect of the L5-S1 facet joint or superior aspect of the S1 neural foramen (for communicating branches between S1 and the L5-S1 facet joint).
2. Insert the needle along the course of the x-ray beam far enough so that it is anchored.
3. Check position with C-arm fluoroscopy.
4. Adjust and advance the needle so that the tip is along the superior margin of the transverse process at the base of the superior articular process. One can accomplish this by making contact between the needle tip and the transverse process and walking the needle up the dorsal aspect of the transverse process until it can be advanced forward, but the position should be checked with lateral fluoroscopy.
5. Inject 0.1 to 0.3 mL of nonionic contrast material and document a nonvascular location of the injected material. The needle tip position should be in an ideal or nearly ideal relationship to bony structures prior to injection. If a vascular injection results, reposition the needle tip until a nonvascular injection results.
6. Inject 0.5 to 0.8 mL of local anesthetic and 0.1 to 0.3 mL of steroid (optional).
7. Repeat with additional levels until the target joints have been anesthetized.
8. Monitor for pain response and record percentage of pain relief at 30 minutes.
9. Release patient when stable. Provide patient with a telephone number to call if there is persistent or increased pain or numbness or if fever, swelling, or redness develops.

Lumbar Medial Branch Block

In patients who come for evaluation of facet joint pain in the lower lumbar spine, because of considerations noted in "Patient Selection" above, it is usually most expeditious simply to block the L4-5 and L5-S1 joints. This is accomplished by injecting along the L3 medial branch on the superior aspect of the L4 transverse process, the L4 medial branch on the superior aspect of the L5 transverse process, the L5 dorsal ramus in the notch of the sacrum, and the communicating branch of S1 at the inferior aspect of the L5-S1 facet joint. Given that two of the four structures blocked are not really medial branches at all, a more accurate name for this procedure is *facet joint nerve block*,

although this risks confusion with the nerve blocks discussed in Chapter 3.

Table 5–4 describes and Figures 5–5 and 5–6 illustrate L4-5 and L5-S1 facet joint nerve blocks. With respect to the illustrated injection, note that the needle insertion route follows that described and illustrated by van Kleef (1999) and Schellhas (2000), although other authors describe a more oblique path to the target point (Dreyfuss 1995, Gray 2001). Extensive degenerative change may make needle positioning quite challenging (Fig. 5–7). In addition, note that 0.5 to 0.8 mL is adequate to anesthetize a relatively large area (Fig. 5–8, and see Fig. 5–6).

A report for the procedure illustrated in Figure 5–6 follows:

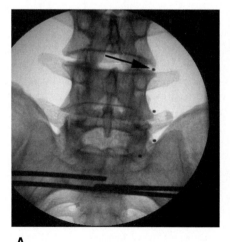

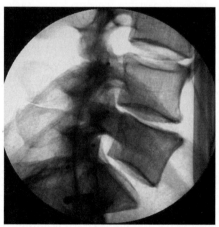

A   **B**

FIGURE 5–5

Skeletal Specimen Radiographs Demonstrating Appropriate Position of Needles for L4-5 and L5-S1 Facet Joint Nerve Blocks. *A,* Frontal view of skeletal specimen with metallic beads marking the L3 medial branch (along the L4 transverse process), L4 medial branch (along the L5 transverse process), L5 dorsal ramus (in the notch of the sacrum and superior articular process of S1), and S1 contributors to the L5-S1 facet joint, as indicated. (The metallic bars through the pelvis hold the sacrum and pelvis together in this specimen.) *B,* Lateral skeletal radiograph with metallic beads marking the L3 medial branch (along the L4 transverse process), L4 medial branch (along the L5 transverse process), L5 dorsal ramus (in the notch of the sacrum and superior articular process of S1) and S1 contributors to the L5-S1 facet joint, as indicated.

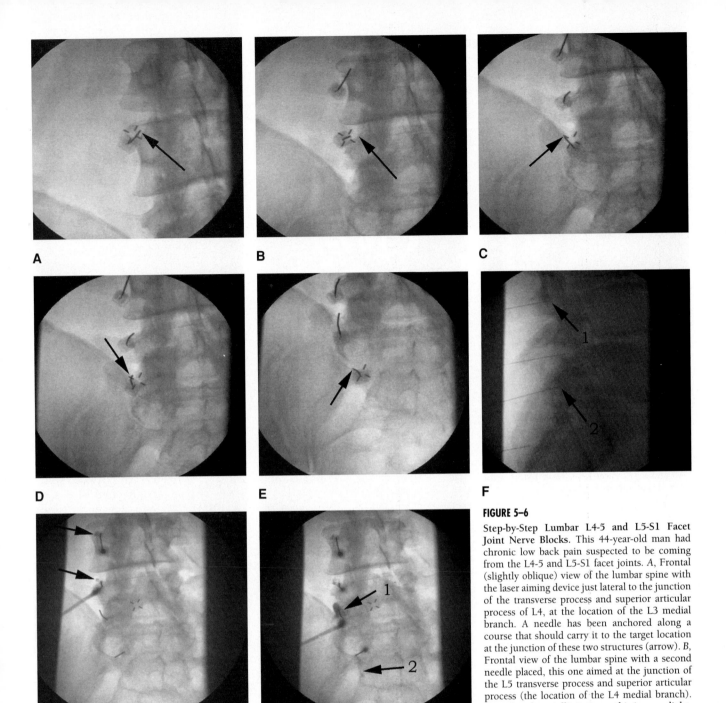

A

B

C

D

E

F

G

H

FIGURE 5–6

Step-by-Step Lumbar L4-5 and L5-S1 Facet Joint Nerve Blocks. This 44-year-old man had chronic low back pain suspected to be coming from the L4-5 and L5-S1 facet joints. *A,* Frontal (slightly oblique) view of the lumbar spine with the laser aiming device just lateral to the junction of the transverse process and superior articular process of L4, at the location of the L3 medial branch. A needle has been anchored along a course that should carry it to the target location at the junction of these two structures (arrow). *B,* Frontal view of the lumbar spine with a second needle placed, this one aimed at the junction of the L5 transverse process and superior articular process (the location of the L4 medial branch). Note that the needle tip is, on this image, slightly lateral to ideal position (marked by the arrow). Since the needle still needs to be advanced,

directing the bevel of the needle superiorly and to the left will help to bring the needle toward the target. Also note that when initially performing these procedures, it may be better to check with lateral fluoroscopy at each level as the procedure is performed. However, with experience, all needles may be placed using frontal fluoroscopy prior to switching to the lateral view to adjust position. *C,* Frontal view of the lumbar spine after placement of the third needle, directed at the L5 dorsal ramus location. The needle (arrow) is slightly lateral to ideal position: the cross-hairs of the laser aiming device indicate the target. Directing the bevel laterally should bring the needle into a better position. *D,* Frontal view of the lumbar spine after the needle directed at the L5 dorsal ramus has been advanced with the bevel directed laterally. Note that the tip of the needle (arrow) is angling toward the target location. *E,* Frontal view of the lumbar spine following introduction of the needle directed to the position of the S1 contributors to the L5-S1 facet joint. The needle tip is in a position to target the inferior aspect of the joint. The tip (arrow) is slightly lateral to ideal position, and the bevel should be directed laterally prior to advancing the needle tip into final position. *F,* Lateral radiograph following placement of the four needles as described above. The needles are at or posterior to ideal position, with the L4 medial branch (top) needle (arrow 1) at least 3 to 4 mm posterior to ideal position, and the L5 dorsal ramus needle (arrow 2) also at least 2 to 3 mm posterior to ideal position. The needles were adjusted prior to final injection. *G,* Frontal radiograph following injection of 0.2 mL of nonionic contrast material through the superior-most two needles demonstrates small collections of contrast material along these needles (arrows). Contrast is used to document a nonvascular location of the needle tip prior to injection of anesthetic. *H,* Frontal radiograph following injection through the two more inferior needles. At the location of the L5 dorsal ramus (arrow 1), 1.0 mL of nonionic contrast material has been injected. Note the much larger area of "coverage" with this amount of injectate. This should approximate the area infiltrated with 1.0 mL of local anesthetic (the typical injection volume for facet joint nerve blocks). At the location of the S1 contributors of the L5-S1 joint, 0.2 mL of nonionic contrast material has been injected. The contrast spreads relatively widely, despite the small volume (arrow 2). Without direct comparison to a pre-injection image (see part *G*), this small amount of contrast would be difficult to appreciate. This patient had bilateral L4-5 and L5-S1 facet joint nerve blocks using 1.0% lidocaine with excellent, transient relief of pain lasting 1 hour. Subsequent blocks performed with 0.5% bupivacaine provided between 2 and 3 hours of pain relief. The patient underwent rhizotomy with excellent long-term pain relief.

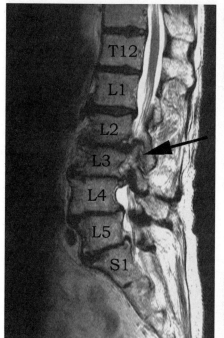

A

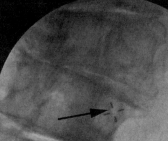

B

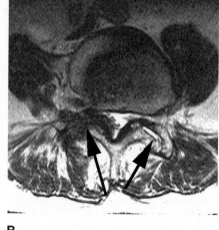

C

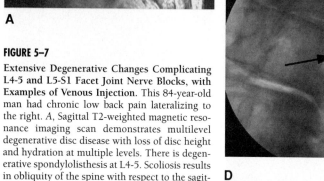

D

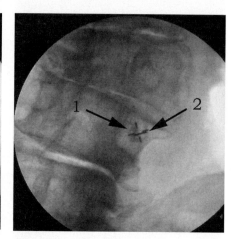

E

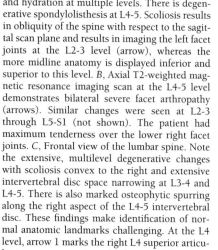

F

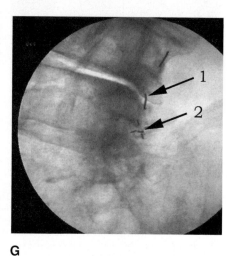

G

FIGURE 5–7

Extensive Degenerative Changes Complicating L4-5 and L5-S1 Facet Joint Nerve Blocks, with Examples of Venous Injection. This 84-year-old man had chronic low back pain lateralizing to the right. *A*, Sagittal T2-weighted magnetic resonance imaging scan demonstrates multilevel degenerative disc disease with loss of disc height and hydration at multiple levels. There is degenerative spondylolisthesis at L4-5. Scoliosis results in obliquity of the spine with respect to the sagittal scan plane and results in imaging the left facet joints at the L2-3 level (arrow), whereas the more midline anatomy is displayed inferior and superior to this level. *B*, Axial T2-weighted magnetic resonance imaging scan at the L4-5 level demonstrates bilateral severe facet arthropathy (arrows). Similar changes were seen at L2-3 through L5-S1 (not shown). The patient had maximum tenderness over the lower right facet joints. *C*, Frontal view of the lumbar spine. Note the extensive, multilevel degenerative changes with scoliosis convex to the right and extensive intervertebral disc space narrowing at L3-4 and L4-5. There is also marked osteophytic spurring along the right aspect of the L4-5 intervertebral disc. These findings make identification of normal anatomic landmarks challenging. At the L4 level, arrow 1 marks the right L4 superior articular process, arrow 2 marks the top of the transverse process, and the laser aiming device aims at the target position at the junction of these two structures. *D*, Frontal view after enabling the magnification feature of the C-arm fluoroscopic device. Magnification allows easier identification of the landmarks, including the target location at the junction of the L4 transverse and superior articular processes (indicated by the cross-hairs of the laser aiming device) (arrow). *E*, Frontal view after placing the needle. The relative position of the needle hub (slightly opaque and marked by arrow 1) and needle tip (arrow 2) indicate that the needle is tracking from medial and inferior to lateral and superior. The needle tip appears to be in good position at the target location. *F*, Frontal view after moving the C-arm so that the cross-hairs of the laser aiming device now aims at the target location at the junction of the L5 transverse and superior articular processes (arrow). Note that degenerative changes makes visualization of landmarks much more difficult at this level, but that comparison to the level above is somewhat helpful. *G*, Frontal view after placement of a needle at the L5 level targeting the L4 medial branch (arrow 1), repositioning of the C-arm to target the L5 dorsal ramus, and positioning of a needle at this location (arrow 2).

(figure continues on following page)

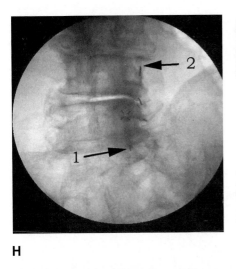

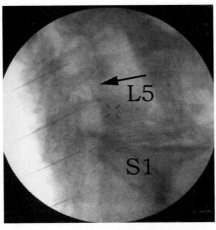

H   **I**

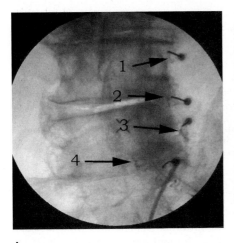

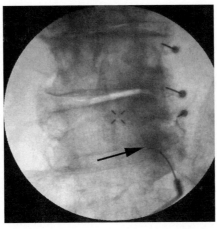

J   **K**

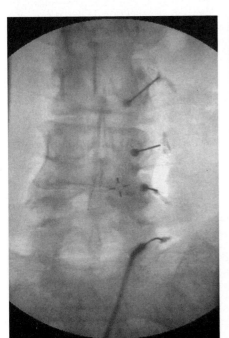

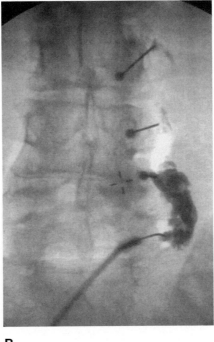

A   **B**

FIGURE 5–7 CONTINUED

H, Frontal view after placing a needle at the expected position of the S1 contributors to the L5-S1 facet joint (arrow 1). The C-arm has been returned to a non-magnified mode to better demonstrate the entire region and has also been adjusted to straighten the patient's scoliosis. Note that the central ray of the x-ray beam (indicated by the cross-hairs of the laser aiming device) is now at the level of the right L5 pedicle. The top needle (arrow 2), targeting the L3 medial branch, because of this slightly different angulation, now appears to project slightly superior to ideal position. This shift of apparent position frequently accompanies changes of angulation of the C-arm and demonstrates that single plane imaging of structures may be misleading. *I*, Lateral view demonstrates that the needle tips are in good position along the expected location of the transverse processes (compare with Figure 5–5B). Because of scoliosis and degenerative changes, landmarks are difficult to identify, but the posterior margin of the L5 vertebral body is relatively well seen (arrow). *J*, Frontal view following injection of 0.2 mL of contrast material through the needle targeting the L3 medial branch (arrow 1), L4 medial branch (arrow 2), and L5 dorsal ramus (arrow 3) demonstrates small collections of contrast material along these needles. Injection through the needle targeting the S1 contributors of the L5-S1 joint demonstrates a tubular appearance (arrow 4), consistent with vascular injection. *K*, Frontal view after manipulation and re-injection through the needle targeting the S1 contributors of the L5-S1 facet joint demonstrates contrast along this joint (arrow). The patient had minimal immediate relief of low back pain on the right side following injection with ongoing left-sided pain. He was scheduled for a return visit in 1 week with a plan to block both sides, as well as to extend the level of blocks proximally on the right side. He did not return to the clinic and a follow-up call 3 weeks later revealed that he had excellent pain relief starting a few days after the diagnostic blocks. This response is occasionally reported and may represent a "placebo" benefit of diagnostic blocks.

FIGURE 5–8

Injection Demonstrating the Extensive Area Covered by 1.0 mL of Injectate. *A*, Frontal view of medial branch block study with needles in place at the positions of the L2, L3, and L4 medial branches and the L5 dorsal ramus following injection of 0.1 to 0.2 mL of nonionic contrast material at each location shows a small amount of contrast at each location (arrows). Note that the needle at the L5 dorsal ramus notch position is 2 mm superior to ideal position along the bony margin. *B*, Continued injection to a total volume of 1.0 mL through the lowest needle demonstrates extensive contrast (arrow). Note the large area of tissue covered by injection of only 1.0 mL.

Facet Blocks

INTRODUCTION

The patient is a 44-year-old man with chronic low back pain suspected to be originating from the L4-5 and L5-S1 facet joints.

TECHNICAL INFORMATION

The procedure and possible complications were explained to the patient. Informed consent was obtained.

Using sterile technique and fluoroscopic guidance, 22-gauge spinal needles were placed bilaterally in a position to anesthetize the L4-5 and L5-S1 facet joints. The nonvascular location of the needle tips was confirmed via injection of 0.2 mL of iohexal (Omnipaque) 240 mg/mL through each needle. Films documented needle tip position and contrast flow. Following this, 1.0 mL of 2% lidocaine was injected at each level.

The patient tolerated the procedure well and there were no immediate complications.

Initial response to the injection was excellent pain relief for the duration of the local anesthetic procedure.

IMPRESSION

1. Technically successful fluoroscopically directed blocks of the L4-5 and L5-S1 facet joints bilaterally.
2. Initial response to injected local anesthetic was excellent pain relief.
3. The plan is to have the patient return in 1 week for facet joint nerve blocks with Sensorcaine. If these also provide temporary pain relief, a rhizotomy may be performed.

Lumbar Intra-articular Injection

One can evaluate lumbar facet joints by blocking the nerves serving them or by intra-articular injection. Facet joint nerve blocks work well as a diagnostic tool and to predict response to rhizotomy. There are occasions when intra-articular facet injection is preferred. These occasions

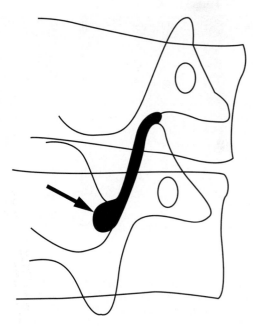

FIGURE 5–9

Diagram of Posterior Approach to Lumbar Facet Injection. With the patient placed prone (facing right) with a bolster under the abdomen, the posterior and inferior aspect of the joint will distend (arrow). This allows relatively easy access to the joint space from a posterior approach. (Figure modified from Sarazin L, Chevrot A, Pessis E, Minoui A, Drape JL, Chemla N, Godefroy D. Lumbar facet joint arthrography with the posterior approach. Radiographics 1999; 19:93–104.)

include when patients cannot undergo rhizotomy because of an indwelling cardiac pacer, when patients have undergone rhizotomy with minimal benefit and intra-articular steroids may provide additional benefit, and for injection and rupture of synovial cysts (see later). Whereas oblique approaches to the facet joint were described first (Carrera 1980a, Dory 1981), Sarazin and associates (Sarazin 1999) describe a superior method of injection (Fig. 5–9). Table 5–5 describes and Figures 5–10 and 5–11 illustrate lumbar intra-articular facet joint injection using the technique of

TABLE 5–5. Step-by-Step Description of Lumbar Intra-articular Facet Injection

1. Place the patient prone on the procedure table with bolsters under the abdomen to flex the lumbar spine. Target the inferior aspect of the joint with the lesion. With practice, this can done directly, but initially it may be necessary to go to an ipsilateral oblique view to visualize the inferior tip of the inferior articular process and then to return to a frontal view.
2. Insert the needle along the course of the x-ray beam far enough so that it is anchored.
3. Check position with the C-arm fluoroscope.
4. Adjust and advance until the needle either encounters bone, feels as if it has entered the joint, or demonstrates a curve in its distal aspect.
5. Visualize the joint with an ipsilateral oblique view and document that the needle tip is in the inferior aspect of the joint. If necessary, adjust the needle tip.
6. Inject 0.1 to 0.3 mL of nonionic contrast material and document the intra-articular location of the needle tip. Reposition the needle if necessary. Remember that any extra-articular contrast material injected will quickly obscure the joint margins and prevent completion of the procedure.
7. Once the needle is definitely intra-articular, inject anesthetic and steroid agents as desired. If strict intra-articular injection is required, injection volumes will need to be low (e.g., 0.5–1.0 mL of local anesthetic and 0.5–1.0 mL of steroid). Take frontal and lateral images and document contrast flow and (if desired) an intact joint capsule at the end of injection. Larger volumes of material will usually need to be injected if joint capsule rupture is desired.
8. Repeat with additional levels until the target joints have been injected.
9. Monitor for pain response and record percentage of pain relief at 30 minutes.
10. Release patient when stable. Provide patient with a telephone number to call if there is persistent or increased pain or numbness or if fever, swelling, or redness develops.

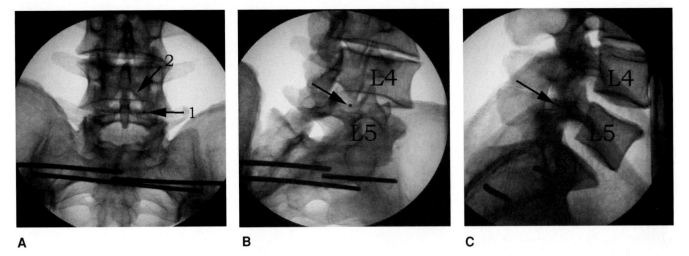

A   **B**   **C**

FIGURE 5–10

Skeletal Radiographs with a Metallic Bead Placed at the Tip of the L4 Inferior Articular Process, Marking the Lower Margin of the L4-5 Facet Joint.
A, Frontal view demonstrates the metallic bead (arrow 1) at the tip of the inferior articular process. This position may be located by following the inferior margin of the right L4 lamina (arrow 2) inferiorly and laterally. (The metallic bars through the pelvis hold the sacrum and pelvis together in this specimen.) *B,* Oblique view demonstrates the metallic bead at the inferior aspect of the L4 inferior articular process (arrow). A relatively large recess just below the bead forms an excellent entrance point into the L4-5 facet joint. *C,* Lateral view demonstrates the metallic bead at the inferior aspect of the L4 inferior articular process once more (arrow). On the lateral study, the bead is somewhat more difficult to see secondary to the superimposition of the left and right facet joints.

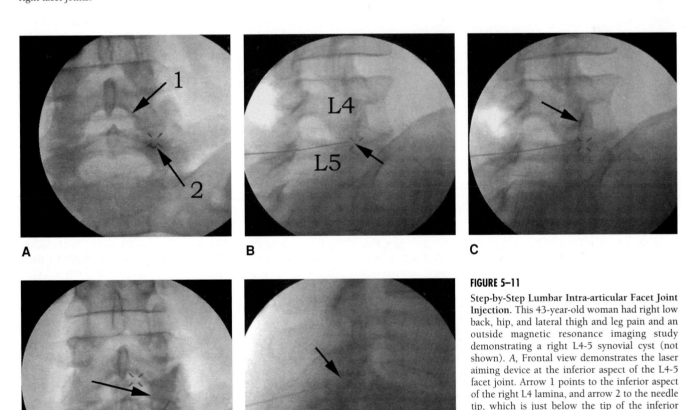

A   **B**   **C**

D   **E**

FIGURE 5–11

Step-by-Step Lumbar Intra-articular Facet Joint Injection. This 43-year-old woman had right low back, hip, and lateral thigh and leg pain and an outside magnetic resonance imaging study demonstrating a right L4-5 synovial cyst (not shown). *A,* Frontal view demonstrates the laser aiming device at the inferior aspect of the L4-5 facet joint. Arrow 1 points to the inferior aspect of the right L4 lamina, and arrow 2 to the needle tip, which is just below the tip of the inferior articular process. The needle was advanced until it rested on bone. Note that in this procedure, unlike in epidural steroid injection or medial branch blocks (other than at the level of the S1 contributors), the needle may be advanced without fear of damage. *B,* Oblique view demonstrates that the needle projects at the lower margin of the L4-5 facet joint (arrow). The needle tip should lie within the inferior recess of the joint (see Fig. 5–9). Note that the patient has a somewhat transitional level, with a very low "L5." *C,* Oblique view following injection of 0.2 mL of nonionic contrast material demonstrates a clear arthrogram, with contrast tracking superiorly into the joint (arrow). *D,* Frontal view following injection of a total of 0.5 mL of contrast material demonstrates contrast material in the right L4-5 facet joint (arrow). Note that due to the oblique orientation of the joint space with respect to the x-ray beam on the frontal view, the contrast material assumes a relatively ill-defined, ovoid shape. *E,* Lateral view in this somewhat obese patient shows that it is difficult to demonstrate the needle tip or contrast with confidence (arrow). Additional contrast was injected to cause synovial cyst rupture (not shown), and the patient had dramatic relief of pain for approximately 2 months, but her pain returned and she eventually underwent fusion surgery with relief of symptoms.

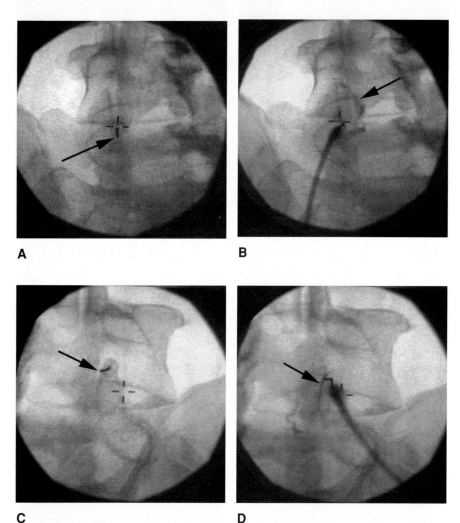

A

B

C

D

FIGURE 5–12

Bilateral Intra-articular L4-5 Facet Joint Injections Demonstrating an Oblique Approach. This 49-year-old woman had low back and bilateral hip pain, left greater than right. Left intra-articular hip joint injection provided little pain relief. *A,* Oblique view demonstrates the left L4-5 facet joint. The laser aiming device targets the inferior aspect of the joint. Although difficult to see because it overlaps the inferior aspect of the cross-hairs of the laser aiming device, there is a needle in place (arrow). *B,* Oblique view following injection of 0.3 mL of nonionic contrast material demonstrates an arthrogram (arrow). Note that the area of contrast has an oval, rather than a linear, appearance because the joint surfaces are not exactly parallel with the x-ray beam. This makes entrance to the apparent joint at its midpoint difficult, because the joint space may be covered by bone. *C,* Oblique view of the right L4-5 facet joint demonstrates a needle directed toward the superior aspect of the joint (arrow). *D,* Oblique view following injection of 0.3 mL of nonionic contrast material demonstrates contrast flow along the joint in a relatively linear fashion (arrow). As demonstrated by these injections, targeting the superior and inferior aspects of the facet joint results in the most reliable success, because the curved nature of the joint makes entry at its midpoint difficult. In general, the posterior approach to the lower recess of the joint (as illustrated in Figure 5–11) is preferred. This patient had moderately good pain relief from bilateral intra-articular facet joint injections.

Sarazin and colleagues. In addition, see the section on Lumbar Synovial Cyst Rupture/Injection for more examples of intra-articular lumbar facet joint injections. If an oblique approach, rather than the posterior approach, is used, it often works well to target the superior (Fig. 5–12) or inferior aspect of the joint, since this results in the best chance of intra-articular needle placement given the curved nature of the joint surfaces.

TABLE 5–6. Step-by-Step Description of Cervical Medial Branch Block

1. Identify the groove along the lateral mass (the midpoint between the articular margins) using anterior-posterior fluoroscopy. Significant cranial angulation may be helpful in identifying the groove and in placing the needle in the same plane as the facet joint margins.
2. Insert the needle along the course of the x-ray beam far enough so that it is anchored.
3. Check position with the C-arm fluoroscope.
4. Adjust and advance the needle until the tip is along the lateral aspect of the lateral mass. This can be accomplished by making contact between the needle tip and the dorsal aspect of the lateral mass and walking the needle laterally off the lateral mass until it can be advanced forward. Lateral fluoroscopy should be used to check position as the needle is advanced. In the lower cervical spine, it may be necessary to substitute oblique for lateral viewing.
5. Once the needle is in the appropriate position at the midpoint of the parallelogram formed by the margins of the lateral mass, return to the frontal view.
6. Inject 0.1 to 0.3 mL of nonionic contrast material and document a nonvascular location of injected material. The needle tip position should be in an ideal or nearly ideal relationships to bony structures prior to injection. If a vascular injection results, reposition the needle tip until a nonvascular injection results.
7. Inject 0.5 to 0.8 mL of local anesthetic and 0.1 to 0.3 mL of steroid (optional).
8. Repeat with additional levels until the target joints have been anesthetized.
9. Monitor for pain response and record percentage of pain relief at 30 minutes.
10. Release patient when stable. Provide patient with a telephone number to call if there is persistent or increased pain or numbness or if fever, swelling, or redness develops.

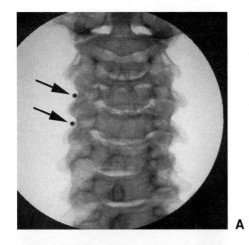

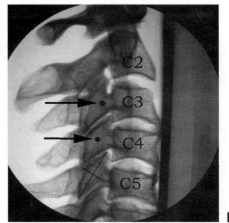

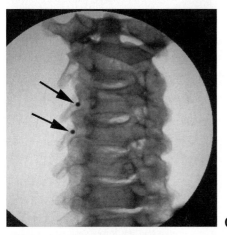

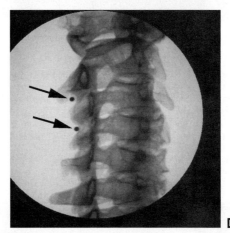

A

B

C

D

FIGURE 5–13

Skeletal Specimen Radiographs with Metallic Beads Placed Along the Lateral Masses of the C3 and C4 Vertebrae, Marking the Target Points for Injection and Rhizotomy for Pain Originating from the C3-4 Facet Joint *A*, Frontal view demonstrates the metallic beads in place along the lateral aspects of the C3 and C4 lateral masses (arrows). *B*, Lateral view demonstrates the metallic beads in approximately the midportion of the C3 and C4 lateral masses (arrows). The C3 bead is approximately 1 mm anterior to ideal position. Note that the beads should form the midpoint (the intersection of lines drawn from the margins, as seen at the C5 level) of the parallelogram formed by the margins of the lateral mass. *C*, Oblique view with the C-arm rotated toward the side with the metallic beads (arrows). *D*, Oblique view with the C-arm rotated away from the side with the metallic beads (arrow).

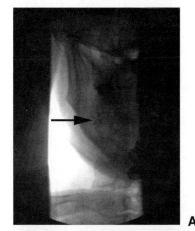

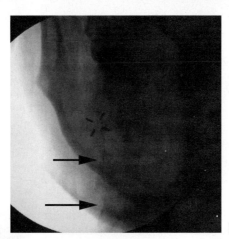

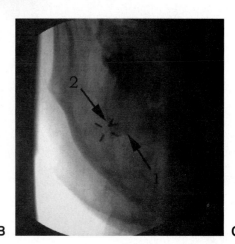

A

B

C

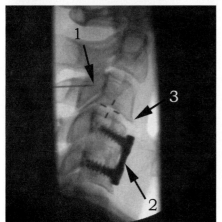

D

FIGURE 5–14

Step-by-Step Lumbar Cervical Medial Branch Blocks. This 30-year-old woman had undergone prior C4-5 fusion surgery for a disc herniation secondary to a motor vehicle accident. She had had several years of pain relief with the return of left-sided neck pain following a second motor vehicle accident. The new neck pain was slightly higher than the pain the patient recalled prior to her surgery. Epidural steroid injections were of little benefit, and it was decided to proceed with medial branch blocks on the basis of location of the patient's pain, which matched the C3-4 level. *A*, Frontal view demonstrates the cross-hairs of the laser aiming device directed at the concavity formed by the C3 lateral mass midportion (arrow). These landmarks are difficult to discern on frontal radiography, particularly at first. *B*, Frontal view following magnification demonstrates the cross-hairs of the laser aiming device directed at the concavity along the lateral aspect of the C3 lateral mass. This feature is difficult to discern even on the magnified view, although the C4 and C5 concavities are more readily demonstrated (arrows). *C*, Frontal radiograph following introduction of a needle at the C3 level. The hub of the needle (arrow 1) projects slightly medially and inferiorly to the tip (arrow 2), and the tip appears to be directed at the correct location. *D*, Lateral view demonstrates the needle tip centered at the level of the C3 lateral mass (arrow 1). Note the fixation plate at C4-5 (arrow 2) with solid-appearing union and degenerative osteophytic spurring along the anterior C2 vertebral body (arrow 3).

(figure continues on following page)

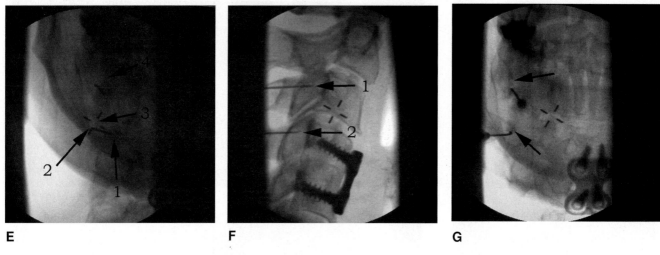

E

F

G

FIGURE 5–14 CONTINUED

E, Frontal view following insertion of a second needle. The needle hub (arrow 1) is medial and slightly inferior to the needle tip (arrow 2), which is slightly below the concavity of the lateral portion of the C4 left lateral mass (arrow 3). Advancing the needle with the bevel directed inferiorly should bring the needle tip into a more optimal position. Note that the needle at C3 (arrow 4) is slightly inferior and lateral to ideal position on this view, although the lateral examination demonstrated ideal position (see part *D*). *F,* Lateral view with the needles in position at the C3 (arrow 1) and C4 (arrow 2) level. Both needle tips are at or quite near the target position of the midpoint of the parallelogram formed by the lateral mass margins (see Fig. 5–13). *G,* Frontal view following injection of 0.2 mL of nonionic contrast material at the C3 and C4 levels demonstrates small collections of contrast material (arrows) in nonvascular locations. The patient had excellent, transient pain relief for approximately 1 hour following the injection of 0.8 mL of lidocaine at each of the target locations. An additional set of blocks performed with 0.8 mL of bupivacaine provided approximately 3 hours of excellent pain relief. This was followed by a rhizotomy with ongoing excellent pain relief.

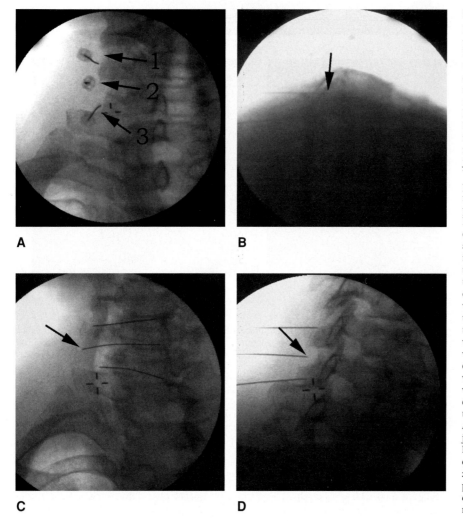

A

B

C

D

FIGURE 5–15

Lower Cervical Medial Branch Blocks. This 42-year-old man had left lower neck pain, particularly with rotation and extension. Left C5-6 and C6-7 medial branch blocks (not shown) provided incomplete relief of pain. Because the patient's residual neck pain was perceived as lower than the location of the blocks, the C6-7 and C7-T1 levels were blocked on the patient's return. *A,* Frontal magnification view demonstrates needles in or near the groove formed by the C6 lateral mass (arrow 1), C7 lateral mass (arrow 2), and just over the T1 transverse process (arrow 3). The C7 level needle was slightly lateral to ideal position. The patient had a great deal of difficulty maintaining a constant position during needle placement, making ideal needle positioning challenging. *B,* Lateral view. Because of the extreme density differences between the cervical spine above and below the level of the shoulders, imaging this region is very difficult. The needle tip at the C6 level (arrow) is barely visible and appears to be in appropriate position. The two lower needle tips cannot be confidently located on this view. The best course of events in this situation is usually to pull the patient's shoulders down until the lateral masses are well seen. This maneuver was not successful in this individual. Oblique views may be helpful. *C,* Ipsilateral oblique view demonstrates the needles in comparable position with the middle (C7) needle tip (arrow) somewhat lateral and anterior to the other two needles. *D,* Contralateral oblique view demonstrates the needle tips along the left lateral masses. Again, the middle (C7) needle tip (arrow) projects somewhat dorsolateral to the lateral mass. However, the needle tip appears to be close enough to the lateral mass to achieve anesthetization with 1.0 mL of local anesthetic. Needle positioning for rhizotomy needs to be more precise and should be placed exactly on the lateral mass for optimal effect.

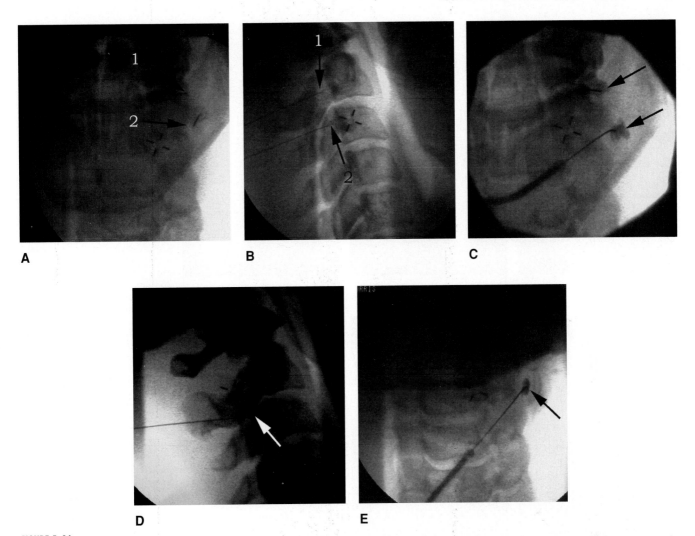

FIGURE 5–16

C3 Dorsal Ramus (Third Occipital Nerve) Block. This 27-year-old woman had severe unilateral headaches and right-sided upper neck pain that was not throbbing in nature. She was sent for evaluation of possible C2-3 facet joint origin of pain. *A,* Frontal view demonstrates needles in place at the level of the C2 (arrow 1) and C3 (arrow 2) masses. *B,* Lateral view demonstrates the needle tips at the C2 (arrow 1) and C3 (arrow 2) levels, appropriately positioned at the midpoints of the parallelograms formed by the lateral masses. *C,* Frontal view following injection of 0.3 mL of contrast material at each level demonstrates contrast pooling at the needle tips (arrows), consistent with a nonvascular location of the needles. *D,* Lateral view following placement of a third needle after removal of the first two needles. Placement of the third needle simultaneously with the first two is technically difficult given the limited space in the region. The needle tip is along the lateral aspect of the C2-3 facet joint (arrow). *E,* Frontal view following injection of 0.2 mL of nonionic contrast material confirms the nonvascular location of the needle tip (arrow). At each level, 0.6 mL of 2.0% lidocaine was injected. The patient had approximately 60% of her pain relieved, with some ongoing, more superior neck pain following the injection.

Cervical Medial Branch Block

Table 5–6 describes and Figures 5–13, 5–14, and 5–15 illustrate cervical medial branch blocks. Note that the C3 dorsal ramus, also known as the third occipital nerve, is blocked by placing needles not only along the lateral masses of C2 and C3 but along the joint line as well (Fig. 5–16), and that, as noted in the Literature Review section, third occipital nerve (C3 dorsal ramus) rhizotomy has a high technical failure rate (Lord 1995).

Cervical Intra-articular Facet Joint Injection

As in the lumbar spine, one can evaluate the cervical spine facet joints by blocking the nerves serving them or by intra-articular injection. Also as in the lumbar spine, facet joint nerve blocks work well as a diagnostic tool and to predict response to rhizotomy. In the cervical spine, intra-articular injection may be preferred if the patient has a pacer in place and therefore cannot undergo rhizotomy. In addition, the atlanto-occipital (O-C1) and lateral atlanto-axial (C1-2) joints have no associated rhizotomy, so intra-articular injection is the method of choice for diagnosis and therapy of these joints. Table 5–7 describes and Figures 5–17, 5–18, and 5–19 illustrate lower (C2-3 through C7-T1) cervical intra-articular facet joint injection. Table 5–8 describes and Figures 5–20, 5–21, and 5–22 illustrate atlantoaxial joint injection. For a description of atlanto-occipital injection (O-C1), see the paper by Dreyfuss and colleagues (Dreyfuss 1994). A description of the injection illustrated in Figure 5–22 follows:

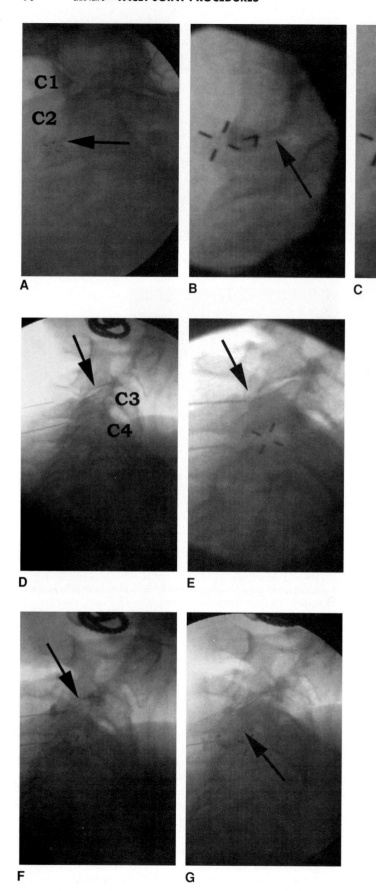

A

B

C

D

E

F

G

FIGURE 5–17

Intra-articular Cervical Facet Joint Injection. This 75-year-old woman had an indwelling pacemaker in place and so was not a candidate for rhizotomy. She had left-sided upper neck pain corresponding in position to the C2-3 and C3-4 levels. *A*, Frontal view, moderate cranial angulation of the C-arm fluoroscope. The C1 and C2 levels are labeled. Note that while the anterior aspect of the C2-3 joint projects somewhat more superiorly, the posterior (target) aspect of the joint projects at the level of the arrow. *B*, Frontal, cone-down, magnified view of the C2-3 (arrow) and C3-4 joints. The cross-hairs of the laser aiming device project along the left lateral aspect of the joint, whereas a 25-gauge needle is placed so that it is tracking toward the joint (arrow). *C*, A second needle has been inserted. The needle tip projects just below the apparent C3-4 joint space (arrow). *D*, Lateral view demonstrates that the more superior needle is on track for the C2-3 facet joint (arrow) but is still well posterior to the joint. The C3-4 needle, on the other hand, is near the posterior margin of the joint. *E*, Cone-down, magnified lateral view demonstrates that the C2-3 needle has been advanced so that the posterior aspect of the joint (arrow) has been entered. *F*, Contrast material flows in a thin line along the joint (arrow), as well as collecting in discrete pockets in the superior/anterior and posterior/inferior recesses. *G*, The C2-3 needle has been removed, and injection through the C3-4 needle demonstrates contrast in the C3-4 joint (arrow). The patient achieved good pain relief for several months following intra-articular injection of a small amount of anesthetic and steroid.

TABLE 5–7. Step-by-Step Description of Intra-articular Cervical Facet Joint Injection

1. Identify the target joint using anterior-posterior fluoroscopy. Counting down from the C1 level is usually easiest. Significant anterior-to-posterior craniocaudal angulation may be helpful in placing the needle along the course of the facet joint.
2. Insert the needle along the course of the x-ray beam far enough so that it is anchored.
3. Check position with the C-arm fluoroscope.
4. Adjust and advance the needle until the tip is near the posterior joint margin. It is better to err on being shallow rather than deep to the joint, because it is possible to cross directly through the joint and impale the vertebral artery. Switching to lateral C-arm positioning, both to document that the needle is heading toward the appropriate joint and also to document that the needle tip is posterior to the joint, should be done relatively early during needle placement.
5. Advance the needle until it is within the posterior aspect of the joint or until it feels as if it has entered the joint capsule. Penetrating the joint capsule may provide a characteristic "bottle-stopper" sensation.
6. Inject 0.1 to 0.3 mL of nonionic contrast material and document the intra-articular location of the needle tip. Reposition the needle if necessary. Remember that any extra-articular contrast material injected will quickly obscure the joint margins and prevent completion of the procedure.
7. Once the needle is definitely intra-articular, inject anesthetic and steroid agents as desired. If strict intra-articular injection is required, injection volumes will need to be low (e.g., 0.5–1.0 mL of local anesthetic and 0.5–1.0 mL of steroid). Take frontal and lateral images and document contrast flow and (if desired) an intact joint capsule at the end of injection.
8. Repeat with additional levels until the target joints have been injected.
9. Monitor for pain response and record percentage of pain relief at 30 minutes.
10. Release patient when stable. Provide patient with a telephone number to call if there is persistent or increased pain or numbness or if fever, swelling, or redness develops.

CERVICAL FACET JOINT INJECTION

INTRODUCTION

The patient is a 55-year-old woman with left-sided neck pain and headaches. Recent CT examination demonstrates relatively striking asymmetric atlantoaxial joint arthropathy worse on the left than on the right.

TECHNICAL INFORMATION

The procedure and possible complications were explained to the patient. Informed consent was obtained.

Using sterile technique and fluoroscopic guidance, and a 25-gauge spinal needle, the needle tip was placed in the left lateral atlantoaxial joint. A dose of 0.5 mL of iopamidol 300 mg/mL (Isovue-M 300) was injected that showed flow along the joint and what appeared to be along the medial aspect of the joint and lateral aspect of the dens. A dose of 1.0 mL of Depo-Medrol 40 mg/mL was injected.

The patient found the injection painful. She could not state precisely whether this was the normal pain that she has originating from her neck.

Because of contrast tracking into the medial aspect of the joint and along the C2 lateral mass, no lidocaine was administered. At no charge to the patient and with her consent, a CT scan was performed through this region. The CT scan demonstrates, again, asymmetric atlantoaxial joint arthropathy along with contrast material in the joint and also what appears to be contrast extravasation around both sides of the dens and along the anterior aspect of the spinal canal.

IMPRESSION

1. Technically successful left atlantoaxial intra-articular injection with 0.5 mL of Isovue-M 300 and 1.0 mL of Depo-Medrol 40 mg/mL.
2. No lidocaine was injected. See above.
3. CT performed at no charge to the patient demonstrated contrast extravasation along the medial aspect of the joint.

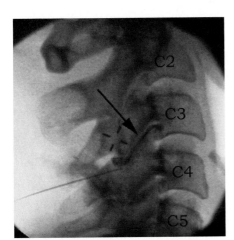

FIGURE 5–18

Intra-articular Cervical Facet Injection at C3-4. This 76-year-old woman had right-sided neck pain that had been successfully but transiently relieved by C3 and C4 medial branch blocks. An intra-articular diagnostic/therapeutic injection was performed to confirm the C3-4 facet joint origin of the pain and to provide possible long-term benefit with steroid injection. Lateral view demonstrates the needle at the posterior, inferior aspect of the C3-4 facet joint. Contrast flows in a linear fashion along the joint (arrow), with pools of contrast along its anterior-superior and inferior-posterior margins. The patient received transient pain relief from the intra-articular injection, but her pain returned in approximately 3 hours. However, a rhizotomy provided excellent, long-term pain relief.

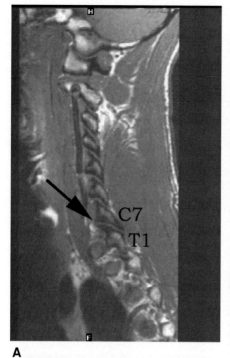

A

B

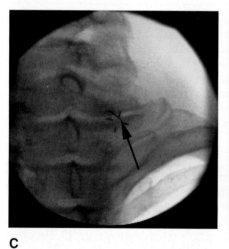

C

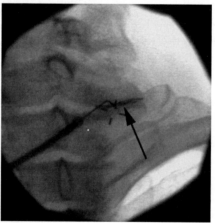

D

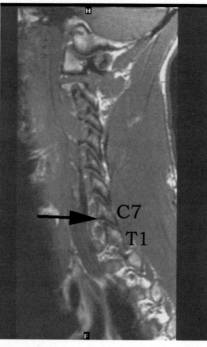

E

FIGURE 5–19

Intra-articular Cervical Facet Injection at C7-T1. This 35-year-old man had right-sided neck pain following trauma. Initial plain films (not shown) were unremarkable. *A*, Right parasagittal T1-weighted magnetic resonance imaging examination at the level of the right facet joints demonstrates anterior to posterior joint widening and anterior osteophytic spurring (arrow) of the C7-T1 facet joint. *B*, Left parasagittal T2-weighted magnetic resonance imaging examination at the level of the left facet joints for comparison. Note that the C7-T1 facet joint (arrow) does not demonstrate the morphologic abnormalities of the opposite side (see part *A*). *C*, Frontal view demonstrates the cross-hairs of the laser aiming device just below the right C7-T1 facet joint. The joint space appears relatively lucent, indicating a more horizontal orientation of the joint compared to the more superior levels. The needle tip (arrow) projects at the inferior margin of the joint space. *D*, Frontal view following injection of 0.3 mL of contrast material demonstrates an arthrogram of the C7-T1 joint (arrow). *E*, Oblique view demonstrates contrast material within the C7-T1 joint (arrow). The patient received 3 to 4 months of excellent pain relief from intra-articular injection of local anesthetic and steroids on two different occasions, then underwent rhizotomy, with long-term pain relief.

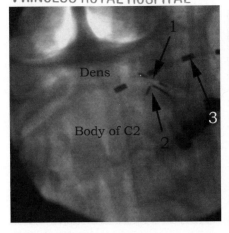

A

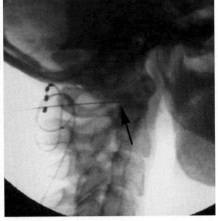

B

FIGURE 5-20

Lateral Atlantoaxial (C1-2) Joint Injection. This 50-year-old woman had undergone craniotomy and stimulator placement for right-sided neck pain and associated headaches. Prior lateral atlantoaxial intra-articular injections had brought moderate prolonged relief of pain. *A,* Frontal view demonstrates the dens and body of C2. The inferior articular margin of the lateral mass of C1 (arrow 1) and superior articular margin of C2 (arrow 2) define the lateral atlantoaxial joint. The needle tip, at the lower aspect of the cross-hairs of the laser aiming device, is in the midportion of the lateral atlantoaxial joint. The patient's stimulator (arrow 3) projects over the joint. Note that the vertebral artery courses along the lateral aspect of the atlantoaxial joint and that the medial aspect of the joint projects at or just medial to the lateral aspect of the spinal canal. Thus, ideal needle position is in the middle portion of the joint, approximately halfway from the medial to the lateral border. *B,* Lateral examination shows the needle tip in the posterior aspect of the lateral atlantoaxial joint (arrow). *C,* Frontal view following injection of 0.2 mL of nonionic contrast material demonstrates flow into the more medial aspect of the joint (arrow). *D,* Lateral view demonstrates contrast flowing along the lateral atlantoaxial joint (arrow). A small volume (0.5 mL) of anesthetic and steroid was injected, and the patient had approximately 6 weeks of excellent pain relief.

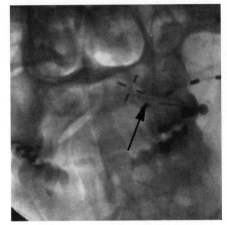

C

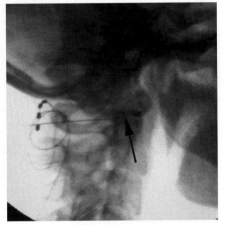

D

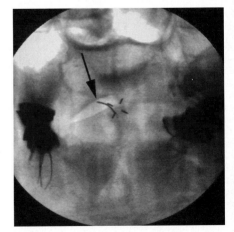

A

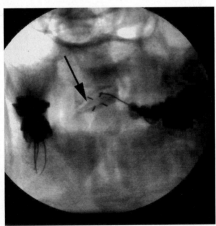

B

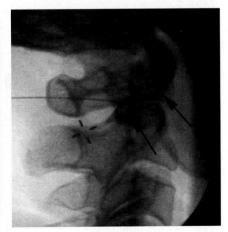

C

FIGURE 5-21

Lateral Atlantoaxial (C1-2) Joint Injection. This 52-year-old man had persistent headaches following an injury. *A,* Frontal view demonstrates the needle in the left C1-2 joint (arrow). *B,* Frontal view following injection of 0.2 mL of nonionic contrast material demonstrates flow into the more lateral aspect of the joint. *C,* Lateral view following contrast injection demonstrates flow along the lateral atlantoaxial joint (arrows). The patient had immediate relief of headache and neck pain following the injection, which lasted for several months.

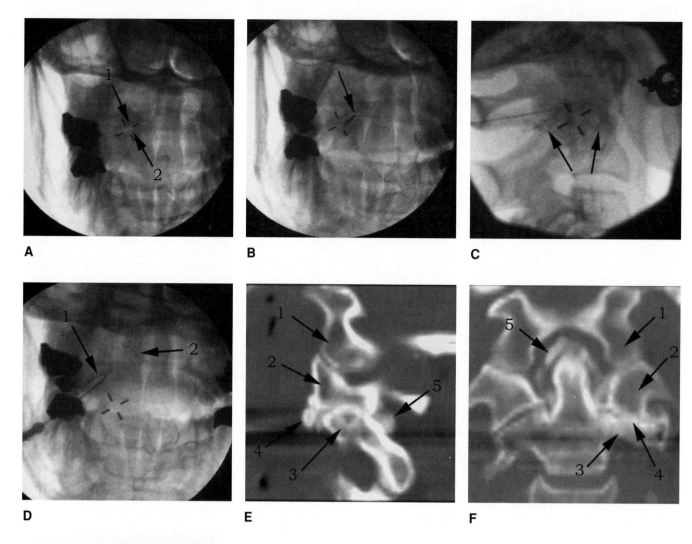

A   B   C

D   E   F

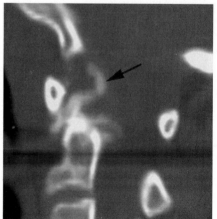

G

FIGURE 5–22

Lateral Atlantoaxial (C1-2) Joint Injection. This 55-year-old woman had left neck pain and headache. A preprocedure CT scan of the cervical spine (not shown) demonstrated extensive, asymmetric degenerative changes of the lateral atlantoaxial joints, with the left joint demonstrating considerably more joint space narrowing and osteophytic spurring than the right. *A,* Frontal view demonstrates the left lateral atlantoaxial joint, defined by the inferior articular margin of the lateral mass of C1 (arrow 1), and the superior articular surface of C2 (arrow 2). The cross-hairs of the laser aiming device target the middle portion of the joint. *B,* Frontal view following insertion of the needle demonstrates that the needle tip (arrow) appears to project within the joint. *C,* Lateral view following injection of 0.3 mL of nonionic contrast material demonstrates contrast flowing through the joint (arrows). *D,* Frontal view demonstrates contrast material flowing into the lateral portion of the joint (arrow 1). However, there is also abnormal density medial to the medial aspect of the joint along the dens (arrow 2). This was unexpected and unusual, so no anesthetic was injected and a CT scan was done through the region. *E,* Left parasagittal reconstruction from a CT study done after contrast injection demonstrates the occipital condyle (arrow 1), left lateral mass of C1 (arrow 2), and body of C2 (arrow 3). Contrast pools along the anterior (arrow 4) and posterior (arrow 5) margins of the lateral atlantoaxial joint. *F,* Coronal reconstruction demonstrates the left occipital condyle (arrow 1), left lateral mass of C1 (arrow 2), and superior articular process of C2 (arrow 3). Note the asymmetry of the left lateral atlantoaxial joint (arrow 4) with the right. Contrast material flows out of the medial joint and surrounds the dens (arrow 5). The material adjacent to the dens was not present on a CT study done 2 weeks previous to this examination. *G,* Left parasagittal reconstruction (medial to part *E*) demonstrates contrast material external to the joint (arrow). Such capsular extravasation is probably secondary to joint damage from degenerative changes. Note that such extravasation is very high in the cervical canal, and that local anesthetic injected in this location could have dramatic consequences. The patient experienced moderate pain relief for several months following injection of steroids into the joint.

TABLE 5–8. Step-by-Step Description of Intra-articular Atlantoaxial (C1-2) Joint Injection

1. Identify the target joint using anterior-posterior fluoroscopy.
2. Insert the needle along the course of the x-ray beam far enough so that it is anchored.
3. Check position with the C-arm fluoroscope.
4. Adjust and advance the needle until the tip is near the posterior joint margin. Switching to lateral C-arm positioning to document that the needle tip is posterior to the joint should be done relatively early during needle placement.
5. Advance the needle until it is within the posterior aspect of the joint or until it feels as if it has entered the joint capsule. Penetrating the joint capsule may provide a characteristic "bottle-stopper" sensation.
6. Inject 0.1 to 0.3 mL of nonionic contrast material and document intra-articular location of the needle tip. Reposition the needle if necessary. Remember that any extra-articular contrast material injected will quickly obscure the joint margins and prevent completion of the procedure.
7. Once the needle is definitely intra-articular, inject anesthetic and steroid agents as desired. Injection volumes will need to be low (e.g., 0.5–1.0 mL of local anesthetic and 0.5–1.0 mL of steroid) to prevent capsular extravasation (not desired in the high cervical spine). Take frontal and lateral images and document contrast flow.
8. Monitor for pain response and record percentage of pain relief at 30 minutes.
9. Release patient when stable. Provide patient with a telephone number to call if there is persistent or increased pain or numbness or if fever, swelling, or redness develops.

Lumbar and Cervical Rhizotomy

Needle positioning for lumbar rhizotomy is identical to needle positioning for medial branch blocks. See Figures 5–6 and 5–14. Table 5–9 describes the procedure.

Lumbar Synovial Cyst Injection/Rupture

As noted in the Patient Selection section, patients undergoing synovial cyst injection/rupture should have radicular pain in an anatomically appropriate location with a corresponding imaging abnormality.

Table 5–10 describes and Figures 5–23 and 5–24 illustrate synovial cyst injection/rupture. As noted earlier (see Lumbar Intra-articular Injection section), the joint access technique is adapted from Sarazin and colleagues (Sarazin 1999) and is markedly superior to attempting to target the visualized "joint space" using an oblique approach. Note that while the best results are reported to follow cyst rupture, some patients receive pain relief with simple intra-articular injection of anesthetic and steroids without cyst rupture (Bureau 2001, Parlier-Cuau 1999). A description of the case illustrated in Figure 5–24 follows:

LUMBAR SYNOVIAL CYST RUPTURE

INTRODUCTION

The patient is a 54-year-old woman with right hip pain and low back pain. A recent magnetic resonance imaging (MRI) examination shows degenerative spondylolisthesis with a right-sided synovial cyst at L4-5.

TECHNICAL INFORMATION

The procedure and possible complications were explained to the patient. Informed consent was obtained.

Using sterile technique, careful fluoroscopic guidance, and a right-sided approach, local anesthesia was obtained with 0.5% bupivacaine (Sensorcaine). A 22-gauge needle was placed into the right L4-5 facet joint. Contrast material was injected into the joint, which filled the joint and entered the synovial cyst. Following this, 3.0 mL of a 2:1 mixture of 0.5% Sensorcaine and 40 mg/mL Depo-Medrol was injected. There was a sudden increase in patient pain accompanied by resistance to injection, followed by a sudden release of resistance to injection, rupture of the synovial cyst with flow into the epidural space, and diminished patient pain.

Films documented contrast entering the epidural space.

The patient had excellent pain relief following rupture of the cyst.

IMPRESSION

Right L4-5 synovial cyst rupture with excellent pain relief.

TABLE 5–9. Step-by-Step Description of Rhizotomy

1. Provide patient analgesia (intravenous or intramuscular narcotics, etc.) and/or sedation.
2. Place needles as they have been placed on prior occasions for successful medial branch blocks. Local anesthetic placed along the planned needle track through a 25-gauge needle may be useful, given the larger size of the rhizotomy needles.
3. When needles are in a radiographically ideal position, test-inject 0.1 to 0.3 mL of nonionic contrast material to document a nonvascular location of the needle tip.
4. Test-stimulate for possible segmental nerve stimulation (check specific voltage and current settings for sensory and motor stimulation on device in use).
5. Inject 1.0 mL of local anesthetic of choice and wait 60 seconds.
6. Create a lesion. In the lumbar spine, 90 seconds at 90°C with two collateral lesions along the long axis of the needle, and in the cervical spine 60 seconds at 80°C with three collateral lesions along the axis of the needle are generally considered adequate.
7. Post-procedure oral narcotic analgesics and muscle relaxants for at least 3 days (and as long as 4 weeks) may be required following rhizotomy.
8. Release patient when stable. Provide patient with a telephone number to call if there is persistent or increased pain or numbness or if fever, swelling, or redness develops.

TABLE 5–10. Step-by-Step Description of Synovial Cyst Injection and Rupture

1. Place a needle into the joint as described in Table 5–5.
2. Once the needle is definitely intra-articular, connect a 3-mL syringe containing a 2:1 mixture of anesthetic and steroid directly to the needle hub (without a connecting tube). Inject forcefully. At this point, either the cyst will fill and not rupture (in which case, the patient will experience a sudden increase in radicular pain), will fill *and* rupture (in which case, the patient will experience a sudden increase and then cessation of pain), or will not fill (with no reproduction of radicular pain). If the cyst has filled but not ruptured, aspirate and reinject repeatedly four or five times. If the cyst does not fill, try adjusting the needle tip. Occasionally, contrast material will simply flow backward along the needle tip, regardless of ideal, intra-articular position.
3. Release patient when stable. Provide patient with a telephone number to call if there is persistent or increased pain or numbness or if fever, swelling, or redness develops.

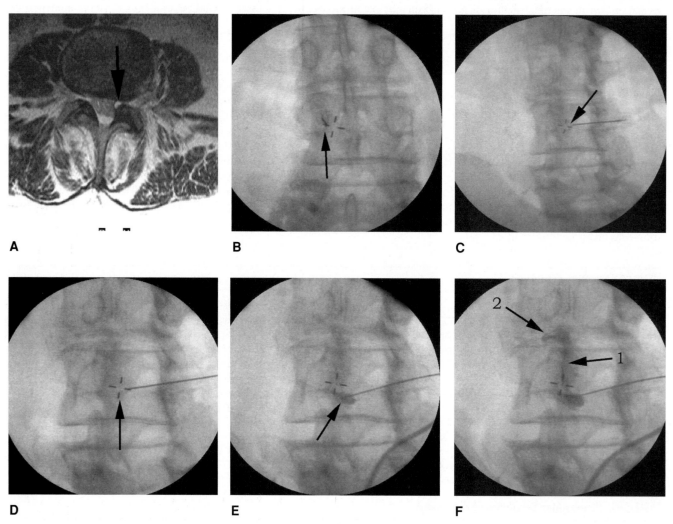

FIGURE 5–23

Step-by-Step Illustration of Synovial Cyst Injection and Rupture. This 78-year-old woman had left hip and leg pain. *A,* Axial T2-weighted magnetic resonance imaging scan at the level of the L3-4 intervertebral disc demonstrates a synovial cyst arising from the left L3-4 facet joint (arrow). The cyst narrows the subarticular recess and compresses the traversing left L4 nerve root. *B,* Frontal view demonstrates the cross-hairs of the laser aiming device at the tip of the left L3 inferior articular process. The needle is located at the same level (arrow). *C,* Oblique view demonstrates the needle tip at the inferior aspect of the left L3-4 facet joint (arrow). *D,* Magnified oblique view somewhat better demonstrates the inferior tip of the left L3 inferior articular process (arrow). Note that even on the magnified view, it is difficult to bring the facet joint into focus secondary to its curved nature and obliquity. However, there was a distinct "bottle stopper" sensation upon needle placement, and the needle rested on bone, making an intra-articular location likely. *E,* Oblique magnified view following injection of 0.1 mL of nonionic contrast material. The material appears to pool around the needle tip but is probably within the inferior recess of the L3-4 facet joint. *F,* Oblique magnified view after injection of an additional 0.3 mL of nonionic contrast material demonstrates an unequivocal arthrogram, with contrast flowing along the joint (arrow 1) and collecting in the superior recess of the joint (arrow 2). At this point, the connecting tubing was removed and 3 mL of an anesthetic/steroid was forcefully injected (see Table 5–10). The patient had sudden reproduction of symptoms, followed by cessation of symptoms accompanied by loss of resistance to injection. This combination of features is consistent with synovial cyst filling and rupture. The patient had immediate and longstanding pain relief following the injection.

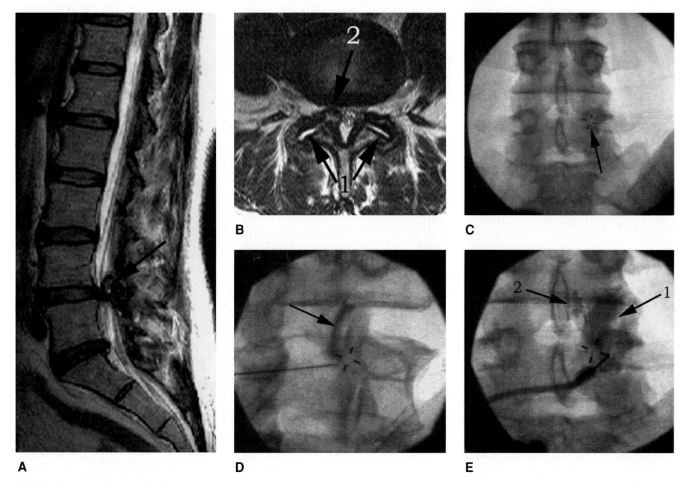

FIGURE 5–24

Synovial Cyst Injection and Rupture. This 54-year-old woman had mild chronic back pain, with the recent onset of right hip and lateral thigh pain. *A,* Right parasagittal T2-weighted magnetic resonance imaging examination demonstrates minimal degenerative spondylolisthesis of L4 on L5. There is a synovial cyst narrowing the spinal canal (arrow). *B,* Axial T2-weighted magnetic resonance imaging scan demonstrates bilateral severe facet arthropathy (arrow 1). On the right side, there is a synovial cyst (arrow 2) narrowing the subarticular recess and compressing the traversing right L5 nerve root. *C,* Frontal view demonstrates the cross-hairs of the laser aiming device at the tip of the right L4 inferior articular process (arrow). A needle was placed and advanced into the joint. *D,* Oblique magnified view demonstrates a needle with its tip in the inferior aspect of the right L4-5 facet joint. The image, taken following injection of 0.2 mL of nonionic contrast material, demonstrates an arthrogram (arrow). *E,* Frontal view after injecting a total of 0.5 mL of nonionic contrast material demonstrates the right L4-5 facet joint (arrow 1) and also filling of the synovial cyst (arrow 2). At this time, the connecting tube was disconnected, and a total volume of 3.0 of a mixture of local anesthetic and steroid was injected (see Table 5–10). The patient had sudden exacerbation of the right leg pain, followed by cessation of this pain, which was accompanied by loss of resistance to injection. The patient had 6 months of excellent pain relief, followed by recurrence of pain. An additional synovial cyst injection and rupture was performed at that time.

Lumbar Pars Defect Injections

One can usually inject pars defects directly by locating the defect using oblique fluoroscopy and advancing the needle until it is in the defect. Table 5–11 describes and Figures 5–25, 5–26, and 5–27 illustrate lumbar pars injection.

TABLE 5–11. Step-by-Step Description of Lumbar Pars Defect Injection

1. Place the patient prone on the procedure table with bolsters under the abdomen to flex the lumbar spine. Identify the pars defect with oblique fluoroscopy.
2. Insert the needle along the course of the x-ray beam far enough so that it is anchored.
3. Check position with the C-arm fluoroscope.
4. Adjust and advance until the needle appears to project within the pars interarticularis defect. Some resistance should be encountered as the needle passes through the proliferative tissue that usually forms along the pars defect margins. A frontal, opposite oblique, or lateral view may help confirm correct needle tip location.
5. Inject 0.1 to 0.3 mL of nonionic contrast material and document flow into the pars interarticularis defect. Reposition the needle if necessary. Remember that any extra-articular contrast material injected will quickly obscure the region and prevent completion of the procedure.
6. Once the needle is definitely within the defect, inject anesthetic and steroid agents as desired.
7. Monitor for pain response and record percentage of pain relief at 30 minutes.
8. Release patient when stable. Provide patient with a telephone number to call if there is persistent or increased pain or numbness or if fever, swelling, or redness develops.

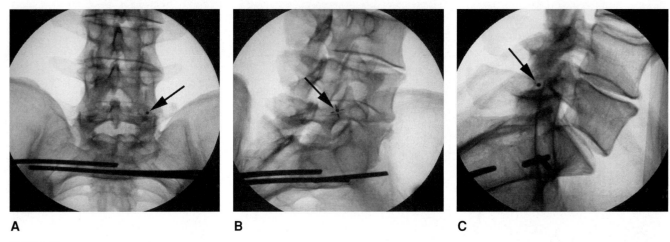

A   B   C

FIGURE 5–25

Skeletal Specimen Radiographs Demonstrating Location of the Pars Interarticularis. *A*, Frontal view of skeletal specimen with a metallic bead (arrow) marking the right L5 pars interarticularis. (The metallic bars through the pelvis hold the sacrum and pelvis together in this specimen.) *B*, Ipsilateral oblique view demonstrating the cross-hairs of the laser aiming device targeting the metallic bead taped to the right L5 pars interarticularis (arrow). The pars interarticularis on this specimen radiograph is intact; in the clinical situation of pars defect injection, a lucency occupies this position (see Figs. 5–26 and 5–27). *C*, Lateral radiograph demonstrating the metallic bead along the posterior aspect of the pars interarticularis at the L5 level (arrow).

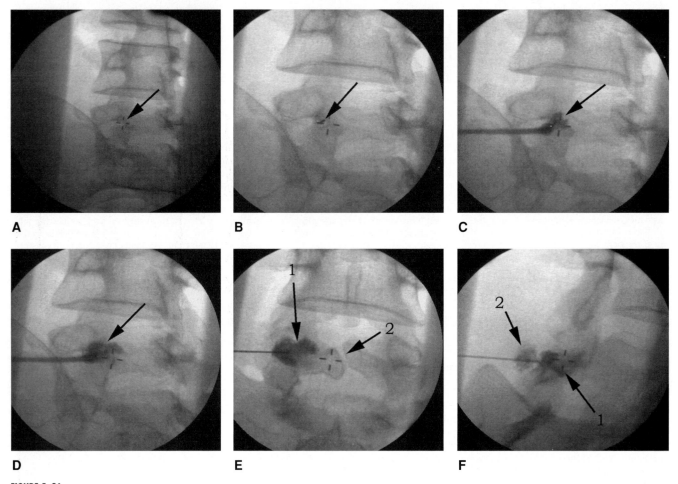

A   B   C

D   E   F

FIGURE 5–26

Pars Interarticularis Injection. This 31-year-old woman had moderate chronic back pain unrelieved by epidural steroid injection. The pars injections were requested for diagnostic and therapeutic purposes. *A*, Oblique view demonstrates the left L5 pars region (arrow). A discrete pars defect is difficult to appreciate but was present on a CT study (not shown). *B*, Magnified view following placement of a needle demonstrates the needle tip near the pars interarticularis (arrow). *C*, Magnified oblique view following injection of 0.2 mL of contrast material demonstrates contrast collecting locally around the needle tip (arrow). *D*, Magnified oblique view following injection of a total volume of 0.5 mL of contrast material shows filling of the left L5 pars defect (arrow). *E*, Frontal view demonstrates contrast at the level of the left L5 pars interarticularis (arrow 1). Note failure of complete ossification of the posterior neural arch at the level of the pars defect (arrow 2). *F*, Opposite oblique view demonstrates contrast material in the pars defect (arrow 1) as well as some posterior extravasation within the soft tissues (arrow 2). Following injection of small amounts of local anesthetic and steroids, the patient had complete transient pain relief, following by moderate long-term pain relief.

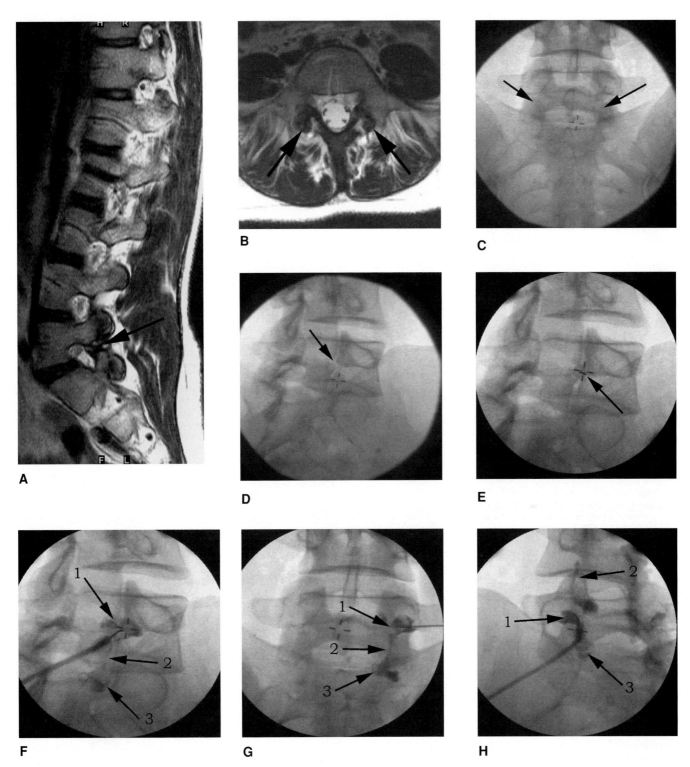

FIGURE 5–27

Bilateral Pars Interarticularis Injections with Flow into Adjacent Facet Joints. This 40-year-old woman had 6 months of low back pain with no significant pain relief from epidural steroid injection. *A,* Right parasagittal T2-weighted magnetic resonance imaging examination demonstrates a pars defect (arrow). Left parasagittal studies (not shown) showed a similar defect in the left pars. *B,* Axial T2-weighted magnetic resonance imaging scan through the level of the L5 pars interarticularis demonstrates bilateral pars defects (arrows). *C,* Frontal view with the cross-hairs of the laser aiming device centered at the L5-S1 intervertebral disc. Note that on this frontal view, the pars defects cannot be identified: arrows mark the general region of the pars interarticularis. *D,* Oblique view demonstrates the right L5 pars defect (arrow). *E,* Oblique view demonstrates the right L5 pars defect with a needle directed toward the defect. The needle is well aligned with the central ray of the x-ray beam, with the tip at the lower margin of the pars defect (arrow). *F,* Oblique view following injection of 0.3 mL of nonionic contrast material demonstrates contrast at the level of the pars defect (arrow 1) as well as faint contrast between the inferior articular process of L5 and the superior articular process of S1 (arrow 2). There is also contrast in the inferior recess of the L5-S1 facet joint (arrow 3). *G,* Frontal view demonstrates contrast along the L5 pars defect (arrow 1), within the L5-S1 facet joint (arrow 2), and in the inferior recess of the L5-S1 facet joint (arrow 3). *H,* Contralateral oblique view following injection of the contralateral pars defect. Contrast flows not only into the pars defect (arrow 1) but also into the ipsilateral L4-5 facet joint (arrow 2) above the defect and the ipsilateral L5-S1 facet joint (arrow 3) below the defect. Such filling of facets above and below the level of the injection is not uncommon. The patient had much better pain relief following pars injections than with epidural injections.

References

Aprill C, Dwyer A, Bogduk N. Cervical zygapophyseal joint pain patterns II: a clinical evaluation. Spine 1990; 15:458–461.

Apostolaki E, Davies AM, Evans N, Cassar-Pullicino VN. MR imaging of lumbar facet joint synovial cysts. Eur Radiol 2000; 10:615–623.

Awwad EE, Martin DS, Smith KR, Bucholz RD. MR imaging of lumbar juxtaarticular cysts. J Comput Tomogr 1990; 14:415–417.

Benzon HT. Epidural steroid injections for low back pain and lumbosacral radiculopathy. Pain 1986; 24:277–295.

Bjorkengren AG, Kurz LT, Resnick D, Sartorius DJ, Garfin SR. Symptomatic intraspinal synovial cysts: opacification and treatment by percutaneous injection. AJR 1987; 149:105–107.

Bureau NJ, Kaplan PA, Dussault RG. Lumbar facet joint synovial cyst: percutaneous treatment with steroid injections and distention—clinical and imaging follow-up in 12 patients. Radiology 2001; 221:179–185.

Carette S, Marcoux S, Truchon R, Grondin C, Gagnon J, Allard Y, Latulippe M. A controlled trial of corticosteroid injections into facet joints for chronic low back pain. N Engl J Med 1991; 325:1002–1007.

Carrera GF. Lumbar facet joint injection in low back pain and sciatica: description of technique. Radiology 1980a; 137:661–664.

Carrera GF. Lumbar facet joint injection in low back pain and sciatica: preliminary results. Radiology 1980b; 137:665–667.

Davis R, Iliya A, Roque C, Pampati M. The advantage of magnetic resonance imaging in diagnosis of a lumbar synovial cyst. Spine 1990; 15:244–246.

Derby R, Bogduk N, Schwarzer A. Precise percutaneous blocking procedures for localizing spinal pain. Part I: The posterior lumbar compartment. Pain Digest 1993; 3:89–100.

Dory MA. Arthrography of the lumbar facet joints. Radiology 1981; 140:23–27.

Dreyfuss P. Practice guidelines and protocols: sacroiliac joint blocks. In International Spinal Injection Society Syllabus for the 9th Annual Scientific Meeting, Orlando, FL, February 2002. San Francisco, ISIS, 2002.

Dreyfuss P, Halbrook B, Pauza K, Joshi A, Mclarty J, Bogduk N. Efficacy and validity of radiofrequency neurotomy for chronic lumbar zygapophysial joint pain. Spine 2000; 25:1270–1277.

Dreyfuss P, Lagattuta FP, Kaplansky B, Heller B. Zygapophyseal joint injection techniques in the spinal axis. In Lennard TA (ed). Physiatric Procedures in Clinical Practice. Philadelphia, Hanley & Belfus, 1995.

Dreyfuss P, Michaelsen M, Fletcher D. Atlanto-occipital and lateral atlanto-axial joint pain patterns. Spine 1994; 19:1125–1131.

Duprez T, Mailleaux P, Bodart A, Coulier B, Malghem J, Maldague B. Retrodural cysts bridging a bilateral lumbar spondylolysis: a report of two symptomatic cases. J Comput Assist Tomogr 1999; 23:534–537.

Dwyer AB, Aprill C, Bogduk N. Cervical zygapophyseal joint pain patterns. I: A study in normal volunteers. Spine 1990; 15:453–457.

Esses SI, Moro JK. The value of facet joint blocks in patient selection for lumbar fusion. Spine 1993; 18:185–190.

Gallagher J, Petriccione di Vadi PL, Wedley JR, Hamann W, Ryan P, Chikanza I, Kirkham B, Price R, Watson MS, Grahame R, Wood S. Radiofrequency facet joint denervation in the treatment of low back pain: a prospective controlled double-blind study to assess its efficacy. Pain Clin 1994; 7:193–198.

Ghelman B, Doherty JH. Demonstration of spondylolysis by arthrography of the apophyseal joint. AJR 1978; 130:986–987.

Ghormley RK. Low back pain with special reference to the articular facets, with presentation of an operative procedure. JAMA 1933; 101:1773–1777.

Goldthwait JE. The lumbosacral articulation: an explanation of many cases of lumbago, sciatica, and paraplegia. Boston Med Surg J 1911; 164:365–372.

Gray DP, Bajwa ZH, Warfield CA. Facet block and neurolysis. In Waldman SD (ed). Interventional Pain Management, 2nd ed. Philadelphia, W.B. Saunders, 2001.

Guyer DW, Wiltse LL, Eskay ML, Guyer BH. The long-range prognosis of arachnoiditis. Spine 1989; 14:1332–1341.

Haldeman S, Dagenais S. Cervicogenic headaches: a critical review. Spine J 2001; 1:31–46.

Hemminghytt S, Daniels DL, Williams AL, Haughton VM. Intraspinal synovial cysts: natural history and diagnosis by CT. Radiology 1982; 145:375–376.

Hirsch C, Ingelmark BE, Miller M. The anatomical basis for low back pain: studies on the presence of sensory nerve endings in ligamentous, capsular and intervertebral disc structures in the human lumbar spine. Acta Orthop Scand 1963; 33:1–17.

Howington JU, Connolly ES, Voorhies RM. Intraspinal synovial cysts: 10-year experience at the Ochsner Clinic. J Neurosurg 1999; 91(2 suppl):193–199.

Jackson DE, Atlas SW, Mani JR, Norman D. Intraspinal synovial cysts: MR imaging. Radiology 1989; 170:527–530.

Jackson RP, Jacobs RR, Montesano PX. Facet joint injection in low-back pain: a prospective statistical study. Spine 1988; 13:966–971.

Kaplan M, Dreyfuss P, Halbrook B, Bogduk N. The ability of lumbar medial branch blocks to anesthetize the zygapophyseal joint: a physiologic challenge. Spine 1998; 23:1847–1852.

van Kleef M, Barendse GAM, Kessels A, Voets HM, Weber WEJ, de Lange S. Randomized trial of radiofrequency lumbar facet denervation for chronic low back pain. Spine 1999; 24:1937–1942.

Kurz LT, Garfin SR, Unger AS, Thorne RP, Rothman RH. Intraspinal synovial cyst causing sciatica. J Bone Joint Surg Am 1985; 67:865–871.

Leclaire R, Fortin L, Lambert R, Bergeron YM, Rossignol M. Radiofrequency facet joint denervation in the treatment of low back pain: a placebo-controlled clinical trial to assess efficacy. Spine 2001; 26:1411–1417.

Lilius G, Laasonen EM, Myllynen P, Harilainen A, Gronlund G. Lumbar facet joint syndrome: a randomised clinical trial. J Bone Joint Surg Br 1989; 71:681–684.

Liu SS, Williams KD, Drayer BP, Spetzler RF, Sonntag VKH. Synovial cysts of the lumbosacral spine: diagnosis by MR imaging. AJR 1990; 154:163–166.

Lord S, Barnsley L, Bogduk N. Percutaneous radiofrequency neurotomy in the treatment of cervical zygapophyseal joint pain: a caution. Neurosurgery 1995; 36:732–739.

Lynch MC, Taylor JF. Facet joint injection for low back pain: a clinical study. J Bone Joint Surg Br 1986; 68:138–141.

Lyons MK, Atkinson JL, Wharen RE, Deen HG, Zimmerman RS, Lemens SM. Surgical evaluation and management of lumbar synovial cysts: the Mayo Clinic Experience. J Neurosurg 2000; 93(1 suppl):53–57.

Maldague B, Mathurin P, Malghem J. Facet joint arthrography in lumbar spondylolysis. Radiology 1981; 140:29–36.

Modic MT, Ross JS, Obuchowski NA, Browning KH, Cianflocco AJ, Mazanec DJ. Contrast-enhanced MR imaging in acute lumbar radiculopathy: a pilot study of the natural history. Radiology 1995; 195:429–435.

Mooney V, Robertson J. The facet syndrome. Clin Orthop Rel Res 1976; 115:149–156.

Moran R, O'Connell D, Walsh MG. The diagnostic value of facet joint injections. Spine 1988; 13:1407–1410.

Nelson DA, Vates TS, Thomas RB. Complications from intrathecal steroid therapy in patients with multiple sclerosis. Acta Neurol Scand 1973; 49:176–188.

Parlier-Cuau C, Wybier M, Nizard R, Champsaur P, Le Hir P, Laredo JD. Symptomatic lumbar facet joint synovial cysts: clinical assessment of facet joint steroid injection after 1 and 6 months and long-term follow-up in 30 patients. Radiology 1999; 210:509–513.

Raskin NH. Lumbar puncture headache: a review. Headache 1990; 30:197–200.

Raymond J, Dumas JM. Intraarticular facet block: diagnostic test or therapeutic procedure? Radiology 1984; 151:333–336.

Roy-Camille R, Mazel CH, Husson JL, Saillant G. Symptomatic spinal epidural lipomatosis induced by a long-term steroid treatment: review of the literature and report of two additional cases. Spine 1991; 16:1365–1371.

Sabo RA, Tracy PT, Weinger JM. A series of 60 juxtafacet cysts: clinical presentation, the role of spinal instability, and treatment. J Neurosurg 1996; 85:560–565.

Sarazin L, Chevrot A, Pessis E, Minoui A, Drape JL, Chemla N, Godefroy D. Lumbar facet joint arthrography with the posterior approach. Radiographics 1999; 19:93–104.

Schellhas KP. Facet nerve blockade and radiofrequency neurotomy. Spine Interventions 2000; 10:493–501.

Schwarzer AC, Aprill CN, Derby R, Fortin J, Kine G, Bogduk N. The false-positive rate of uncontrolled diagnostic blocks of the lumbar zygapophysial joints. Pain 1994a; 58:195–200.

Schwarzer AC, Aprill CN, Derby R, Fortin J, Kine G, Bogduk N. Clinical features of patients with pain stemming from the lumbar zygapophyseal joints: is the lumbar facet syndrome a clinical entity? Spine 1994b; 19:1132–1137.

Schwarzer AC, Wang SC, O'Driscoll D, Harrington T, Bogduk N, Laurent R. The ability of computed tomography to identify a painful zygapophyseal joint in patients with chronic low back pain. Spine 1995; 20:907–912.

Shealy C. Percutaneous radio frequency denervation of spinal facets. J Neurosurg 1975; 43:448–451.

Silbergleit R, Gebarski SS, Brunberg JA, McGillicudy J, Blaivas M. Lumbar synovial cysts: correlation of myelographic, CT, MR, and pathologic findings. Am J Neurorad 1990; 11:777–779.

Silbergleit R, Mehta BA, Sanders WP, Talati SJ. Imaging-guided injection techniques with fluoroscopy and CT for spinal pain management. Radiographics 2001; 21:927–942.

Silvers HR. Lumbar percutaneous facet rhizotomy. Spine 1990; 15:36–40.

Sjaastad O, Fredriksen TA, Pfaffenrath V. Cervicogenic headache: diagnostic criteria. Headache 1998; 38:442–445.

Stambough JL, Booth RE, Rothman RH. Transient hypercorticism after epidural steroid injection. J Bone Joint Surg Am 1984; 66:1115–1116.

Suh PB, Esses SI, Kostuik JP. Repair of pars interarticularis defect: the prognostic value of pars infiltration. Spine 1991; 16:S445–S448.

van Suijlekom HA, van Kleef M, Barendse GAM, Sluijter ME, Sjaastad O, Weber WEJ. Radiofrequency cervical zygapophyseal joint neurotomy for cervicogenic headache: a prospective study of 15 patients. Funct Neurol 1998; 13:297–303.

Victory RA, Hassett P, Morrison G. Transient blindness following epidural analgesia. Anaesthesia 1991; 46:940–941.

Yuh WTC, Drew JM, Weinstein JN, McGuire CW, Moore TE, Kathol MH, El-Khoury GY. Intraspinal synovial cysts: magnetic resonance evaluation. Spine 1991; 16:740–745.

6 Discography

DONALD L. RENFREW

Definition

Discography is puncture of the intervertebral disc with introduction of contrast material into the nucleus. A test result is considered positive if injection into the nucleus reproduces the patient's typical pain. Some authorities also require contrast to extend to the outer third of the annulus (as best seen on computed tomography [CT]-discography) to consider a test result positive (Bogduk 1997).

Literature Review

The following discussion reviews the literature on discography in four sections: early reports and descriptions; evaluation of false-positive results; magnetic resonance imaging (MRI) and discography; and clinical studies using outcome measurements. This review is not exhaustive but highlights a few of the more historically and clinically pertinent articles. Following the literature review is a brief discussion of research methodology.

EARLY REPORTS AND DESCRIPTIONS

In a 1948 paper, Lindblom stated, "Diagnostic disk puncture with injection of opaque medium demonstrates disk ruptures and protrusions and tells if the patient's symptoms originate from the punctured disk. The method seems to be of great practical value" (Lindblom 1948). Lindblom based this statement on a study of 13 patients with low back and leg pain who had failed to improve with conservative therapy and who had negative myelographic findings. He used a posterior approach with serial plain films guiding disc puncture and injected water-soluble (ionic) contrast material and novocaine. Lindblom also stated, "If the punctured disk is the cause of the symptoms of lumbago and sciatica, then pains caused by the injection will remind the patient of his usual complaints. If his usual sciatic pains become worse by the injection this means that the punctured disk is the ruptured one responsible for the root or nerve compression."

Also in 1948, Hirsch studied 16 patients with recurrent low back pain and noted that "a transdural puncture of one or both of the two lowest lumbar discs produced pain identical with the patient's spontaneous pain. Pain occurred either at the moment of puncture or when the intra-discal pressure was increased by introducing normal saline under

pressure. It rapidly diminished, and the Lasegue sign was either markedly reduced or abolished, with the injection of 1/2 cc of 1% Novocain into the disc" (Hirsch 1948). Hirsch also noted, "It must be admitted that it is sometimes difficult to place the needle correctly, but the procedure becomes easier with practice."

In 1960, Fernstrom published a lengthy treatise on discography, which included an extensive literature review, study of 13 cadavers, and reports of 386 discograms and correlative information from 182 operations (Fernstrom 1960). He found two types of annular ligament ruptures in degenerated discs: ruptures with nerve root compression (which he called "herniated discs"); and ruptures without nerve root compression (which he called "simple ruptured discs"). He found the discographic appearance similar in both entities, and that the "simple ruptured disc" may cause symptoms without signs. He stated, "Pain on injection is identical with experienced pain no matter whether the operation revealed nerve root compression or not. For that reason simple ruptured disc is considered to be of importance as a pain provoking factor." Fernstrom's "simple ruptured disc" would later be called "internal disc disruption" (Crock 1986).

Incidentally, although early reports of intradiscal injection of steroids reported favorable results (Feffer 1956, Feffer 1969, Leao 1960), later reports (Graham 1976, Simmons 1992, Wilkinson 1980) were not as encouraging, and the procedure appears to be little used.

EVALUATION OF FALSE-POSITIVE RESULTS

In 1968, Holt published a paper in which he stated, "The inescapable conclusion is that lumbar discography is unreliable as a diagnostic test" (Holt 1968). He based this conclusion on a study of 26 volunteers from a prison population, 21 to 41 years of age, with no history of back pain or sciatica. Using plain films to guide injections, he performed transdural punctures using a coaxial technique, with a 24-gauge needle advanced through a 20-gauge needle used to inject 1.0 to 2.0 mL of ionic contrast material. He found that 27 of 72 injections produced "severe pain." Simmons and colleagues (Simmons 1988) published a reassessment of Holt's data in 1988, noting (among other things) that the study population and technology (and hence technique) called into question both the validity of the results and the ability to generalize the results to other settings.

In 1990, Walsh and colleagues (Walsh 1990) conducted another study of volunteers (as well as patients) and concluded, "With current techniques and in conjunction with standardized methods for assessment of pain, lumbar discography is a highly reliable and specific diagnostic test." An experienced injectionist (Dr. Charles Aprill) injected the 10 volunteers and seven patients in Walsh's study. Blinded observers reviewed the videotaped responses and CT images from the injections. Five of the 10 volunteers (5 of 30 discs injected) had morphologically abnormal discs, but none of these was associated with substantial pain upon injection and thus using the criteria of abnormal morphology and pain reproduction, there were no false-positive study results. On the other hand, all seven of the symptomatic patients demonstrated morphologically abnormal discs, with six of the seven patients having substantial pain associated with disc injection.

Since 1999, Carragee and colleagues have published a series of papers (Carragee 1999, Carragee 2000a, Carragee 2000b, Carragee 2000c, Carragee 2000d, Carragee 2002) summarized in a review by Carragee and Alamin (Carragee 2001). The first of these (Carragee 1999) studied eight patients 2 to 4 months following iliac bone graft harvesting for non-spine orthopedic surgery with 24 disc injections and found that 14 injections were painful (5 "nonconcordant," 7 "similar," and 2 "exact"). Ten discs were found to have full-thickness annular fissures, and 5 of these injections produced "similar or exact pain" compared to the pain experienced by the patients originating from their iliac bone graft harvest site. The authors noted, "By the usual criteria of positive discography, 4 of the 8 patients (50%) would have been classified as positive. In these patients, the pain on a single disc injection was very painful, and the pain quality was noted to be exact or similar to the usual discomfort. All subjects had a normal control disc."

In another study, Carragee and colleagues (Carragee 2000d) examined pain responses of 26 individuals, 10 of whom were pain free, 10 of whom had chronic arm and neck pain without low back symptoms, and 6 of whom had somatization disorders without low back symptoms. Using criteria of pain and abnormal morphology, they found "positive" results in 1 of the 10 subjects in the pain-free group, 4 of the 10 chronic arm and neck pain group, and 5 of the 6 somatization disorder group. They noted that many pain score reports of 3, 4, or 5 out of 5 were given upon injection of discs with morphologic abnormality, but that no pain report exceeded 2 out of 5 in normal discs. The authors state, "A low false-positive rate of provocative discography in carefully screened patients with persistent low back pain is tentatively supported by the findings of the present study." They go on to say, however, "In light of the other findings, however, it is questionable how helpful discography would be in evaluation of a group of patients with significantly abnormal psychological profiles or long-standing chronic pain syndromes, especially patients with disability or compensation issues." Bogduk (Bogduk 2001) reevaluated the data in this study. By reclassifying patients without a nonpainful "control" level as "indeterminate" and using different manometric criteria, he found the "no pain" and "chronic pain group" false-positive rates to be much lower, with confidence interval estimates overlapping 0.

In a follow-up study of the same group, Carragee and colleagues (Carragee 2000a) noted that while patients with normal psychometric testing reported no persistent pain, 6 of the 15 patients (40%) with abnormal psychometric test results reported significant new chronic low back pain.

Another report by Carragee and colleagues (Carragee 2000b) compared injections in post-discectomy asymptomatic volunteers and symptomatic patients. Both groups reported pain scores of 3, 4, and 5 on a 5-point scale upon injection of the previously operated disc with equal frequency (about 40% in both the asymptomatic volunteers and symptomatic patients). In yet another study, the same authors (Carragee 2002) evaluated 25 subjects with benign, mild, persistent "backache" who were not seeking treatment. These patients volunteered for discography, and 9 of these 25 patients (36%) had concordant, painful injections and met the criteria published by Walsh and colleagues (Walsh 1990).

MAGNETIC RESONANCE IMAGING AND DISCOGRAPHY

Relatively early in the development of MRI, Gibson and colleagues (Gibson 1986) and Schneiderman and colleagues (Schneiderman 1987) reported a high concordance rate between MRI findings and discography. These reports were followed, however, by studies reporting 18 cases (Zucherman 1988), 4 cases (Kornberg 1989), and 7 cases (Brightbill 1994) wherein MRI results were not predictive of discography. In a series of 108 discs in 33 patients, Osti and Fraser (Osti 1992) found that although all 58 discs found to be abnormal by MRI were also abnormal at discography, 18 of 60 MRI-normal discs were also found to be abnormal by discography. In a similar study, Horton and colleagues (Horton 1992) found some general patterns of correspondence between positive discograms but concluded, "In many cases MRI does not reliably predict or replace discography."

In 1992, Aprill and Bogduk coined the term *high intensity zone* (HIZ) to denote a focus of high signal intensity on T2-weighted images (T2 prolongation) "located in the substance of the posterior annulus fibrosus, clearly dissociated from the signal of the nucleus pulposus in that it is surrounded superiorly, inferiorly, posteriorly, and anteriorly by the low-intensity (black) signal of the annulus fibrosus and is appreciably brighter than that of the nucleus pulposus" (Aprill 1992). Such HIZs could occur in an otherwise normal annulus but could also be found in a "bulging annulus": "it may be located superiorly or inferiorly behind the edge of the vertebral body in a severely bulging annulus."[1] They stated, regarding the HIZ, "Its sensitivity as a sign of either annular disruption or pain was modest but its specificity was high, and its positive predictive value for a severely disrupted, symptomatic disc was 86%. This sign is diagnostic of painful internal disc disruption." Subsequent investigations have both supported (Milette 1999, Saiffudin 1998, Schellhas 1996a) and contested (Carragee 2000c, Rankine 1999, Ricketson 1996, Smith 1998) this contention.

Two studies (Ito 1998, Weishaupt 2001) have correlated not only HIZs and disc degeneration but also subchondral marrow degenerative change with response at discography,

---

[1]This article was written in 1992, prior to the attempted standardization of nomenclature offered by the North American Spine Society, the American Society of Spine Radiology, etc. The abnormality described by Aprill and Bogduk as a "severely bulging annulus" would be termed a disc extrusion (a subset of disc herniation) in the NASS/ASSR terminology.

with no finding having more than moderate accuracy. Disc degeneration (evidenced by narrowing and dehydration) appears to be somewhat more sensitive (98% in Weishaupt et al's study) and subchondral degenerative changes somewhat more specific (76% in Weishaupt et al's study and 95% in Ito et al's study). Similarly, Schellhas and colleagues (Schellhas 1996b, Schellhas 2000) have found little correlation with MRI evaluation of disc morphology and response to discography (particularly at C2-3).

CLINICAL STUDIES USING OUTCOME MEASUREMENTS

Given the lengthy history and widespread use of discography, outcome studies evaluating the utility of the examination are scarce. Colhoun and colleagues (Colhoun 1988) published a large series and concluded, "In patients with low back and leg pain but no nerve root compression, operation at disc levels identified as symptomatic by discography gives a significantly better chance of a good result than surgery on asymptomatic discs." They based their conclusion on evaluation of 195 patients studied 2 to 10 years (average 3.6 years) after surgery; 182 had undergone fusion and 13 laminectomy/discectomy. They defined success as the combination of three outcomes: complete relief or significant improvement of pain, resumption of work (or normal duties), and no analgesics. Of the 195 patients, 137 had painful, abnormal discs, 25 had nonpainful, abnormal discs, 27 had "disc resorption" with no discogram performed, and 6 had three-level normal discograms. Eighty-nine percent of the 137 patients with positive (symptom-producing and morphologically abnormal) discography had a successful outcome; only 52% of patients without pain (but with abnormal morphology) on discography had a successful outcome. Interestingly, of 43 patients who had adjacent segment morphologically abnormal (but nonpainful to injection) discs, 41 of 43 operations (95%) were a success as defined here, which provides evidence to answer the question, "Can you fuse to a morphologically abnormal but pain-free level?"

In an uncontrolled study, Rhyne and colleagues (Rhyne 1995) followed 25 patients with low back pain, no psychiatric disease, and single-level disease on discography for a minimum of 3 years (mean 4.9 years). They found 17 of the 25 (68%) improved, 2 (8%) unchanged, and 6 (24%) worsened. Although the authors did not include a control group, they argued that their results were comparable to operative treatment (however, see above study by Colhoun and colleagues [Colhoun 1988]).

Madan and colleagues (Madan 2002) compared the outcome (using modified Oswestry scoring) of two groups of patients who had undergone fusion surgery. The first group comprised 41 patients who underwent surgery without discography, and the second group comprised 32 patients who underwent surgery with discography. Both groups had comparable rates of satisfactory outcomes (75.6% for the first group and 81.2% for the second group). However, all the discography patients who underwent fusion surgery were "positive." The paper did not include analysis of patients who underwent discography, were "negative," but then nonetheless underwent surgery. The paper suggests that if a patient who is to undergo surgery on the basis of data other than discography has a positive discogram, the chances of a good outcome do not improve. However, the paper does not answer the question of whether the chances of a good outcome decrease if a patient who is to undergo surgery on the basis of data other than discography has a negative discogram.

Research Methodology

One issue relating to research in discography is whether injection of normal volunteers can be extrapolated to patients who are candidates for fusion surgery. For some laboratory tests (e.g., measurement of serum cholesterol), it is difficult to see how a patient's attitude toward and tolerance of pain would have much of an effect. For other variables, including pain response, this is not the case. Extrapolation from "normal volunteers" must be done carefully (and may not be possible). It may be reasonable to ask a patient undergoing discography the following question: "If you were 25 years old, needed cash, and were paid a moderate amount of money,[2] would you undergo this test?" If the answer is "Are you kidding? I hate needles, and I'm scared to death of this test!", then it is reasonable to question whether the test results are as meaningful in this patient as in a patient who answers, "How much money? Oh. Yeah, probably."

Another issue relating to research in discography is the criteria used for a positive test. Recent proposals have suggested that manometric criteria be included in an analysis of discography (Bogduk 2001, Bogduk 2002). Using a minimum pressure below which a disc is considered "negative" even though concordant pain is produced upon injection of that disc risks classifying as negative those patients with "chemical sensitivity" (Derby 1999). Creating an "indeterminate" category (including patients who had intermediate levels of pain upon injection, no normal control level of injection, or experienced pain at intermediate levels of pressurization) complicates evaluation of diagnostic efficacy and may also discourage use of the test by resulting in a large number of patients being placed in the intermediate category (with an expensive and painful procedure having been done with little to show for it).

Finally, with respect to evaluation of discography results, a logistical difficulty arises in the calculation of measurements of diagnostic efficacy (sensitivity, specificity, predictive value of a positive test, predictive value of a negative test, and accuracy). Bayes' theorem, widely (if mostly intuitively) used in clinical medicine, calculates the post-test odds of a disease based on the pretest odds using sensitivity and specificity:

$$\text{Post-Test Odds} = \text{Pre-Test Odds} \times [\text{Sensitivity} \div (1 - \text{Specificity})]$$

This equation assumes that we know or can know the sensitivity and specificity of a test. These numbers are generally derived from the familiar 2 × 2 contingency table:

---

[2]Approximately $150 in 1990.

	Disease Present	Disease Absent	
Test positive	True positive (TP)	False positive (FP)	PVP = TP/(TP + FP)
Test negative	False negative (FN)	True negative (TN)	PVN = TN/(TN + FN)
	Sensitivity = TP/(TP + FN)	Specificity = TN/(TN + FP)	

PVP: Predictive value of a positive test
PVN: Predictive value of a negative test

To create this table, one must have a "reference standard" (also known as a "gold standard" or "criterion standard") to know how to classify patients as "Disease Present" or "Disease Absent." The reference standard is a social convention. Medical scientists decide the reference standard. Pathology results form the reference standard for many diseases. This works particularly well when the disease causes death and the pathologist immediately performs an autopsy. In much of the scientific literature, a proxy for the pathology standard is used, because the pathology standard (e.g, autopsy) may not be available, but the proxy has been shown in studies to be a reasonable substitute. For example, the diagnostic efficacy for detection of pulmonary nodules of a new, digital method of obtaining a chest radiograph (the test) could be compared to CT results (the reference standard, substituting for pathology results).

When we study back pain, the first issue that arises is that pain is a symptom and not a disease. This problem arises elsewhere: for example, in acute chest pain. With chest pain, a differential diagnosis immediately comes to mind: myocardial infarction, gastroesophageal reflux, dissecting thoracic aorta, rib fracture, and so on. With chest pain, each of the diseases listed has a recognized and accepted reference standard, as well as methods of achieving the diagnosis with tests of known diagnostic efficacy with respect to the reference standard. Cardiologists recognize myocardial infarction as a cause of chest pain, accept the reference standard of pathologic examination at autopsy, and evaluate the diagnostic efficacy of their tests (electrocardiogram results, serum enzyme studies, nuclear examinations of the heart, etc.) based on comparison to the reference standard (or an acceptable proxy). Similarly, gastroenterologists recognize gastroesophageal reflux disease as a cause of chest pain, accept prolonged pH monitoring of the distal esophagus as the reference standard for gastroesophageal reflux disease, and evaluate the diagnostic efficacy of their tests based on comparison to the reference standard.

In cases of axial spine pain, what are the diseases that may cause the symptom? Some of these diseases, like myocardial infarction and gastroesophageal reflux disease in cases of chest pain, have widely recognized reference standards. Spine tumors have the reference standard of autopsy or biopsy results, and infections have the reference standard of culture. However, these processes account for only a small minority of those patients who present for evaluation of axial back pain.[3] Most of these patients have diagnoses *that have no widely accepted reference standard.*

The two most frequently cited culprits are internal disc disruption[4] and facet arthropathy. Neither of these entities has a recognized pathology standard. Many autopsy specimens, upon direct examination, and normal volunteers, upon imaging examination, demonstrate morphologic findings without associated pain. Therefore, the definition of the diseases rests not on findings of morphology but on functional test results. Presumably (given our materialist assumptions about disease), there is "something" about patients with internal disc disruption and facet arthropathy (microstructural changes? chemical alterations?) that is present in patients with pain from these diseases but absent in patients without pain but with similar morphologic findings. However, to date, this "something" has not been discovered; that is to say, no reference standard demonstrating the "something" has been proposed and accepted. Therefore, we have a situation wherein a disease has no universally recognized standard, which is the same thing as saying we have a disease that is not universally recognized, for in one sense a disease is defined in terms of its reference standard. For those investigators who accept internal disc disruption and facet arthropathy as diseases that cause pain, they must either accept discography as the reference standard for internal disc disruption (and, similarly, response to facet blocks as the reference standard for facet arthropathy), or admit that there is no accepted reference standard for the disease in question. In either case, discussion of evaluation of the diagnostic efficacy of "discography" and "facet blocks" is complicated. Either discography and facet blocks *are* the reference standard, in which case it makes no sense to talk about measuring their diagnostic efficacy (sensitivity, specificity, etc.), or there is no reference standard, in which case we cannot talk meaningfully about diagnostic efficacy because we cannot complete the above contingency table.

Note that while lack of an accepted reference standard prevents completion of the left ("Disease Present") column of the above table, a study on suitable volunteers should allow completion of the right ("Disease Absent") column. For further discussion of this topic, see the section Evaluation of False-Positive Results. Note that even evaluating this column is problematic. What constitutes a "normal" subject? As noted earlier, are (relatively young) men who willingly undergo discography for money representative of the patient population being studied? With respect to the 2002 study by Carragee and colleagues on patients with mild backache who were not candidates for spine fusion (see under Evaluation of False-Positive Results), were those patients with positive discograms simply in the "preclinical" phase of disease, and within a few more years would they have developed

---

[3]This discussion focuses on axial back pain and somatic referred pain. Radicular pain is a different subject and probably fits much better with the "chest pain" model, with a differential diagnosis of herniated disc, synovial cyst, stenosis, nerve root sheath tumor, etc.

[4]Herniated discs as a cause of axial back pain (rather than radiculopathy) are included in this category.

TABLE 6–1. Equipment and Supplies for Discography

C-arm fluoroscope
Surgical scrub solution
Needles
Syringes
Connecting tube
Nonionic contrast material
Anesthetic agent
Antibiotics
Manometer (if pressure measurement is desired)
Computed tomography scanner

clinically severe back pain requiring evaluation for fusion surgery? The concluding line of Carragee and colleagues' 2002 study summarizes the present state of affairs well: "At this point, the root cause of this modern epidemic [severe chronic low back pain illness] remains obscure and the evidence cannot confirm a specific pathoanatomic process of the spine as a primary lesion."

Rationale for Procedure

The "provocation" aspect of injection (embodied in Fundamental Assumption 1; see Table 1–1) provides the rationale for discography: although early investigators (Hirsch 1948, Lindblom 1948) advocated a role for symptom amelioration in the diagnosis of disc disease, this is not currently part of the diagnostic regimen for most investigators. Brodsky and Binder (Brodsky 1979) proposed five mechanisms whereby discography might produce pain: stretching of fibers within an abnormal annulus; extradural extravasation of contrast with nerve irritation; pressure on nerves secondary to disc distention; hyperflexion of posterior joints secondary to disc distention; and vascular granulation tissue with ingrowth of pain fibers. In an interesting animal study, Weinstein and colleagues (Weinstein 1988) found increased levels of substance P in the dorsal root ganglia and discs of dogs injected with contrast material versus those injected with contrast and anesthetic agents.

Equipment and Supplies[5]

Table 6–1 lists equipment required for nerve root blocks.

A C-arm fluoroscope is necessary to obtain ideal positioning for discography. A laser aiming device (an attachment that shows a cross-hair on the fluoroscopic screen corresponding in position to a red dot on the skin surface) is extremely helpful for proper needle placement. Selection of needle type varies with the operator; a 22-gauge spinal needle for most lumbar injections and a 25-gauge spinal needle for thoracic and cervical injections work well. These needles are inexpensive, are readily available, and can usually be inserted without prior local anesthetic. Everything injected into the patient must be as safe as possible and preferably safe for intrathecal use, since there will be occasions when some of the injected materials will reach the epidural space and possibly the thecal sac. For this reason, nonionic contrast material and an anesthetic agent approved for intrathecal injection should be used.

In addition to the equipment listed in Table 6–1, a crash cart should be readily available to handle medical emergencies (e.g., contrast media and drug reactions).

Informed Consent Issues[6]

Informed consent issues can be divided into three topics: description of the procedure, warning the patient about possible drug side effects, and delineation of material risks. Informed consent also implies that alternatives to the proposed treatment have been described; for a general description of such alternatives, see Chapter 1.

Either the performing physician or a trained subordinate should completely explain the entire procedure in detail to the patient prior to performance of the procedure. Patients who know what to expect are much less anxious than those who do not. A step-by-step description of the procedure will apprise the patient of what to expect during the test. Many patients are frightened at the prospect of discography, and reassurance that the procedure usually takes about 15 minutes (in experienced hands) and that narcotic analgesics may be used immediately following the procedure may calm the patient. Oral antianxiety medication (e.g., oral liquid Valium 5 to 10 mg) can be used to allay anxiety. Narcotics and other analgesics may alter the patient's pain response and, as a rule, should be avoided.

The performing physician or a trained subordinate should also explain that local anesthetic placed along the course of the needle during lumbar discography may cause numbness and weakness of the leg. Patients should be warned that the injection may recreate or exacerbate their pain, and that this exacerbation may last 2 or 3 days following the procedure.

Complications can be subdivided into two categories: occasional (but inevitable) and rare but reported in the literature. Vasovagal reactions (treated with time, intravenous fluids, and atropine as necessary) and "post-tap headaches" following thecal puncture constitute the first category. Treatment of a post-tap headache includes bedrest, caffeine, analgesics, and an epidural "blood patch" (or saline injection) (Raskin 1990). The epidural blood patch is applied as indicated in Chapter 2 for an interlaminar epidural steroid injection, with injection of 10 to 15 mL of freshly drawn venous blood from the patient injected into the epidural space.

Table 6–2 lists less frequent complications of discography. Patients should cease taking all anticoagulants and other agents that might increase the risk of hematoma formation prior to performance of discography. With respect to anaphylactic reaction, patients should be screened for sensitivity to contrast media. If a patient has had a prior minor reaction to intravenous contrast agents, either reassurance or oral prednisone prior to the procedure is

---

[5]This section is virtually identical to the Equipment and Supplies section in Chapter 2 and can be skipped if the reader is already familiar with this material.

[6]This section is very similar to the Informed Consent Issues section of Chapter 2 and can be skipped if the reader is already familiar with this material.

TABLE 6–2. Possible Complications of Discography

Reported in discography
Discitis (Osti 1990; Grubb 2000)
Epidural abscess
Epidural hematoma
Anaphylactic reaction to contrast material
Anaphylactic reaction to anesthetic
Anaphylactic reaction to antibiotic
Anaphylactic reaction to latex, surgical scrub solution, etc.
In cervical discography: puncture of carotid vessels, esophagus, and larynx/trachea

advised. For prior major contrast reactions, the best option is probably to perform the procedure with fluoroscopic guidance and to use either saline or gadolinium-based contrast material (Huang 2002). Nonlatex gloves and surgical scrub without iodine may be used as appropriate.

Patient Selection

Indications for the procedure are controversial and are likely to remain so, since the "cure" (fusion surgery) and the "disease" (internal disc disruption) diagnosed by discography are controversial. The ideal patient for discography suffers from incapacitating axial low back or somatic referred pain, has failed conservative therapy, has normal psychometric testing findings, and is a fusion surgery candidate. Given such a patient, the question arises, "Is discography mandatory in the clinical evaluation of this patient?" Many surgeons believe that it is not and advocate either not operating on such patients, or treating them without discography (using clinical information and other imaging data) (Jackson 1997). Although MRI may be moderately predictive of symptoms, it is insensitive and nonspecific using discography as a reference standard (see subsection Magnetic Resonance Imaging and Discography in the

Literature Review section). Stated alternately, discography is inaccurate using MRI as a reference standard. Neither MRI nor discography is a perfect predictor of surgical outcome, and no study comparing MRI findings with fusion surgery success has been forthcoming (to compare, for example, with the study by Colhoun and colleagues [Colhoun 1988], which showed better clinical results for fusion in patients with positive discography).

Consultation with the referring spine surgeon regarding the levels to be injected is mandatory. There appears to be little reason to perform discography unless the patient is a fusion candidate, and this decision is basically in the hands of the spine surgeon. As a generalization, in the lumbar spine, the bottom three discs (L3-4, L4-5, and L5-S1) are usually tested (including any transitional level disc). If injection into all three of these discs provokes severe concordant pain (6 or greater on a 10-point scale), injection into L2-3 follows. Practice patterns vary, but most spine surgeons rarely fuse more than three segments of the lumbar spine for internal disc disruption.

In the cervical spine, studies have demonstrated that MRI is not predictive of discography results, and since any level may be involved in pain generation, it makes sense to study all accessible levels (Grubb 2000, Schellhas 1996b, Schellhas 2000). Somewhat limited work has been published regarding thoracic discography, but in general, injection of MRI-abnormal levels (with adjacent levels as controls) appears to form an acceptable starting point (Schellhas 1994).

Procedure Description

LUMBAR DISCOGRAPHY

Table 6–3 describes and Figures 6–1 and 6–2 illustrate lumbar discography. The reports for the discogram and discogram-CT scan illustrated in Figure 6–2 follow:

TABLE 6–3. Step-by-Step Description of Typical Lumbar Discography

1. Position C-arm fluoroscope for a clear view of the L3-4 disc. An oblique position with the superior articular process approximately halfway between the anterior and posterior visualized disc margins is ideal. The target point lies just anterior to the superior articular process, along the lower aspect of the disc. The C-arm fluoroscope should be angled in the cranial or caudal direction until the superior and inferior vertebral bony margins along the disc are distinct and the disc is well defined.
2. Insert needle along the course of the x-ray beam far enough so that it is anchored.
3. Check position with C-arm fluoroscope.
4. Adjust and advance the needle until it is within the central portion of the disc. If radicular pain is encountered, adjust needle localization or anesthetize with 1 to 2 mL of lidocaine.
5. Check position with frontal and lateral fluoroscopy.
6. Repeat for L4-5.
7. Repeat for L5-S1. The target may be quite small and require considerable caudal and oblique angulation. The target will be a triangle formed by the superior articular process posteriorly, the iliac crest anteriorly, and the inferior bony margin of the L5 vertebral body. The needle may need to be arced for ideal placement.
8. When needle placement is completed and checked for position in frontal and lateral planes, change gloves and instruct the patient again in the purpose of the examination. Tell the patient to ignore all pain caused by needle placement and concentrate on any new pain with each injection.
9. Inject under lateral fluoroscopic visualization and ensure that the needle is intranuclear. Injection material should be 10:1 nonionic contrast (safe for intrathecal use) and antibiotic (Osti 1990). Query patient for pain responses. Record pain on a 0 (no pain at all) to 10 (severe pain) scale and as concordant or discordant. Record location of pain. Record pressure at which pain is experienced, if desired. Record volume of contrast material. Record images in frontal and lateral projections. Note contrast pattern of injection.
10. Perform CT with 3.0-mm slices and the gantry angled to the intervertebral disc space.
11. Release patient when stable. Oral narcotic analgesics and/or muscle relaxants for a two- to three-day period may be prescribed. Provide patient with a telephone number to call if there is persistent or increased pain or numbness or if fever, swelling, or redness develops.

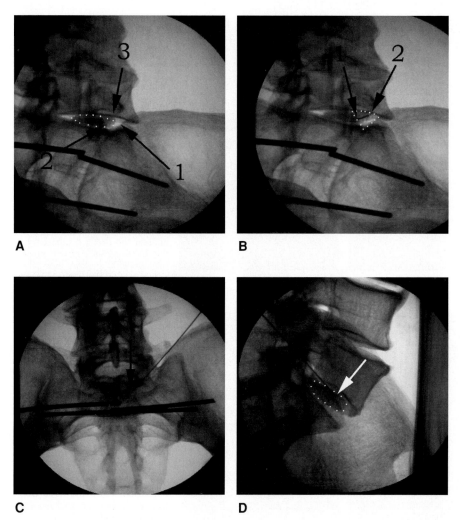

A   **B**

C   **D**

FIGURE 6-1

Skeletal Specimen Radiograph Demonstrating Target Position for Lumbar Discography. *A*, Oblique specimen radiograph with optimal position for needle placement at the L5-S1 level. A small amount of modeling clay has been placed in the location of the nucleus pulposus (surrounded by white dots). Three sides form the target triangle for needle placement: the iliac crest (arrow 1) anteriorly, the S1 superior articular process (arrow 2) posteriorly, and the inferior end plate of L5 (arrow 3) superiorly. Ideally, a needle should pass from anterior to posterior en route to the intervertebral disc. (The metallic bars through the pelvis hold the sacrum and pelvis together in this specimen.) *B*, The borders of the target triangle have been marked with white dots. Oblique view following placement of needle with the needle tip (arrow 1) in the central portion of the "nucleus" (modeling clay). The hub of the needle (arrow 2) is faintly seen and projects anterior to the needle tip, indicating an anterior-to-posterior direction of needle passage. *C*, Frontal view following needle placement. The needle demonstrates a marked cranial-to-caudal angle secondary to the necessity of aligning the needle with the intervertebral disc. The needle tip is substantially to the right of midline (arrow tip). While advancing the needle might result in a more midline position, review of the lateral image is necessary first. If the needle is in the peripheral portion of the disc, advancing the needle may result in passage through the anterior disc margin and into the pelvic viscera. *D*, Lateral view following needle placement. The "nucleus" (modeling clay) has been marked by white dots. Note that this representation of the nucleus is very generous and the actual nucleus may be substantially smaller; however, in most patients coming for discography, L5-S1 has annular degeneration and injection in a relatively peripheral portion of the disc

will still result in nuclear filling (and a valid test). The needle tip (arrow) in this case is in the midportion of the intervertebral disc, and, considering the location to the right of midline on the frontal examination (see part C), the needle tip may or may not be intranuclear in a clinical case with this needle position. The best way to proceed at this time would usually be to inject a small amount of contrast material and evaluate the contrast injection pattern. Generally speaking, free flow away from the needle tip with relatively "fuzzy" margins or a "cotton ball" appearance represents an intranuclear injection, whereas small, sharply defined contrast collections represent intra-annular injections.

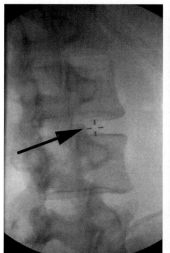 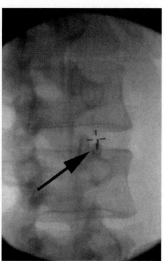

A   **B**

FIGURE 6-2

Step-by-Step Illustration of Typical Lumbar Discography. This 30-year-old man had persistent central low back pain and degenerative changes at L5-S1 on magnetic resonance imaging examination (not shown). *A*, Oblique view of the lumbar spine with the laser pointing device aimed at the L3-4 intervertebral disc. The cross-hair is just anterior to the L4 superior articular process (arrow). *B*, A 22-gauge needle has been inserted. The needle is tracking slightly superiorly, with the hub (arrow) slightly below the tip (projecting just to the right of center in the laser aiming device). The needle bevel could be turned anteriorly during advancement, since there is 1 to 2 mm of space anterior to the superior articular process of L4.

(figure continues on following page)

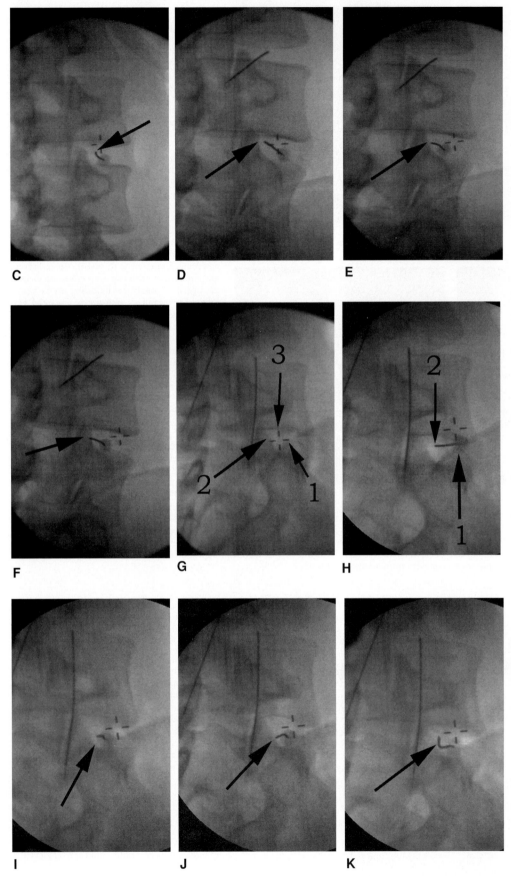

C D E

F G H

I J K

FIGURE 6–2 CONTINUED

C, Advance of the needle resulted in the typical "bottle stopper" feeling as the needle penetrated the intervertebral disc. The tip deflected minimally anteriorly (arrow), but overall the position appears acceptable (at least on this view). *D,* A second needle has been advanced along a course toward the L4-5 disc. The needle tip is coursing anteriorly to posteriorly and aimed just anterior to the L5 superior articular process (arrow). Note that repositioning of the C-arm with the central ray at the L4-5 level disc results in an oblique appearance of the L3-4 needle. *E,* Further advance of the needle brought the needle to the level of the L5 superior articular process (arrow) with a slight increase in resistance felt. The needle bevel was directed posteriorly (to slide past the superior articular process) before advance. *F,* The needle was advanced into the disc. The needle tip actually overlaps the superior articular process (arrow), and if it were superficial to the superior articular process, the needle could not penetrate the disc from this angle. However, the needle tip was actually on the far side of the articular process (as shown on later frontal and lateral examinations), and the familiar "bottle stopper" feeling of passing into the disc was encountered. *G,* The C-arm has been positioned for ideal visualization of the L5-S1 level. The cross-hairs of the laser aiming device are centered within the target triangle, formed by the iliac crest anteriorly (arrow 1), the superior articular process of S1 posteriorly (arrow 2), and the inferior bony margin of L5 superiorly (arrow 3). *H,* A third needle has been inserted. The needle is running in an anterolateral to posteromedial direction, as the hub (arrow 1) projects anterior to the needle tip (arrow 2) on this oblique view. This is ideal needle course, since the needle is running from anterior to posterior, which is important to place the needle in the posterior aspect of the intervertebral disc at L5-S1. The only issue will be whether the needle will penetrate the disc before engaging the S1 superior articular process.

I, The needle has been advanced and continues to project within the target triangle, albeit in the inferior aspect (arrow). *J,* The needle was further advanced and resistance was encountered. The needle tip rests against the S1 superior articular process (arrow). At this point, the bevel was directed inferiorly and the needle advanced. *K,* The needle has deflected off the S1 superior articular process, with a change of course (arrow). The needle entered the disc at this time.

(figure continues on following page)

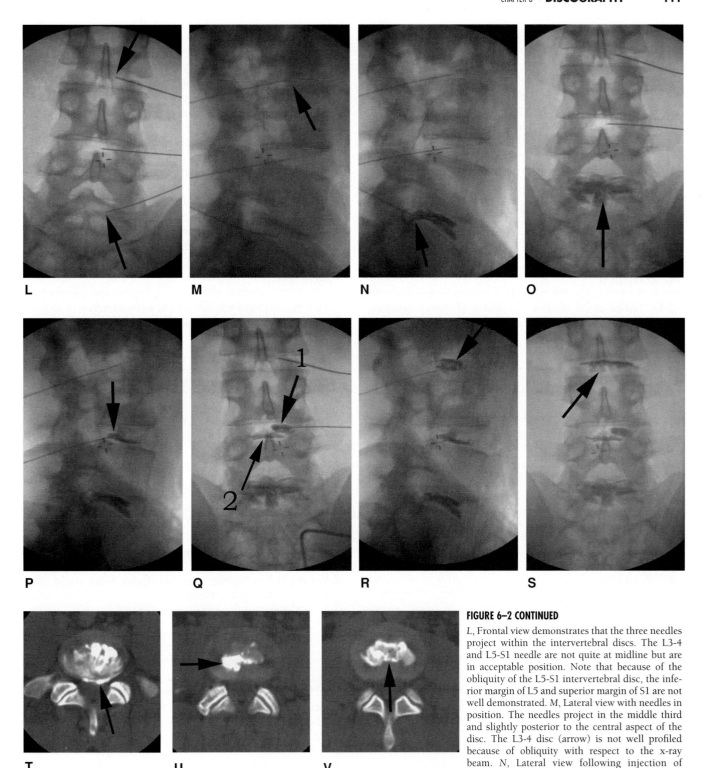

FIGURE 6–2 CONTINUED

L, Frontal view demonstrates that the three needles project within the intervertebral discs. The L3-4 and L5-S1 needle are not quite at midline but are in acceptable position. Note that because of the obliquity of the L5-S1 intervertebral disc, the inferior margin of L5 and superior margin of S1 are not well demonstrated. *M*, Lateral view with needles in position. The needles project in the middle third and slightly posterior to the central aspect of the disc. The L3-4 disc (arrow) is not well profiled because of obliquity with respect to the x-ray beam. *N*, Lateral view following injection of 2.6 mL of nonionic contrast material and antibiot-

ic agent into the L5-S1 intervertebral disc. Contrast flows through the posterior aspect of the disc through a full-thickness annular fissure and into the anterior vertebral canal (probably the epimembranous space). This injection produced concordant low back pain scored at 9 on a 10-point scale. *O*, Frontal view demonstrates contrast at the L5-S1 level (arrow). *P*, Lateral view following injection of 2.0 mL of contrast material at L4-5 demonstrates a linear collection paralleling the superior margin of L5 and a round collection more posteriorly (arrow). The appearance is consistent with an intranuclear injection. This injection caused no pain. *Q*, Frontal view shows a combination of inner annular (arrow 1) and intranuclear (arrow 2) injection at this level. The inner annular injection is not centered within the disc space, has sharply defined margins, and is relatively small. The intranuclear collection is more central, has relatively less well defined margins, and is relatively large. *R*, Lateral view following injection at L3-4 with 2.2 mL of the contrast/antibiotic mixture demonstrates a normal-appearing nucleogram (arrow). This injection produced no additional pain. *S*, Frontal view demonstrates a nucleogram at L3-4. *T*, Axial computed tomography (CT) study done at the level of the L5-S1 disc demonstrates extensive annular fissure formation with contrast leakage into the anterior vertebral canal (arrow), consistent with a full-thickness annular fissure and posterior annular degeneration. *U*, Axial CT study at the level of the L4-5 disc demonstrates a combination of inner annular (arrow) and nuclear contrast material, without annular fissure formation. *V*, Axial CT study at the level of the L3-4 disc demonstrates intranuclear contrast material (arrow) without annular fissure formation.

INTRODUCTION

Central low back pain. Evaluate for internal disc disruption.

The procedure and possible complications as well as alternatives to the procedure were discussed with the patient. Informed consent was obtained.

Oral ciprofloxacin 1000 mg was administered.

TECHNICAL INFORMATION

Using sterile technique and fluoroscopic guidance, and a right-sided extra-pedicular approach, the L3-4, L4-5, and L5-S1 intervertebral discs were punctured with 22-gauge 5-inch spinal needles.

INTERPRETATION

L5-S1: Injection of 2.5 mL of a 10:1 mixture of iohexol (Omnipaque) 240 mg/mL and cefazolin 100 mg/mL without any firm end point produced

gradually increasing concordant low back pain scored at 9 on a 10-point scale. Pain occurred relatively late in injection. A dose of 1.0 mL of 2.0% lidocaine was injected. Accompanying CT scan (see separate report) shows a full-thickness right posterior annular fissure and accompanying disc protrusion.

L4-5: Injection of 1.5 mL of the contrast-antibiotic mixture to a firm end point produced no pain.

L3-4: Injection of 1.8 mL of the contrast-antibiotic mixture to a firm end point produced no pain.

The patient tolerated the procedure well. His responses to injection are felt to be valid.

Meperidine (Demerol) 50 mg IM was given for pain relief.

CONCLUSION

1. L5-S1 concordant back pain scored at 9 on a 10-point scale.
2. L3-4 and L4-5 were not painful upon injection.

INTRODUCTION

Central low back pain. Evaluate for internal disc disruption.

TECHNICAL INFORMATION

The patient underwent discography. See separate report for details, including pain responses. Axial 3-mm slices at 3-mm intervals were obtained through the L3-4, L4-5, and L5-S1 intervertebral discs.

INTERPRETATION

L5-S1: There is an intranuclear injection. There is a full-thickness posterior

annular fissure formation and an accompanying 6-mm disc protrusion, with contact of the traversing left S1 nerve root sleeve.

L4-5: There is an intranuclear injection. No annular fissure or external disc contour abnormality is seen.

L3-4: There is an intranuclear injection. No annular fissure or external disc contour abnormality is seen.

CONCLUSION

1. L5-S1 full-thickness annular fissure formation with accompanying disc protrusion.
2. L3-4 and L4-5 demonstrate intranuclear injection without annular fissure formation or disc contour abnormality.
3. For pain responses at discography, see separate report.

One of the more frequently encountered problems when performing lumbar discography is how to access a low-lying or transitional L5-S1 (or S1-2) disc. Often, the iliac crest blocks the best route to the middle to posterior portion of the intervertebral disc at this level. Fortunately, the L5-S1 level is usually degenerated in those patients undergoing lumbar discography, and therefore injection in any portion of the disc will result in nuclear filling and a valid examination. In some instances, however, the disc may appear normal on MRI and the extrapedicular approach would result in an unacceptably peripheral location of the needle tip. In these cases, a transthecal injection may be performed (Figs. 6–3 and 6–4).

Computed tomography following discography may be helpful for three reasons. First, although almost all patients referred for discography will have had MRI performed, this imaging may have been done on a low-field, open unit with very poor signal-to-noise ratio. In such cases, the CT scan

may add additional information regarding disc protrusion, facet arthropathy (Fig. 6–5), and spinal stenosis. Second, in patients who are candidates for the IDET (intradiscal electrothermal annuloplasty) procedure (see Chapter 9), the CT scan will demonstrate the position of any full-thickness annular fissure, which will help plan the side of puncture and catheter positioning (Fig. 6–6). Third, there are times that the contrast material will appear to project at or near the central portion of the intervertebral disc on anterior-posterior and lateral projection radiographs, but the CT study shows that the injection is in the inner annulus rather than the nucleus (Figs. 6–7 and 6–8).

Patients occasionally come for evaluation by discography following fusion surgery. In general, there are two scenarios in which this occurs. First, note that some patients appear to benefit from combined anterior-posterior fusion, particularly those who have dramatic, positive responses to minimal injection volumes at low pressure (Derby 1999). When these

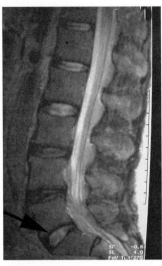

A

FIGURE 6–3

Transthecal Approach at L5-S1. This 42-year-old man had chronic central back pain. *A*, Sagittal T2-weighted magnetic resonance imaging scan demonstrates a very low-lying L5-S1 disc, which appears normally hydrated (compare with L3-4 and L4-5, both of which demonstrate moderate loss of disc height and hydration). *B*, Slightly oblique view centered at the L5-S1 intervertebral disc. Needles have already been placed in the L3-4 and L4-5 levels using a right-sided, extrapedicular approach. At L4-5, needle placement was challenging secondary to a very high-riding iliac crest. Fluoroscopy demonstrated no clear extrapedicular path to the L5-S1 intervertebral disc. In this view, a needle has been anchored in the skin, aimed at the lucency of the L5-S1 disc. The needle must pass inferior to the L5 laminae (marked on the contralateral side with an arrow). *C*, Lateral view following needle penetration of the disc. The needle tip (arrow) is in the central portion of the intervertebral disc. *D*, Frontal view following needle insertion at L5-S1. Note the markedly oblique course taken by the L5-S1 needle (arrow) to reach the angled disc. *E*, Oblique view taken to demonstrate extremely limited access to the L5-S1 intervertebral disc via the extrapedicular approach. The cross-hairs of the laser aiming device project over the S1 superior articular process, and an arrow marks the iliac crest. Only a tiny portion of the peripheral-most aspect of the disc could be accessed from the route. Even if the needle could be placed in this portion of the disc, given the normal-appearing hydration on magnetic resonance imaging examination (see part A), it would be unlikely that the nucleus could be filled. *F*, Lateral view following injection of contrast material at L5-S1. Injection of 2.2 mL of contrast material into the nucleus of the disc (arrow) resulted in concordant low back pain scored at 9 on a 10-point scale. *G*, Frontal view demonstrates centrally located contrast within the L5-S1 disc (arrow).

(figure continues on following page)

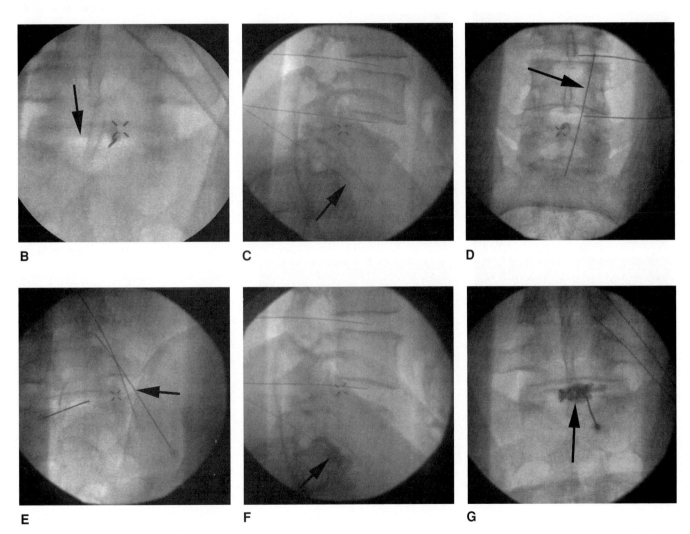

B   **C**   **D**

E   **F**   **G**

patients undergo only posterior fusion, they may return for discography (Fig. 6–9). Patients undergoing anterior fusion surgery, particularly with interbody fusion cages, may also come for evaluation. In these patients, the goal is to place the needle directly beside the cage (Fig. 6–10). If an injection at this location is accompanied by pain, particularly if there is contrast extravasation along the cage-vertebral interface, this is evidence of pseudarthrosis.

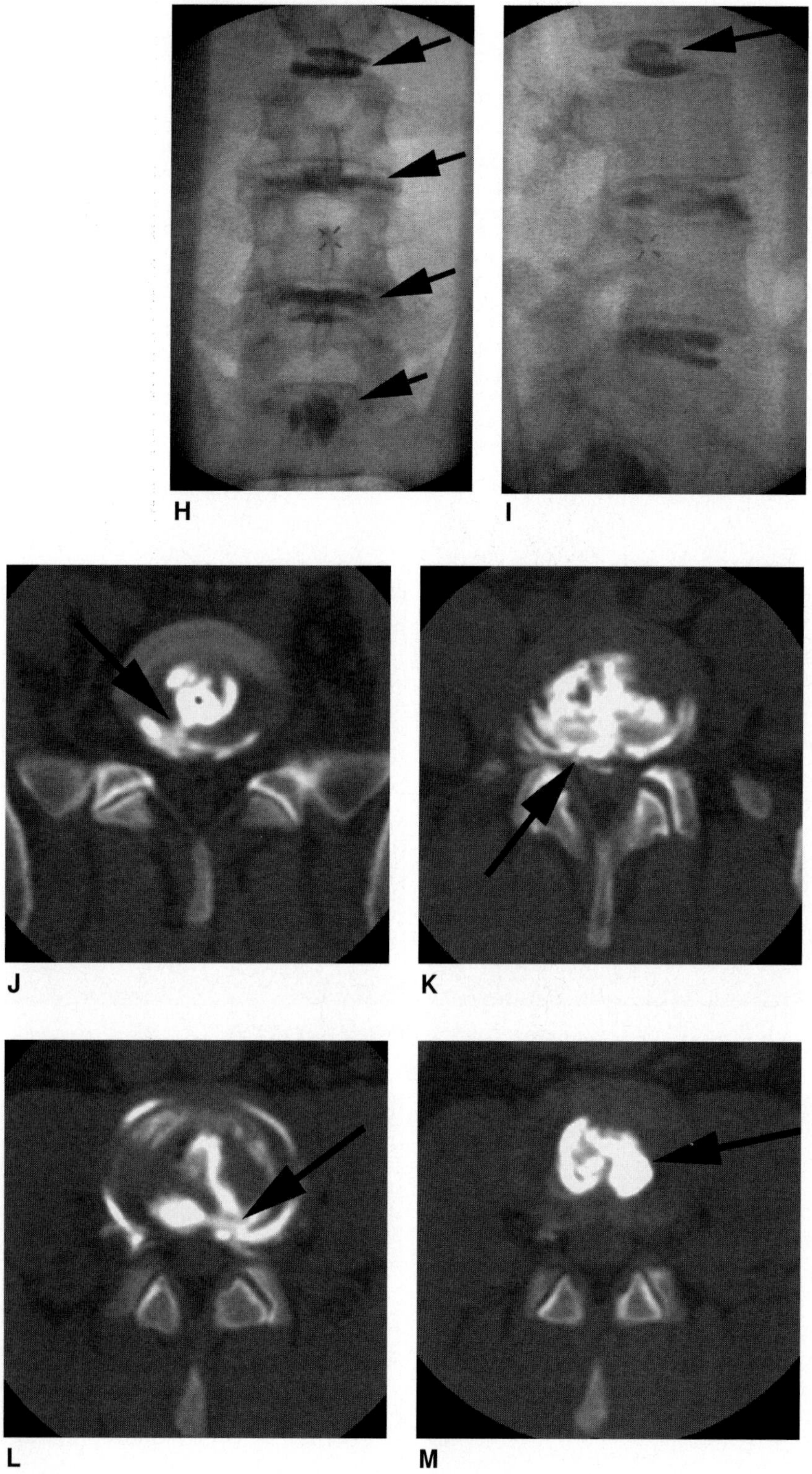

FIGURE 6–3 CONTINUED

H, Frontal view following injection at L4-5 (concordant pain score of 10), L3-4 (concordant pain score of 9), and L2-3 (painless injection). Injection at L2-3 was done because no control had been found after the bottom three discs were injected. Arrows mark contrast material within the intervertebral discs. *I*, Lateral view following four-level discography. The L5-S1 disc is at the inferior margin of the image. The L2-3 intervertebral disc has a normal "pac-man" configuration, with the other discs demonstrating annular degeneration. *J*, Axial computed tomographic (CT) scan at the L5-S1 level following discography. There is a full-thickness annular fissure leading to the right central aspect of the disc (arrow). *K*, Axial CT scan at the L4-5 level following discography. There is annular degeneration, and contrast reaches the dorsal disc margin and anterior vertebral canal (arrow). *L*, Axial CT scan at the L3-4 level following discography. There is annular degeneration with contrast spread throughout the annulus and along the peripheral disc margins, as well as through what appears to be a more discrete fissure in the left posterior aspect of the disc (arrow). *M*, Axial CT scan at the L2-3 level following discography. There is contrast within the nucleus (arrow) without annular fissure formation or contrast extravasation.

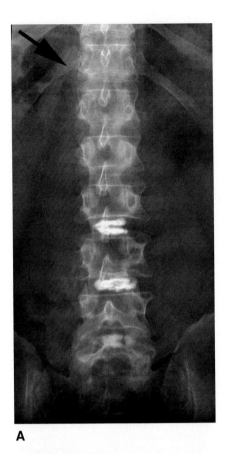

A

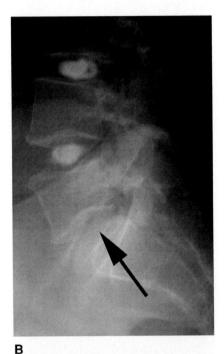

B

FIGURE 6-4

Transthecal Approach at S1-2. This 40-year-old man had low back pain. *A*, Frontal plain film following discography. This examination was performed following discography at L3-4, L4-5, and L5-S1 by rib count on fluoroscopy, and was done to document the six lumbar-type vertebral bodies and transitional anatomy. None of the three injections caused pain. Note contrast at the L3-4, L4-5, and L5-S1 levels using the lowest rib (arrow) as the T12 level. *B*, Lateral view demonstrating a well-developed S1-2 disc (arrow). At this time, the patient was returned to the C-arm fluoroscopy room for discography at S1-2. *C*, Oblique view at the S1-2 level, taken earlier (while the needles were still in place for the L3-4, L4-5, and L5-S1 discograms). The arrow marks the anterior margin of the S1 superior articular process, and the crosshairs of the laser aiming device are on the iliac crest. There is a very small target representing the peripheral-most aspect of the intervertebral disc visible. Because of the small target for needle placement, a transthecal approach was used to inject this disc (similar to Fig. 6–3). *D*, Lateral view with needle in the S1-2 disc (arrow). *E*, Anterior-posterior view demonstrates contrast at the L5-S1 level (arrow). This injection was also not painful. Note the extreme angulation of the needle necessary to reach the intervertebral disc.

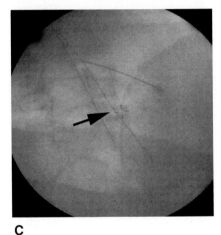

C

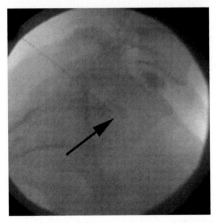

D

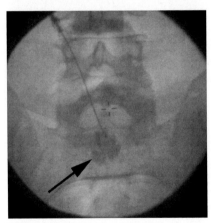

E

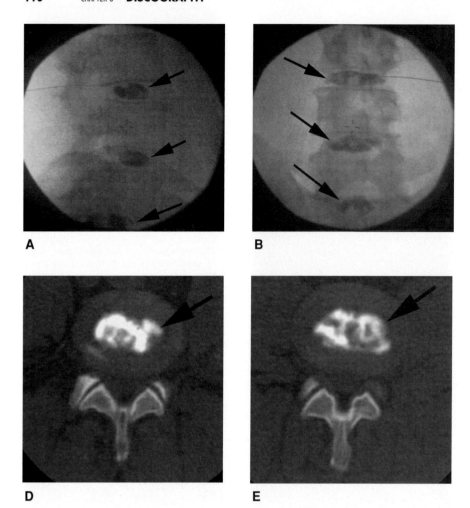

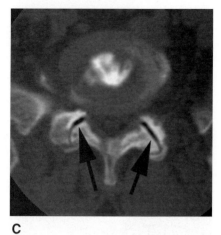

FIGURE 6–5

Computed Tomography-Discography Demonstrating Ancillary Pathology. This 48-year-old man had intermittent, chronic low back pain. *A,* Lateral view of lumbar spine following L3-4, L4-5, and L5-S1 discography (arrows). *B,* Frontal view of lumbar spine following L3-4, L4-5, and L5-S1 discography (arrows). None of these injections caused pain. *C,* Axial computed tomographic (CT) scan at L5-S1 following discography demonstrates bilateral facet arthropathy with vacuum phenomena and osteophytic spurring (arrows). There is intranuclear contrast material without full-thickness annular fissure formation or contrast extravasation. *D,* Axial CT scan at L4-5 demonstrates intranuclear contrast (arrow) without full-thickness annular fissure formation or contrast extravasation. Note the more normal appearance of the facet joints. *E,* Axial CT scan at the L3-4 level demonstrates intranuclear contrast (arrow), again without full-thickness annular fissure formation or contrast extravasation.

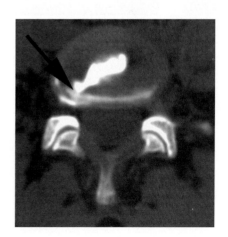

FIGURE 6–6

Computed Tomography-Discography Allowing Planning for IDET Procedure. This 29-year-old woman had low back pain. An axial computed tomographic (CT) scan was done at the L5-S1 level following discography. Injection at this level produced concordant pain scored at 10 on a 10-point scale. The CT scan demonstrates a full-thickness annular fissure tracking to the right neural foramen. Documentation of the location of the fissure is helpful for planning the route of entrance into the disc. In addition, given this image, the heating catheter should pass along the posterolateral, right corner of the disc.

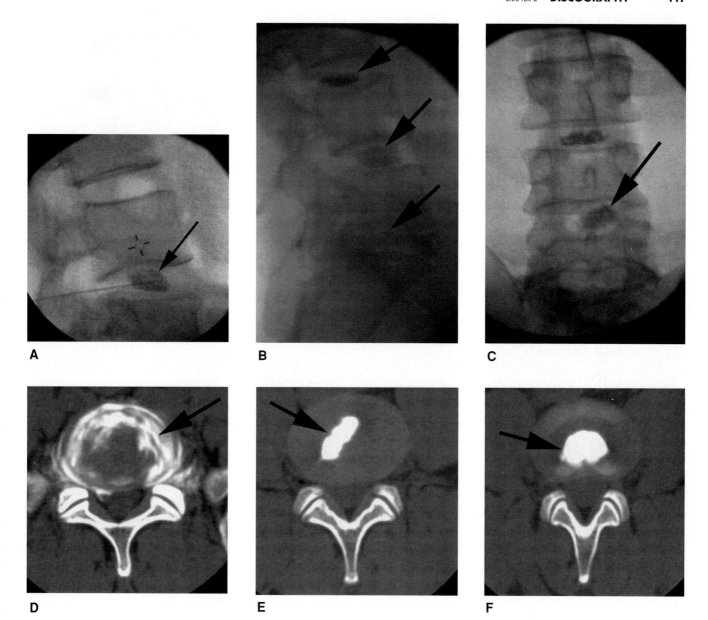

A

B

C

D

E

F

FIGURE 6–7

Computed Tomography-Discography Revealing Non-nuclear Location of Injection Despite Adequate Appearance at Fluoroscopy. This 48-year-old man had low back and bilateral leg pain. *A,* Lateral cone-down view taken during injection at the L4-5 level shows contrast flowing freely away from the needle tip in the central portion of the disc. *B,* Lateral study following L3-4, L4-5, and L5-S1 "discography" (arrows). There is annular degeneration at L5-S1. Contrast is more posteriorly located at L3-4 than at L4-5. *C,* Frontal view following "discography" at L3-4, L4-5, and L5-S1. The contrast material at L4-5 appears slightly to the left of midline but does cross midline and has somewhat "feathered" edges (arrow). *D,* Axial computed tomographic (CT) scan at L5-S1 following discography demonstrates annular degeneration (arrow). *E,* Axial CT scan at L4-5 following discography demonstrates contrast (arrow) in the inner annulus rather than in the nucleus. *F,* Axial CT scan at L3-4 following discography demonstrates an intranuclear injection with no annular fissure or external disc contour abnormality (arrow). The injection at L4-5 should be considered inadequate to evaluate the disc, because an intranuclear injection may demonstrate annular fissure formation not demonstrated by an inner annular injection. In addition, the pain response from inner annular injection is not necessarily representative of the pain response from an intranuclear injection.

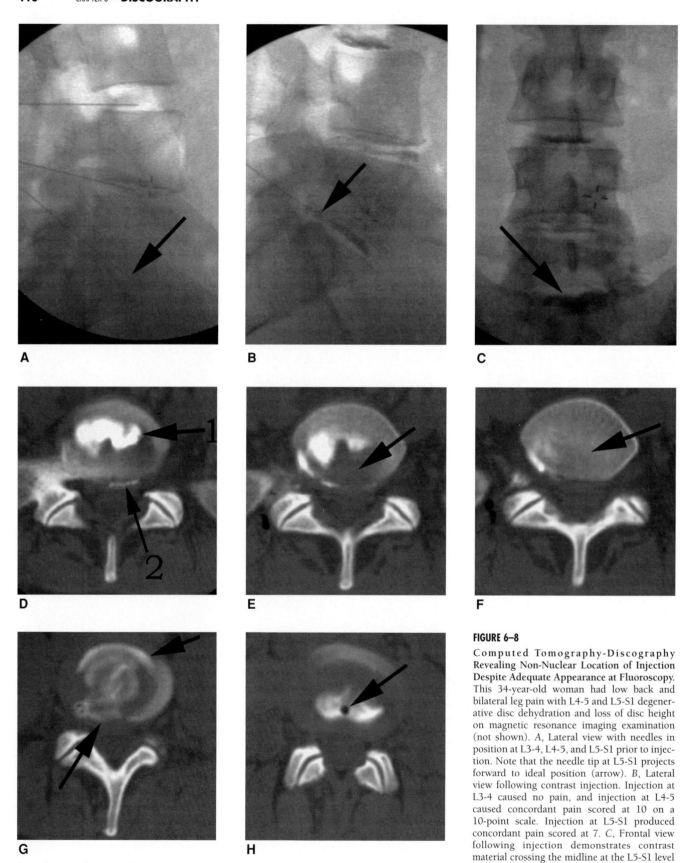

FIGURE 6–8

Computed Tomography-Discography Revealing Non-Nuclear Location of Injection Despite Adequate Appearance at Fluoroscopy. This 34-year-old woman had low back and bilateral leg pain with L4-5 and L5-S1 degenerative disc dehydration and loss of disc height on magnetic resonance imaging examination (not shown). *A,* Lateral view with needles in position at L3-4, L4-5, and L5-S1 prior to injection. Note that the needle tip at L5-S1 projects forward to ideal position (arrow). *B,* Lateral view following contrast injection. Injection at L3-4 caused no pain, and injection at L4-5 caused concordant pain scored at 10 on a 10-point scale. Injection at L5-S1 produced concordant pain scored at 7. *C,* Frontal view following injection demonstrates contrast material crossing the midline at the L5-S1 level (arrow). *D,* Axial computed tomographic (CT) scan following injection at L5-S1 shows contrast in the anterior aspect of the disc (arrow 1). A small amount of contrast also projects along the left central aspect of the posterior disc (arrow 2). *E,* Axial CT scan following injection at L5-S1, 3 mm superior to image D. Because of the obliquity of the L5-S1 disc, the entire disc is not on a single slice, even with maximal gantry tilt. This image, through the more posterior aspect of the intervertebral disc, fails to show contrast material in the expected position of the nucleus (arrow). The injection at this level was inner annular, rather than nuclear. *F,* Axial CT scan following injection at L5-S1 (next most superior cut). This image displays the inferior aspect of the L5 vertebral body (arrow) and proves that there was no contrast in the posterior margin of the L5-S1 intervertebral disc. *G,* Axial CT scan following L4-5 discography demonstrates annular degeneration, with contrast spreading to the periphery of the disc (arrows). *H,* Axial CT scan following L3-4 discography demonstrates intranuclear injection of contrast (and air) (arrow) without annular fissure formation.

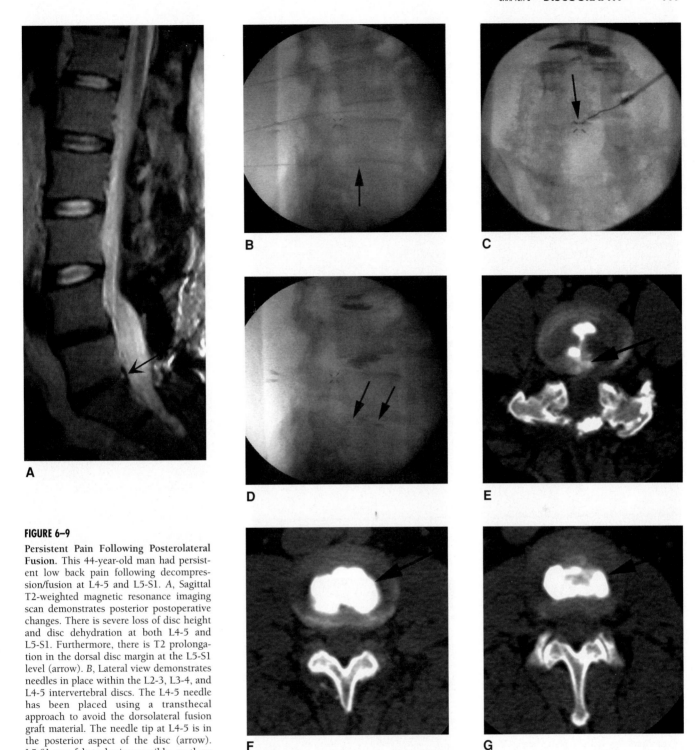

FIGURE 6–9

Persistent Pain Following Posterolateral Fusion. This 44-year-old man had persistent low back pain following decompression/fusion at L4-5 and L5-S1. *A*, Sagittal T2-weighted magnetic resonance imaging scan demonstrates posterior postoperative changes. There is severe loss of disc height and disc dehydration at both L4-5 and L5-S1. Furthermore, there is T2 prolongation in the dorsal disc margin at the L5-S1 level (arrow). *B*, Lateral view demonstrates needles in place within the L2-3, L3-4, and L4-5 intervertebral discs. The L4-5 needle has been placed using a transthecal approach to avoid the dorsolateral fusion graft material. The needle tip at L4-5 is in the posterior aspect of the disc (arrow). L5-S1 was felt to be inaccessible, as there was no dorsolateral or dorsal approach route. *C*, Frontal view following injection on nonionic contrast material and antibiotic mixture at L2-3 and L3-4 (both producing no pain). A small amount of contrast is seen at the L4-5 level (arrow). This injection was intensely painful, producing concordant pain scored at 10 on a 10-point scale. *D*, Lateral view following injection at L2-3, L3-4, and L4-5 demonstrates intranuclear injection without gross full-thickness annular fissure formation at L2-3 and L3-4. Contrast at the L5-S1 level spreads along the degenerated disc. *E*, Axial computed tomographic (CT) scan following discography at the L4-5 level demonstrates contrast within the nucleus as well as along the dorsal full-thickness annular fissure (arrow). *F*, Axial CT scan following discography at the L3-4 level demonstrates an intranuclear injection (arrow) without annular fissure or disc contour abnormality. *G*, Axial CT scan following discography at the L2-3 level also demonstrates an intranuclear injection (arrow) without annular fissure or disc contour abnormality.

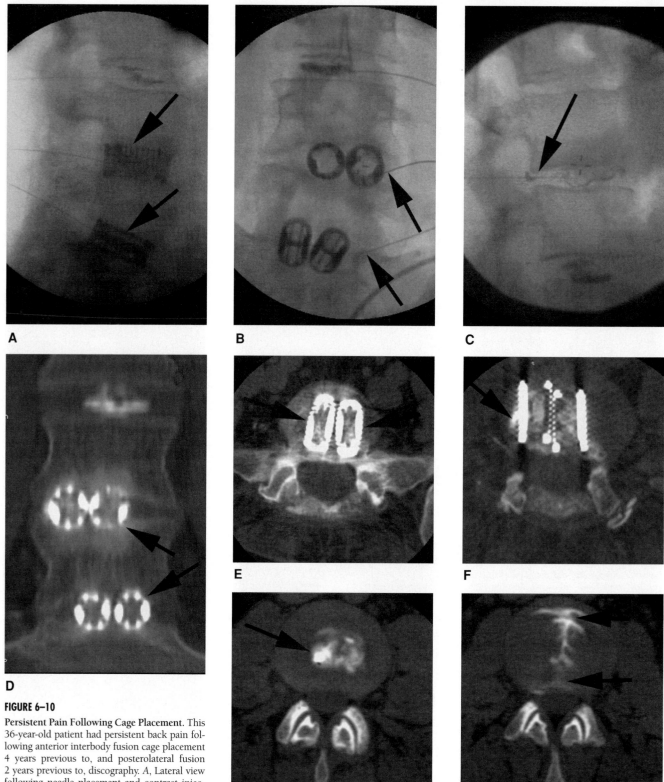

A **B** **C**

D

E **F**

G **H**

FIGURE 6–10

Persistent Pain Following Cage Placement. This 36-year-old patient had persistent back pain following anterior interbody fusion cage placement 4 years previous to, and posterolateral fusion 2 years previous to, discography. *A,* Lateral view following needle placement and contrast injection at L3-4, L4-5, and L5-S1. The interbody fusion cages at L4-5 and L5-S1 (arrows) obscure the needle tips. Contrast is seen at the L3-4 level.

B, Frontal view following needle placement and contrast injection. The needle tips (arrows) at L4-5 and L5-S1 are within the discs, although the L5-S1 needle tip is somewhat lateral to the cage. Injections at these three levels caused no pain. *C,* Lateral study with a needle placed at the L2-3 level. Upon injection at this level, the patient experienced concordant back pain scored at 9 on a 10-point scale, simultaneous with filling of a full-thickness annular fissure (arrow). *D,* Coronal reconstruction computed tomographic (CT) scan done following contrast injection. Thin cuts (1 mm slice thickness) are required to create the detail seen on this reconstruction view. No lucency at the cage/vertebral interface is seen at L4-5 or L5-S1 (arrows). *E,* Axial CT scan at the L5-S1 level following injection demonstrates no lucency at the cage/vertebral interface (arrows), nor is there contrast material along the cage margins. *F,* Axial CT scan at the L4-5 level following injection again demonstrates no lucency at the cage/vertebra junction. There is a small amount of contrast within the disc adjacent to the right cage (arrow), but this does not track along the cage/vertebra interface. The CT scan and discography results at L5-S1 and L4-5 are consistent with solid interbody fusion without pseudarthrosis or other cause of persistent or recurrent pain. *G,* Axial CT scan at the L3-4 level following discography demonstrates an intranuclear injection (arrow) without annular fissure formation. *H,* Axial CT scan at the L2-3 level following discography demonstrates both anterior and posterior annular fissure formation (arrows). On the basis of the discography evidence, the patient's persistent pain is likely coming from internal disc disruption at the L2-3 level rather than the fused L4-5 and L5-S1 levels.

Thoracic Discography

Thoracic discography (Fig. 6–11) resembles lumbar discography, with the added burden of difficult needle placement, particularly in the middle and upper thoracic spine (Schellhas 1994, Schellhas 1995). The usual needle route just anterior to the superior articular process may be blocked by the rib. A too-lateral approach risks lung puncture and attendant pneumothorax.

Cervical Discography

Table 6–4 describes and Figures 6–12 and 6–13 illustrate cervical discography.

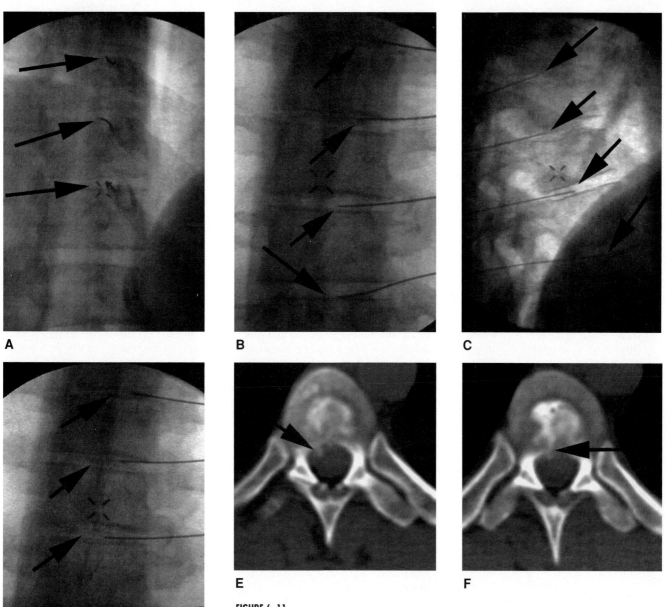

FIGURE 6–11

Thoracic Discography. This 35-year-old man presented with back pain and right-sided chest pain radiating into the anterior chest wall. *A,* Oblique view demonstrates needles (arrows) in place at the T7-8, T8-9, and T9-10 levels. Note the challenging access route for thoracic discography. *B,* Frontal view demonstrates needles (arrows) at T7-8 through T10-11. *C,* Lateral view demonstrates needles (arrows) at T7-8 through T10-11. The needles are at the middle to posterior aspects of the discs in all cases, in a good position for injection. *D,* Frontal view following injection at T7-8 (which did not produce any pain) and T8-9 and T9-10 (both of which produced concordant pain scored at 10 on a 10-point scale). Injection at T10-11 followed, which produced nonconcordant pain scored at 9. *E,* Axial computed tomographic (CT) scan at T7-8 following discography demonstrates nuclear contrast with contrast in the right side of the vertebral canal consistent with full-thickness annular fissure formation and disc protrusion (arrow). *F,* Axial CT scan at T8-9 following discography shows nuclear contrast with a full-thickness annular fissure (arrow) leading to a right central disc protrusion.

(figure continues on following page)

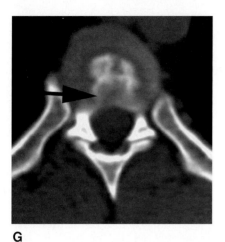

G

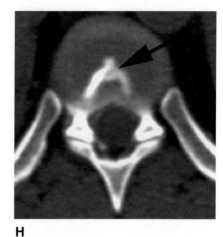

H

FIGURE 6–11 CONTINUED

G, Axial CT scan at T9-10 following discography shows nuclear contrast with posterior annular fissure formation (arrow). *H*, Axial CT scan at T10-11 following discography shows nuclear contrast material (arrow).

TABLE 6–4. Step-by-Step Description of Typical Cervical Discography

1. Position C-arm fluoroscope for a clear view of the target disc. A position that is slightly right anterior oblique is ideal. The C-arm fluoroscope should be angled in the craniocaudad direction until the superior and inferior vertebral bony margins along the disc are perfectly distinct.
2. Palpate the neck with the index and long fingers of the nondominant hand. With gentle pressure, it should be possible to feel the vertebral bodies. Use the long finger to move the carotid sheath laterally and the index finger to move the esophagus and trachea/larynx medially.
3. Insert the needle under direct visualization until it is anchored in the disc. Be sure not to pass the needle completely through the disc, as it is possible to traverse the entire disc and enter the cervical spinal cord.
4. Check position with C-arm fluoroscope in both frontal and lateral planes.
5. Adjust and advance the needle until it is within the central portion of the disc.
6. When needle placement is completed and checked for position in frontal and lateral planes, instruct the patient again in the purpose of the examination. Tell the patient to ignore all pain caused by needle placement and concentrate on any new pain with each injection.
7. Inject under lateral fluoroscopic visualization and ensure that the needle is intranuclear. Injection material should be 10:1 nonionic contrast (safe for intrathecal use) and antibiotic (Osti 1990). Query patient for pain responses. Record pain on a 0 (no pain at all) to 10 (severe pain) scale and as concordant or discordant. Record pressure at which pain is experienced, if desired. Record volume of contrast material. Record images in anterior-posterior and lateral projections. Note contrast pattern of injection.
8. Repeat for additional levels.
9. Perform 1 mm slice thickness computed tomographic cuts through cervical discs if desired.
10. Release patient when stable. Oral narcotic analgesics and/or muscle relaxants for a two- to three-day period may be prescribed. Provide patient with a telephone number to call if there is persistent or increased pain or numbness or if fever, swelling, or redness develops.

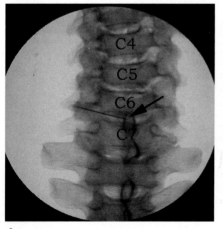

A

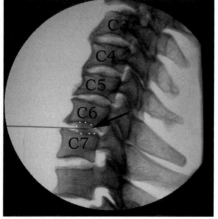

B

FIGURE 6–12

Skeletal Specimen Radiograph Demonstrating Target Position for Cervical Discography. *A*, Frontal view with a needle placed at the C6-7 level in the central portion of the disc from a right-sided approach. The needle is located in the middle third of the disc (arrow). *B*, Lateral view with the needle tip (arrow) appropriately located in the posterior third of the C6-7 intervertebral disc. The approximate position of the nucleus has been marked by white dots.

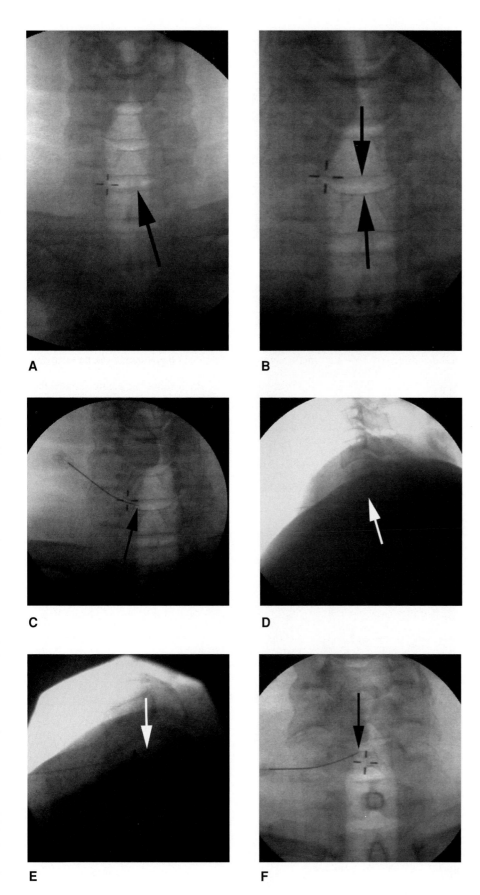

A

B

C

D

E

F

FIGURE 6–13

Step-by-Step Cervical Discography. This 53-year-old man had persistent cervical and upper middle back pain. *A,* Frontal view for orientation. The cross-hairs of the laser aiming device are positioned at the right margin of the C5-6 intervertebral disc (arrow). The C-arm has been rotated in a craniocaudal direction so that the vertebral body margins at this level are optimally visualized. *B,* Magnified view demonstrates crisp margins of the inferior C5 and superior C6 vertebrae (arrows). *C,* Frontal view following insertion of a 25-gauge needle. The needle tip is within the disc but is well lateral to ideal position (arrow). *D,* Lateral view with the needle in position at C5-6. As often happens, particularly in broad-shouldered and thick-necked men (this individual was both), the lower cervical levels are very difficult to adequately visualize on lateral examination. *E,* With magnification and coning to lessen scatter, the C5-6 intervertebral disc can be visualized on the lateral study. The needle tip (arrow) projects at the junction of the middle and posterior thirds of the intervertebral disc. *F,* Because of the initial placement to the right of midline, a return to frontal fluoroscopy was performed prior to injection to make sure that the needle was not located too far laterally within the disc. On the frontal view, the needle tip (arrow) is just to the right of midline, and while not ideal, this is probably acceptable at least for a trial injection.

(figure continues on following page)

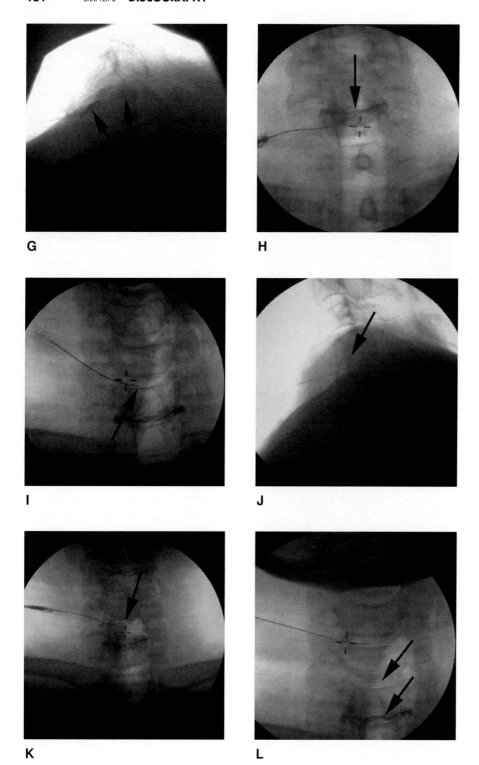

G

H

I

J

K

L

FIGURE 6–13 CONTINUED

G, Lateral view during injection of contrast material. Contrast flows both anteriorly and posteriorly along the intervertebral disc (arrows). *H*, Frontal view demonstrates contrast along the abnormal, degenerated C5-6 disc (arrow). Injection produced concordant lower neck and bilateral shoulder pain scored at 6 on a 10-point scale. *I*, Following examination of the C5-6 level, the study proceeded to the C4-5 level. The first 25-gauge needle has been removed, and a second needle has been placed at the C4-5 level (arrow). *J*, Lateral view again suffers from poor penetration because of the patient's large size. The needle tip is difficult to see but projects at the mid-disc level. Contrast collects at the level of the needle tip (arrow). *K*, Frontal view demonstrates contrast flow along the C4-5 disc (arrow). Injection at this level produced no pain. *L*, Frontal view demonstrates residual contrast at the C4-5 and C5-6 levels (arrows) and a needle at the C3-4 level. Injection at this level produced concordant low neck and upper back pain scored at 7 on a 10-point scale.

(figure continues on following page)

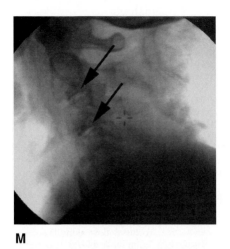

M

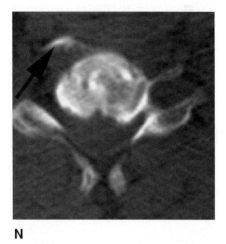

N

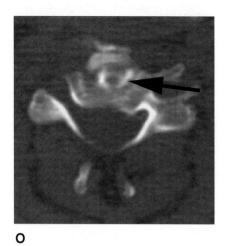

O

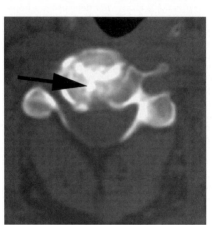

P

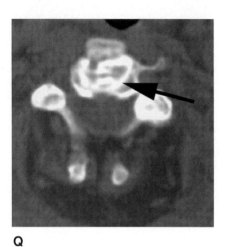

Q

FIGURE 6–13 CONTINUED

M, Lateral view after injection of C3-4 and C2-3 (arrows). Injection at this level produced concordant midback and upper cervical spine pain scored at 7. *N,* Axial computed tomographic (CT) scan at C5-6 done following injection demonstrates contrast within the disc as well as anterior to the disc (arrow). *O,* Axial CT scan at C4-5 done following injection demonstrates contrast within the central portion of the disc without annular fissure formation. *P,* Axial CT scan at C3-4 done following injection demonstrates contrast in the central and anterior portion of the disc (arrow). *Q,* Axial CT scan at C2-3 done following injection of contrast material demonstrates a degenerated annulus (arrow).

References

Aprill C, Bogduk N. High-intensity zone: a diagnostic sign of painful lumbar disc on magnetic resonance imaging. Br J Radiol 1992; 65:361–369.

Bogduk N. Clinical Anatomy of the Lumbar Spine, 3rd ed. New York, Churchill Livingstone, 1997.

Bogduk N. An analysis of the Carragee data on false-positive discography. Int Spinal Injection Soc Sci Newslett 2001; 4:3–10.

Bogduk N. Practice guidelines and protocols: sacroiliac joint blocks. In International Spinal Injection Society Syllabus for the 9th Annual Scientific Meeting, Orlando, Florida, February, 2002. San Francisco, ISIS, 2002.

Brightbill TC, Pile N, Eichelberger RP, Whitman M. Normal magnetic resonance imaging and abnormal discography in lumbar disc disruption. Spine 1994; 19:1075–1077.

Brodsky AE, Binder WF. Lumbar discography: its value in diagnosis and treatment of lumbar disc lesions. Spine 1979; 4:110–120.

Carragee EJ, Alamin TF. Discography: a review. Spine J 2001; 1:364–372.

Carragee EJ, Alamin TF, Miller J, Grafe M. Provocative discography in volunteer subjects with mild persistent low back pain. Spine J 2002; 2:25–34.

Carragee EJ, Chen Y, Tanner CM, Hayward C, Rossi M, Hagle C. Can discography cause long-term symptoms in previously asymptomatic subjects? Spine 2000a; 25:1803–1808.

Carragee EJ, Chen Y, Tanner CM, Truong T, Lau E, Brito JL. Provocative discography in patients after limited lumbar discectomy: a controlled, randomized study of pain response in symptomatic and asymptomatic subjects. Spine 2000b; 25:3065–3071.

Carragee EJ, Paragioudakis SJ, Khurana S. Lumbar high-intensity zone and discography in subjects without low back problems. Spine 2000c; 25:2987–2992.

Carragee EJ, Tanner CM, Khurana S, Hayward C, Welsh J, Date E, Truong T, Rossi M, Hagle C. The rates of false-positive lumbar discography in select patients without low back symptoms. Spine 2000d; 25:1373–1381.

Carragee EJ, Tanner CM, Yang B, Brito JL, Truong T. False-positive findings on lumbar discography: reliability of subjective concordance assessment during provocative disc injection. Spine 1999; 24:2542–2547.

Colhoun E, McCall IW, Williams L, Pullicino VNC. Provocative discography as a guide to planning operations of the spine. J Bone Joint Surg Br 1988; 70:267–271.

Crock HV. Internal disc disruption: a challenge to disc prolapse fifty years on. Spine 1986; 11:650–653.

Derby R, Howard HW, Grant JM, Lettice JJ, Peteghem PKV, Ryan DP. The ability of pressure-controlled discography to predict surgical and nonsurgical outcomes. Spine 1999; 24:364–372.

Feffer HL. Treatment of low-back and sciatic pain by the injection of hydrocortisone into degenerated intervertebral discs. J Bone Joint Surg Am 1956; 38:585–592.

Feffer HL. Therapeutic intradiscal steroids: a long-term study. Clin Orthop Rel Res 1969; 67:100–104.

Fernstrom U. A discographical study of ruptured lumbar intervertebral discs. Acta Chir Scand 1960; 258(Suppl):1–60.

Gibson MJ, Buckley J, Mawhinney R, Mulholland RC, Worthington BS. Magnetic resonance imaging and discography in the diagnosis of disc degeneration. J Bone Joint Surg Br 1986; 68:369–373.

Graham CE. Chemonucleolysis: a double-blind study comparing chemonucleolysis with intra-discal hydrocortisone. Clin Orthop 1976; 117:179–192.

Grubb SA, Kelly CK. Cervical discography: clinical implications from 12 years of experience. Spine 2000; 25:1382–1389.

Hirsch C. An attempt to diagnose the level of a disc lesion clinically by disc puncture. Acta Orthop Scand 1948; 18:132–140.

Holt EP. The question of discography. J Bone Joint Surg Am 1968; 50:720–726.

Horton WC, Daftari TK. Which disc as visualized by magnetic resonance imaging is actually a source of pain? A correlation between magnetic resonance imaging and discography. Spine 1992; 17:S164–S171.

Huang TS, Zucherman JF, Hsu KY, Shapiro M, Lentz D, Gartland J. Gadopentetate dimeglumine as an intradiscal contrast agent. Spine 2002; 27:839–843.

Ito M, Incorvaia KM, Yu SF, Fredrickson BE, Yuan HA, Rosenbaum AE. Predictive signs of discogenic lumbar pain on magnetic resonance imaging with discography correlation. Spine 1998; 23:1252–1260.

Jackson RP. Lumbar discography. Semin Spine Surg 1997; 9:51–56.

Kornberg M. Discography and magnetic resonance imaging in the diagnosis of lumbar disc disruption. Spine 1989; 14:1368–1372.

Leao L. Intradiscal injection of hydrocortisone and prednisolone in the treatment of low back pain. Rheumatism 1960; 16:72–77.

Lindblom K. Diagnostic puncture of intervertebral disks in sciatica. Acta Orthop Scand 1948; 17:231–239.

Madan S, Gundanna M, Harley JM, Boeree NR, Sampson M. Does provocative discography screening of discogenic back pain improve surgical outcome? J Spine Disord Treatment 2002; 15:245–251.

Milette PC, Fontaine S, Lepanto L, Cardinal E, Breton G. Differentiating lumbar disc protrusions, disc bulges, and discs with normal contour but abnormal signal intensity; magnetic resonance imaging with discographic correlations. Spine 1999; 24:44–53.

Osti OL, Fraser RD. MRI and discography of annular tears and intervertebral disc degeneration: a prospective clinical comparison. J Bone Joint Surg Br 1992; 74:431–435.

Osti OL, Fraser RD, Vernon-Roberts B. Discitis after discography: the role of prophylactic antibiotics. J Bone Joint Surg Br 1990; 72:271–274.

Rankine JJ, Gill KP, Hutchinson CE, Ross ERS, Williamson JB. The clinical significance of the high-intensity zone on lumbar spine magnetic resonance imaging. Spine 1999; 24:1913–1920.

Raskin NH. Lumbar puncture headache: a review. Headache 1990; 30:197–200.

Rhyne AL, Smith SE, Wood KE, Darden BV. Outcome of unoperated discogram-positive low back pain. Spine 1995; 20:1997–2001.

Ricketson R, Simmons JW, Hauser BO. The prolapsed intervertebral disc: the high-intensity zone with discography correlation. Spine 1996; 21:2758–2762.

Saifuddin A, Braithwaite I, White J, Taylor BA, Renton P. The value of lumbar spine magnetic resonance imaging in the demonstration of anular tears. Spine 1998; 23:453–457.

Schellhas KP. Diskography. Spine State Art Rev 1995; 9:27–44.

Schellhas KP, Garvey TA, Johnson BA, Rothbart JP, Pollei SR. Cervical diskography: analysis of provoked responses at C2-3, C3-4, and C4-5. Am J Neuroradiol 2000; 21:269–275.

Schellhas KP, Pollei SR, Dorwart RH. Thoracic discography: a safe and reliable technique. Spine 1994; 19:2103–2109.

Schellhas KP, Pollei SR, Gundry CR, Heithoff KB. Lumbar disc high-intensity zone: correlation with magnetic resonance imaging and discography. Spine 1996a; 21:79–86.

Schellhas KP, Smith MD, Gundry CR, Pollei SR. Cervical discogenic pain. Prospective correlation of magnetic resonance imaging and discography in asymptomatic patients and pain sufferers. Spine 1996b; 21:300–312.

Schneiderman G, Flannigan B, Kingston S, Thomas J, Dillin WH, Watkins RG. Magnetic resonance imaging in the diagnosis of disc degeneration: correlation with discography. Spine 1987; 12:276–281.

Simmons JW, Aprill CN, Dwyer AP, et al. A reassessment of Holt's data on "The question of lumbar discography." Clin Orthop 1988; 237:120–124.

Simmons JW, McMillin JN, Emery SF, Kimmich SJ. Intradiscal steroids: a prospective double-blind clinical trial. Spine 1992; 17:S172–S175.

Smith BMT, Hurwitz EL, Solsberg D, Rubinstein D, Corenman DS, Dwyer AP, Kleiner J. Interobserver reliability of detecting lumbar intervertebral disc high-intensity zone on magnetic resonance and association of high-intensity zone with pain and anular disruption. Spine 1998; 23:2074–2080.

Walsh TR, Weinstein JN, Spratt KF, Lehmann TR, Aprill C, Sayre H. Lumbar discography in normal subjects: a controlled, prospective study. J Bone Joint Surg Am 1990; 72:1081–1088.

Weinstein J, Claverie W, Gibson S. The pain of discography. Spine 1988; 13:1344–1348.

Weishaupt D, Zanetti M, Hodler J, Min K, Fuchs B, Pfirrmann CWA, Boos N. Painful lumbar disk derangement: relevance of endplate abnormalities at MR imaging. Radiology 2001; 218:420–427.

Wilkinson HA, Schuman N. Intradiscal corticosteroids in the treatment of lumbar and cervical disc problems. Spine 1980; 5:385–389.

Zucherman J, Derby R, Hsu K, Picetti G, Kaiser J, Schofferman J, Goldthwaite N, White A. Normal magnetic resonance imaging with abnormal discography. Spine 1988; 13:1355–1359.

7

Percutaneous Needle Biopsy

DONALD L. RENFREW

Definition

Percutaneous needle biopsy is tissue sampling of the bony (usually vertebral body) or soft tissue (usually intervertebral disc) components of the spine by imaging-guided small-bore needles.

Literature Review

In 1952, Mazet and Cozen (Mazet 1952) described a technique for needle biopsy of lumbar and cervical vertebral bodies using a localizing Kirschner wire with plain film radiographic localization. They described a similar technique for the thoracic spine, with surgical resection of the associated rib to allow access to the vertebral body. Of 36 total cases, a positive diagnosis was made in 17, malignancy was excluded in 9, and the material obtained was indeterminate in 10. In 1953, Ray (Ray 1953) described an additional 48 biopsies using trigonometric calculation of the needle path based on plain film evaluation and relying on radiographic documentation of appropriate needle position prior to obtaining the biopsy. In 1954, Frankel (Frankel 1954) reported on an additional 34 biopsies done under radiographic control with the patients anesthetized. In 1956, Craig (Craig 1956) stated that "morbidity due to open biopsy is rarely justified," briefly reviewed two severe complications of open biopsy, and described a new design of needle along with five case reports. In 1965, however, Nagel and colleagues (Nagel 1965) argued that localization "is more accurate with open biopsy and because more material can be obtained for culture and histological study than

TABLE 7–1. Equipment and Supplies for Percutaneous Needle Biopsy

C-arm fluoroscope or computed tomography scanner
Surgical scrub solution
Needles (for anesthetic and biopsy)
Syringes
Connecting tube
Nonionic contrast material
Anesthetic agent
Specimen containers

is possible with needle biopsy, we feel open biopsy is the method of choice in spinal lesions."

Adapon and colleagues (Adapon 1981) described 22 patients undergoing computed tomography (CT)–directed closed biopsy of the spine. Eighteen of the 22 specimens yielded a histologic diagnosis. Stoker and Kissen (Stoker 1985) used radiographic guidance to perform 135 vertebral biopsies, with an overall accuracy of 88.9%. My colleagues and I (Renfrew 1991) described transpedicular biopsy as a modification of the CT-directed technique in 1991. No specific information regarding the diagnostic utility of vertebral biopsies is available, but for musculoskeletal tumors in general, biopsy of infections and metastatic disease has a high diagnostic utility, whereas biopsies of primary tumors, while technically accurate, have lower diagnostic utility because these biopsies tend to be repeated prior to definitive treatment (Fraser-Hill 1992a). Cost-effectiveness for most musculoskeletal lesions (and particularly for infections and metastatic deposits) is high (Fraser-Hill 1992b).

Rationale for Procedure

Unlike the other procedures described in this book, percutaneous biopsy of the spine does not necessarily involve the diagnosis and treatment of spine pain (although frequently spine pain is what brings the patient to the physician's attention when there is a suspected spine tumor or infection). The rationale for the procedure in this case is to obtain tissue in a cost-effective fashion to allow a specific diagnosis and appropriate treatment.

Equipment and Supplies[1]

Table 7–1 lists equipment required for percutaneous needle biopsy.

A standard fluoroscope can be used for percutaneous biopsies, but it is generally much more difficult to obtain ideal positioning than with a C-arm device. A laser aiming device (an attachment that shows a cross-hair on the

---

[1]This section is virtually identical to the Equipment and Supplies section in Chapter 2 and can be skipped if the reader is already familiar with this material.

fluoroscopic screen corresponding in position to a red dot on the skin surface) is extremely helpful for proper needle placement. Selection of needle type varies with the operator. For biopsy of soft tissues with no intervening soft tissues, cutting needles such as those used for liver or other organ biopsies are appropriate. For biopsy through intact bone, a cutting instrument is necessary. Prior to performance of biopsies, it is wise to check with the pathology laboratory responsible for analyzing the specimen to ensure appropriate specimen handling. CT-directed biopsies obviously require a CT scanner for guidance.

In addition to the equipment listed in Table 7–1, a crash cart should be readily available to handle medical emergencies (e.g., contrast media and drug reactions).

Informed Consent Issues

For percutaneous needle biopsy, the issues can be divided into a description of the procedure (and possible alternatives) and delineation of material risks. Patients should know what to expect when undergoing biopsy but should also know that in most cases the discomfort of having the biopsy done is minimal if adequate systemic analgesia and sedation and local anesthesia is provided. Drug side-effects are those of the analgesics, sedatives, and local anesthetics used.

Material risks vary with the location of the biopsy. Generally, the biopsy should be planned to put major vascular structures (including the aorta and vena cava) at minimal risk, to avoid lung puncture, and to avoid the spinal cord and spinal nerves. Radiographic guidance and thoughtful planning should accomplish these goals, but the risk of misadventure always looms when one is using the relatively larger instruments necessary for most biopsies, and patients need to be warned of (1) extensive arterial bleeding, possibly requiring hospital admission, transfusion, and even emergency surgery; (2) pneumothorax in thoracic, high lumbar, or low cervical spine biopsies; (3) infection of the wound, possibly requiring hospitalization, prolonged intravenous antibiotics, and surgery for incision and drainage of abscesses.

Patient Selection

Patients undergoing vertebral biopsy are suspected of having either infection or tumor. Suspicion of infection and tumor is generally based on magnetic resonance imaging findings. Often, biopsy is performed to confirm metastatic disease.

Infections of the spine can be dramatic or subtle. Some patients present with an obvious clinical picture, with, for example, an immunocompromised condition, elevated white blood cell count, fever, and a swollen intervertebral disc with extensive associated marrow changes. Other patients may present in a far more subtle manner, and it is good to keep in mind that half of patients with infectious spondylitis have normal white blood cell counts and no fever. If a patient is not immunocompromised, however, the erythrocyte sedimentation rate and C-reactive protein level are always elevated in cases of infectious spondylitis (Carragee 1997, Hitchon 1992, Sharif 1992).

Most vertebral tumors examined by imaging-directed biopsy are in patients with a known primary tumor and suspected metastatic deposit. Since these patients nearly always have bone scans done or will need one anyway, perusal of the bone scan may reveal a more readily (and more safely) accessed lesion. Chest, abdomen, and pelvis CT may reveal the location of not only metastatic disease but not infrequently the primary tumor as well (if one is not already known) (Heller 1997, Rougraff 1993).

Procedure Description

This section describes two fluoroscopically directed lumbar biopsy techniques (one for suspected discitis and the other for vertebral body abnormality), and one CT technique.

Table 7–2 describes and Figure 7–1 illustrates the lumbar disc aspiration and biopsy procedure. Magnetic resonance imaging findings may be dramatic (see Fig. 7–1), but more subtle findings may also accompany infectious spondylitis (Fig. 7–2), and these findings overlap those of "mechanical" discitis (Fig. 7–3).

TABLE 7–2. Step-by-Step Description of Lumbar Disc Aspiration and Biopsy

1. Obtain sedation and analgesia with drugs of choice.
2. Position the C-arm fluoroscope so that a clear view of the target disc is obtained. Position will be as for lumbar discography (see Chapter 6). An oblique position with the superior articular process projecting approximately halfway between the anterior and the posterior visualized disc margins is ideal. The target point lies just anterior to the superior articular process, along the lower aspect of the disc. The C-arm should be angled until the superior and inferior vertebral bony margins along the disc are perfectly distinct. For the lower lumbar spine, caudal angulation is usually necessary; in the midlumbar spine neutral angulation and in the upper lumbar spine cranial angulation are often required.
3. Insert a 3.5-inch 25-gauge spinal needle along the course of the x-ray beam far enough so that it is anchored.
4. Check position with the C-arm fluoroscope.
5. Adjust and advance until the needle hub is at the skin surface or the needle tip is at the edge of the intervertebral disc, whichever comes first. Inject local anesthetic through the needle while withdrawing it.
6. Place an 18-gauge trocar along the course of the anesthetic needle until the tip is at the disc margin.
7. Coaxially place a 22-gauge spinal needle through the trocar into the disc and aspirate. If pus is removed, send for culture and sensitivity. Inject 1.0 to 3.0 mL of a contrast material/antibiotic mixture and document needle position.
8. If no pus is aspirated from the 22-gauge spinal needle, remove this needle and place a spring-loaded cutting needle through the trocar to the edge of the disc. Obtain three to six samples of the intervertebral disc and send for culture and sensitivity testing.
9. When done with all biopsies, inject 1.0 to 3.0 mL of a contrast material/antibiotic mixture and document needle position.
10. Release patient when stable. Provide patient with a telephone number to call if there is persistent or increased pain or numbness or if fever, swelling, or redness develops.

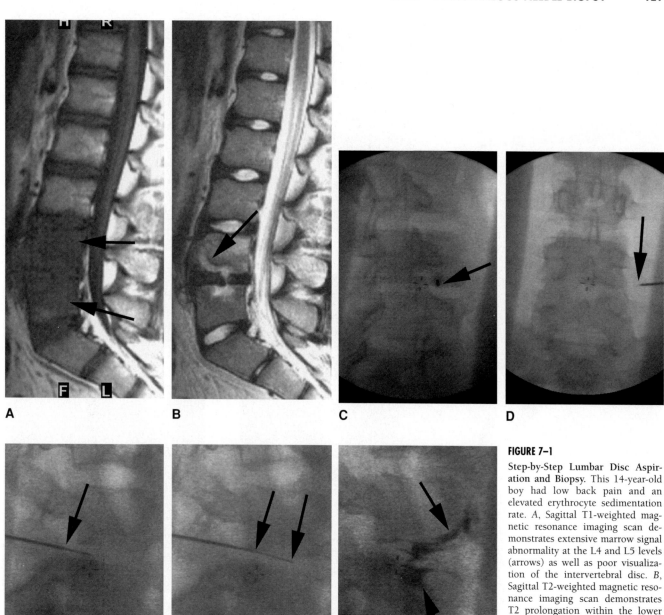

FIGURE 7–1

Step-by-Step Lumbar Disc Aspiration and Biopsy. This 14-year-old boy had low back pain and an elevated erythrocyte sedimentation rate. *A,* Sagittal T1-weighted magnetic resonance imaging scan demonstrates extensive marrow signal abnormality at the L4 and L5 levels (arrows) as well as poor visualization of the intervertebral disc. *B,* Sagittal T2-weighted magnetic resonance imaging scan demonstrates T2 prolongation within the lower half of the L4 and upper half of the L5 vertebral body (arrow). Note the abnormal appearance of the L4-5 intervertebral disc. *C,* Oblique view. Anesthetic has already been infiltrated with a 25-gauge needle. An 18-gauge trocar (arrow) is in place, on course for the L4-5 intervertebral disc. *D,* Anterior-posterior view demonstrates that the trocar is still 1 to 2 cm from the L4-5 disc margin (arrow). The trocar was advanced so that it was directly adjacent to the disc margin. No pus could be aspirated through a coaxially placed 22-gauge spinal needle. *E,* Lateral view. A 22-gauge spring-activated cutting needle has been placed coaxially through the trocar and has engaged the disc edge. The end of the trocar is seen (arrow), with the cutting needle passing through the trocar and into the disc. *F,* The spring-activated cutting needle has been deployed. The length marked by the arrows represents the sample obtained by the device. Five passes were made with this needle. *G,* Lateral view obtained following injection of a contrast material/antibiotic mixture demonstrates flow of contrast through defects in the vertebral endplates and into the inferior L4 and superior L5 vertebral bodies (arrows). *Staphylococcus aureus* was cultured from the aspirate, and the patient was treated with appropriate antibiotics with full recovery. (Parts A and B from Renfrew DL. Atlas of Spine Imaging. Philadelphia, Elsevier Science, 2003.)

Table 7–3 describes and Figure 7–4 illustrates fluoroscopically directed lumbar vertebral body biopsy. Such biopsies may be helpful not only in determining the origin of malignant lesions but also in confirming the diagnosis in cases of benign abnormalities (Fig. 7–5). Occasionally, even very aggressive-appearing processes may yield benign results (Fig. 7–6).

Table 7–4 describes and Figures 7–7 and 7–8 illustrate CT-directed vertebral body biopsy.

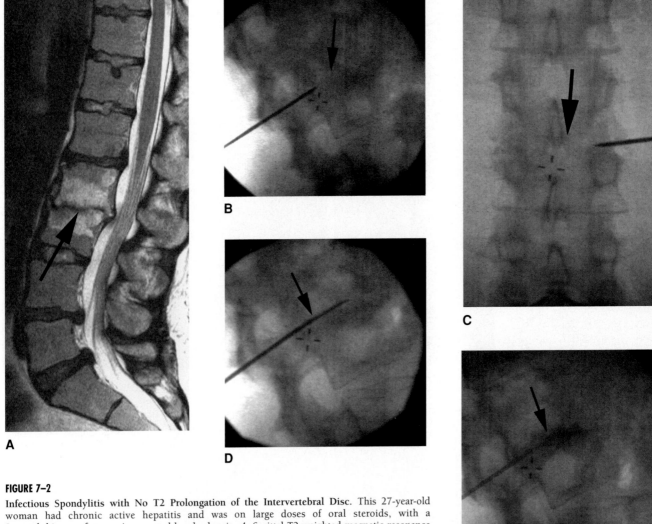

FIGURE 7–2

Infectious Spondylitis with No T2 Prolongation of the Intervertebral Disc. This 27-year-old woman had chronic active hepatitis and was on large doses of oral steroids, with a 2-month history of worsening, central low back pain. *A*, Sagittal T2-weighted magnetic resonance imaging scan demonstrates extensive T2 prolongation of the marrow adjacent to the L2-3 intervertebral disc. However, the disc itself is collapsed with no T2 prolongation (arrow). *B*, Lateral view demonstrates the trocar needle at the margin of the L2-3 intervertebral disc (arrow). Note that collapse of the disc and subchondral erosion makes it difficult to visualize the disc space. *C*, Frontal view demonstrates the trocar at the lateral margin of the L2-3 disc (arrow). Again, the disc itself is difficult to see because of erosion of the vertebral body margins. Aspiration with a coaxial 22-gauge spinal needle provided no pus. *D*, Lateral view following deployment of spring-loaded biopsy needle demonstrates the junction of the trocar and biopsy needle (arrow). Four passes were made, yielding tissue for culture and sensitivity. *E*, Lateral view after injection of a contrast material/antibiotic mixture. Note the disorganized appearance of the intervertebral disc with interdigitation of the contrast material in erosions along the vertebral body margins (arrow). The culture grew gram-positive cocci. The patient was treated with antibiotics, with an uneventful recovery. (Parts A and D from Renfrew DL. Atlas of Spine Imaging. Philadelphia, Elsevier Science, 2003.)

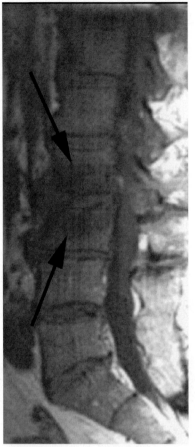

A

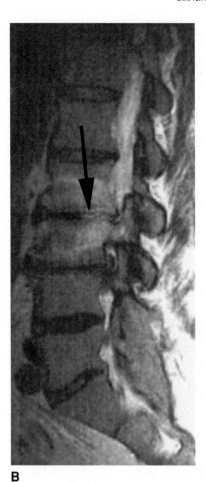

B

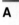

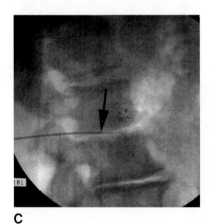

C

FIGURE 7–3

"Mechanical" Discitis with T2 Prolongation of the Disc but No Infection on Biopsy. This 78-year-old man had undergone posterior spine fusion from L4 through S1 many years ago. Three months prior to this biopsy, he underwent transurethral resection of the prostate. Starting a week after the procedure, he has had persistent severe low back pain even at rest. A, Sagittal T1-weighted magnetic resonance imaging scan demonstrates T1 prolongation in the inferior L2 and superior L3 vertebral body (arrows). B, Sagittal T2-weighted magnetic resonance imaging scan demonstrates T2 prolongation of the L2-3 intervertebral disc (arrow). C. Lateral view with spring-loaded biopsy needle in the L2-3 disc. Aspiration through a 22-gauge spinal needle produced no pus. Biopsy revealed no evidence of infectious or inflammatory cells, and cultures were negative. The patient's back pain slowly diminished over the next several months, and approximately 1 year later he was doing well with no evidence of ongoing infection and no constitutional symptoms. (Parts A, B, and C from Renfrew DL. Atlas of Spine Imaging. Philadelphia, Elsevier Science, 2003.)

TABLE 7–3. Step-by-Step Description of Fluoroscopically Directed Lumbar Vertebral Body Biopsy

1. Obtain sedation and analgesia with drugs of choice.
2. Position the C-arm fluoroscope so that a clear view of the target is obtained. If the lesion involves the pedicle or the posterolateral vertebral body immediately anterior to the pedicle, use the pedicle as the target and perform transpedicular biopsy. If the lesion is located more anteriorly in the vertebral body, target the lesion directly. Note that if targeting the lesion directly and if cross-sectional images show that a clear, safe access route is necessary, it is probably better to perform the biopsy under computed tomography guidance.
3. Insert a 25-gauge spinal needle along the course of the x-ray beam far enough so that it is anchored.
4. Check position with fluoroscopy.
5. Adjust and advance until the needle is at the hub or against bone. Inject local anesthetic through the needle while withdrawing it.
6. Place an 11-gauge Cook needle along the anesthetized needle track. It may be helpful to create a nick in the skin measuring 2 to 3 mm. When the Cook needle is at the bone margin, inject additional anesthetic, then penetrate the cortex.
7. Place a 14-gauge Franseen needle coaxially through the 11-gauge Cook needle into the bone marrow. Obtain three to six cores of tissue with the Franseen needle.
8. When done with the Franseen needle biopsies, advance the Cook needle for one additional biopsy.
9. Send samples for pathologic evaluation. Include samples in formalin for anatomic pathology and microbiology collection devices for culture and sensitivity as indicated.
10. Release patient when stable. Provide patient with a telephone number to call if there is persistent or increased pain or numbness or if fever, swelling, or redness develops.

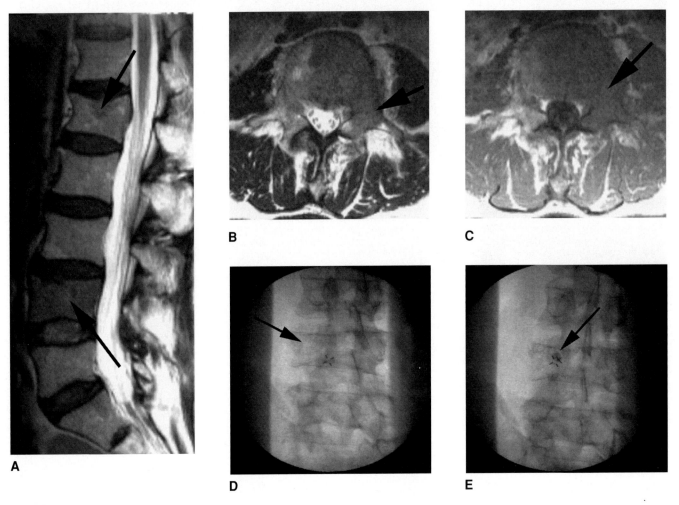

FIGURE 7–4

Fluoroscopically Directed Transpedicular Biopsy of Lumbar Vertebral Body. This 73-year-old man had cervical, thoracic, and lumbar pain. He had lesions on bone scan (not shown). He had no known primary cancer. *A,* Sagittal T2-weighted magnetic resonance imaging scan demonstrates foci of T2 shortening within the L4 and L1 vertebral bodies (arrows). The lesions are atypical, since metastatic deposits usually demonstrate T2 prolongation. *B,* Axial T2-weighted magnetic resonance image demonstrates abnormal marrow signal through the left half of the L4 vertebral body, including the entire pedicle (arrow). *C,* Axial T1-weighted magnetic resonance image demonstrates T1 prolongation matching the T2 shortening seen in part B, including involvement of the pedicle (arrow). *D,* Slightly oblique fluoroscopically directed examination demonstrates destruction of the L4 pedicle margins, with poor visualization of this structure (arrow). The position of the L4 pedicle can be extrapolated by noting the position of the L3 and L5 pedicles. *E,* Slightly oblique view with the cross-hairs of the laser aiming device directed at the L4 pedicle. A 25-gauge spinal needle (arrow) has been placed down the x-ray beam. Anesthetic was administered.

(figure continues on following page)

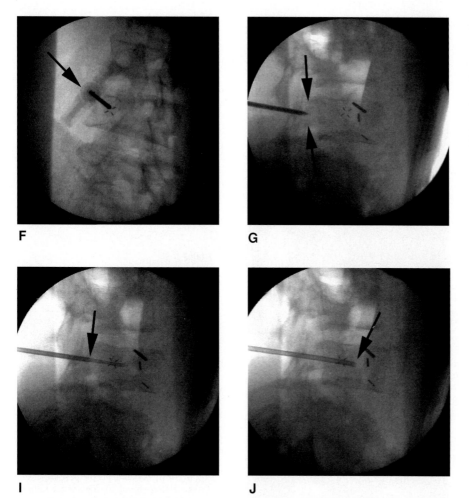

F

G

H

I

J

FIGURE 7–4 CONTINUED

F, Slightly oblique view with the 11-gauge Cook needle directed down the path of the x-ray beam. The hub of the needle (arrow) is readily seen, and the needle has a superolateral to inferomedial course en route to the pedicle. The tip of the needle rests on bone. Anesthetic was administered and the cortex was penetrated. *G,* Lateral view demonstrates the 11-gauge Cook needle with its tip in the posterior aspect of the L4 pedicle (arrows). The visualized pedicle is probably actually the right side, but given the good positioning on this lateral view (note the appearance of the disc margins), the left pedicle should be at the same level. *H,* Frontal view demonstrates the needle course. Because the needle was placed down the x-ray beam in an oblique fashion, the needle courses from posterolateral to anteromedial. The tip projects at the L4 pedicle level (arrow). *I,* Lateral view following coaxial placement of a 14-gauge Franseen needle through the Cook needle. The end of the Cook needle is seen at the posterior margin of the pedicle (arrow). The biopsy sample obtained includes tissue from the junction of the Cook and Franseen needles (at the arrow) to the tip of the Franseen needle, including material from the pedicle and vertebral body. Five passes were obtained, providing extensive tissue. *J,* Following completion of all biopsies with the Franseen needle, the Cook needle is advanced for one final, larger biopsy specimen. Note the teeth seen at the end of this large instrument (arrow). Pathologic analysis demonstrated metastatic adenocarcinoma consistent with colonic origin.

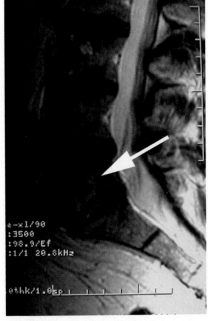

A

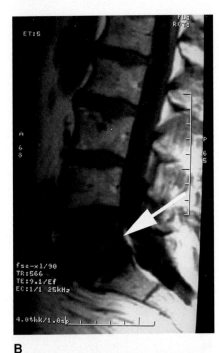

B

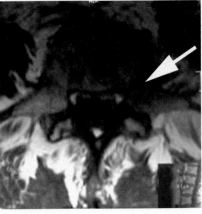

C

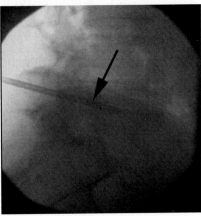

D

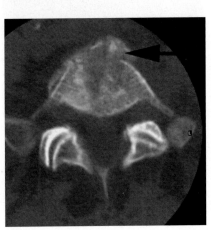

E

FIGURE 7–5

Fluoroscopically Directed Transpedicular Biopsy of L5. This 69-year-old woman presented with persistent low back pain and no history of primary malignancy, weight loss, or other constitutional signs. *A,* Sagittal T2-weighted magnetic resonance imaging scan demonstrates minimal signal intensity abnormality of the L5 vertebral body (arrow). *B,* Sagittal T1-weighted magnetic resonance imaging scan demonstrates much more dramatic signal intensity change in the L5 vertebral body (arrow), with pronounced T1 prolongation. *C,* Axial T2-weighted magnetic resonance imaging scan demonstrates T1 prolongation of the left pedicle. *D,* Lateral view during biopsy. Cores with the 14-gauge Franseen needle had already been obtained, and this image documents the position of the 11-gauge Cook needle (arrow) in the L5 vertebral body. *E,* Axial computed tomographic scan done following completion of the biopsy. The CT examination was performed because of the somewhat unusual characteristics of the lesion, which demonstrated little T2 prolongation. Cortical discontinuity consistent with osteoporotic compression fracture is seen anteriorly (arrow). Biopsy results showed no evidence of malignancy and were consistent with a healing fracture.

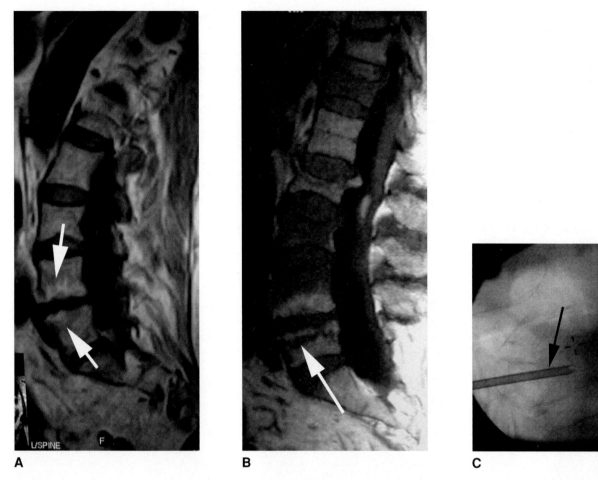

A   B   C

FIGURE 7–6

Fluoroscopically Directed Transpedicular Biopsy in Aggressive Osteoporosis. This 82-year-old woman had low back pain and relatively rapid onset of multilevel extensive marrow abnormality on magnetic resonance imaging examination. *A,* Sagittal T2-weighted magnetic resonance imaging scan demonstrates subchondral degenerative changes at L4-5 (arrow), but vertebral body signal intensity is otherwise unremarkable and vertebral height is maintained. *B,* Sagittal T2-weighted magnetic resonance imaging scan 5 months later shows multiple compression deformities and extensive marrow signal abnormality with T1 prolongation. Note the linear character of the signal intensity within the L5 vertebra, typical of fracture (arrow). Incidentally noted is a lipoma of the filum terminale at the L2 level. *C,* Lateral study with the 11-gauge Cook needle in the L3 vertebral body (arrow). Five passes with the 14-gauge Franseen needle had already been obtained, and tissue obtained was from the abnormal region as seen on the magnetic resonance imaging study. Note the difficulty of visualizing the bony margins in this patient with osteoporosis. Pathologic examination failed to reveal any evidence of malignancy, with normal-appearing bone and bone marrow. Findings are most consistent with healing osteoporotic compression fractures.

TABLE 7–4. Step-by-Step Description of Computed Tomography–Directed Lumbar Vertebral Body Biopsy

1. Obtain sedation and analgesia with drugs of choice.
2. Scan patient and plan needle course to avoid complication. Project back to the skin surface from the location of the lesion along a reasonable path. Measure the distance from midline. Mark the patient's skin at the measured distance from midline at the appropriate level (done by placing the patient in the scanner and activating the positioning laser light). Use a 25-gauge 3.5-inch needle to anesthetize the skin and aim the needle toward the lesion.
3. Scan the patient and judge whether the path of the needle is appropriate. If not, adjust and rescan. If so, place the biopsy needle along the same path. Usually it is best to use an 11-gauge Cook needle so that once it is in place, coaxial samples can be drawn with a 14-gauge Franseen needle. Alternately, if no bone blocks the path to the lesion, an 18-gauge trocar can be placed with coaxial passage of a spring-loaded cutting needle.
4. Once the guiding needle is at the lesion margin, coaxially pass the biopsy needle into the lesion. Document needle position with serial computed tomographic scans. Marking a position on the biopsy needle with a piece of sterile tape can help prevent overzealous entry of the needle past the vertebral body and into anterior vascular structures during lumbar biopsies.
5. Send samples for pathologic evaluation. Include samples in formalin for anatomic pathology and microbiology collection devices for culture and sensitivity as indicated.
6. Release patient when stable. Provide patient with a telephone number to call if there is persistent or increased pain or numbness or if fever, swelling, or redness develops.

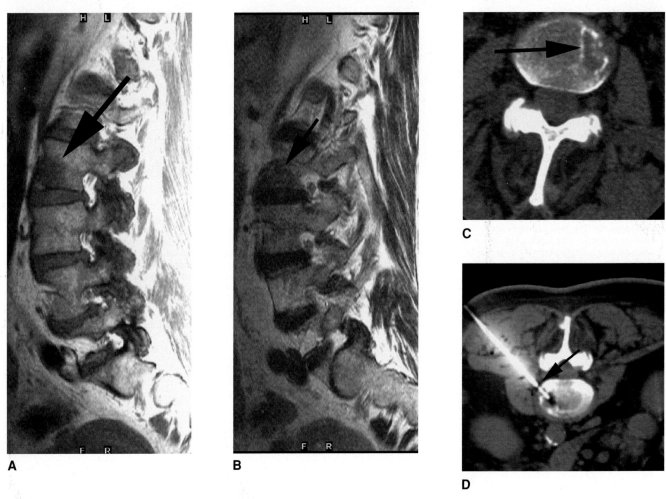

A   **B**   **C**

D

FIGURE 7–7

Computed Tomography–Directed Biopsy. This 73-year-old woman had back pain and a history of breast cancer. *A,* Sagittal T1-weighted magnetic resonance imaging scan demonstrates a focus of T1 prolongation along the left lateral aspect of the L2 vertebral body (arrow). *B,* Sagittal T2-weighted magnetic resonance imaging scan demonstrates T2 shortening matching the T1 prolongation (arrow). *C,* Axial computed tomographic (CT) scan through the lesion demonstrates a relatively sclerotic border and benign appearance (arrow). *D,* Axial CT study with the 11-gauge Cook needle placed to the vertebral body margin, with coaxial introduction of the 14-gauge Franseen needle into the lesion. The border between the Cook needle and the coaxially introduced Franseen needle is visible at the vertebral body margin (arrow). Biopsy demonstrated findings of metastatic breast cancer.

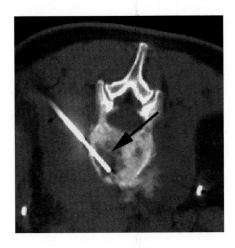

FIGURE 7–8

Computed Tomography–Directed Biopsy. This 44-year-old woman had cervical cancer, back pain, and lesions detected by bone scan (not shown). Axial computed tomographic study shows a 14-gauge Franseen needle passed through an 11-gauge Cook needle, through a vertebral body lesion (arrow). Histologic evaluation demonstrated findings of metastatic cervical carcinoma.

References

Adapon BD, Legada BD, Lim EVA, Silao JV, Dalmacio-Cruz A. CT-guided closed biopsy of the spine. JCAT 1981; 5:73–78.

Carragee EJ. Pyogenic vertebral osteomyelitis. J Bone Joint Surg Am 1997; 79:874–880.

Craig FS. Vertebral-body biopsy. J Bone Joint Surg Am 1956; 38:93–102.

Frankel CJ. Aspiration biopsy of the spine. J Bone Joint Surg Am 1954; 36:69–74.

Fraser-Hill MA, Renfrew DL. Percutaneous needle biopsy of musculoskeletal lesions. 1. Effective accuracy and diagnostic utility. AJR 1992a; 158:809–812.

Fraser-Hill MA, Renfrew DL, Hilsenrath PE. Percutaneous needle biopsy of musculoskeletal lesions. 2. Cost-effectiveness. AJR 1992b; 158:813–818.

Heller JG, Pedlow FX. Tumors of the spine. In Garfin SR, Vaccaro AR (eds). Orthopedic Knowledge Update: Spine. Rosemont, IL: American Association of Orthopedic Surgeons, 1997.

Hitchon PW, Osenbach RK, Yuh WTC, Menezes AH. Spinal infections. Clin Neurosurg 1992; 38:373–387.

Mazet R, Cozen L. The diagnostic value of vertebral body needle biopsy. Ann Surg 1952; 135:245–252.

Nagel DA, Albright JA, Keggi KJ, Southwick WO. Closer look at spinal lesions: open biopsy of spinal lesions. JAMA 1965; 191:975–978.

Ray RD. Needle biopsy of the lumbar vertebral bodies: a modification of the Valls technique. J Bone Joint Surg 1953; 35:760–762.

Renfrew DL, Whitten CS, Wiese JA, et al. CT-guided percutaneous transpedicular biopsy. Radiology 180:574–576, 1991.

Rougraff BT, Kneisl JS, Simon MA. Skeletal metastases of unknown origin: a prospective study of a diagnostic strategy. J Bone Joint Surg Am 1993; 75:1276–1281.

Sharif HS. Role of MR imaging in the management of spinal infections. AJR 1992; 158:1333–1345.

Stoker DJ, Kissen CM. Percutaneous vertebral biopsy: a review of 135 cases. Clin Radiol 36:569–577, 1985.

8 Vertebroplasty and Kyphoplasty

DONALD L. RENFREW • MARK BECKNER • KENT B. REMLEY

Definition

Percutaneous vertebroplasty consists of the introduction of polymethylmethacrylate (PMMA) or bone cement into the vertebral body via a percutaneously placed needle. Kyphoplasty consists of the introduction of a bone tamp and balloon, reduction of kyphosis and tamping of bone via inflation of the balloon, and subsequent placement of PMMA within the cavity created by the balloon. Both techniques utilize image guidance for placement of the instrumentation and bone cement delivery.

Literature Review

Percutaneous vertebroplasty with PMMA was invented in 1984 by Galibert and Deramond (Deramond et al 1998) for the treatment of painful or aggressive vertebral hemangiomas. Most of the early development, research, and clinical applications occurred in Europe, with the results published in the European (primarily French) literature.

In 1996, Cotten and colleagues reported on 37 patients who underwent 40 percutaneous vertebroplasties for metastases (30 cases) and multiple myeloma (10 cases). Thirty-six of the 37 patients obtained partial or complete sustained pain relief. Interestingly, pain relief was not related to the extent of lesion filling in these patients treated for tumor. Because of a lack of cortical margin around the periphery of the lesion, PMMA leakage was frequent (15 epidural, 8 intradiscal, 8 foraminal, and 2 venous leakages). Although most of these leaks were of no clinical consequence, two of the eight foraminal leaks resulted in nerve root compression and radicular pain and required surgery (which rectified the problem).

Deramond and colleagues (1998) published a review of the technique, indications, and results, summarizing the experience of the developers of the method in France. Indications for vertebroplasty included aggressive/painful vertebral angiomas, osteoporotic vertebral collapse, and malignant vertebral tumors. Their series consisted of 50 patients with vertebral angiomas, 80 patients with osteoporotic vertebral collapse, and 101 patients with malignant lesions; in the first two categories, pain relief was achieved in approximately 90% of patients, whereas in patients with malignancies it was achieved in about 80%. Two patients with extensive metastatic lesions died a few days after vertebroplasty from unrelated problems. One immunocompromised patient with breast cancer developed infectious spondylitis requiring prolonged bedrest (this patient did not receive preoperative antibiotics). The authors listed transient increased pain without cement leak, radiculopathy from cement leak, and cord compression from cement leak as complications due to injection itself. Of 11 patients with radiculopathy, 3 (with lumbar radiculopathy) required surgical decompression; several thoracic lesions were treated by injections (usually of anesthetic but one of alcohol). One patient with spinal cord compression after injection (who had compression prior to injection by tumor) underwent emergency surgery without permanent neurologic deficit. The authors pointed out that complications were more frequent in patients undergoing percutaneous vertebroplasty for malignancy (at about 10%) than in patients with vertebral angiomas (2–5%) or osteoporotic collapse (1–3%).

Martin and colleagues (1999) published a report of their experience in Switzerland detailing 68 percutaneous vertebroplasties done in 40 patients. Indications included 11 patients with osteoporotic collapse, 7 with hemangiomas, 19 with metastatic disease, 2 with myeloma, and 1 with primary lymphoma. The authors' results were similar to the results from other series, with pain relief in approximately 80% of patients and a complication rate of 6% per level. One patient experienced radiculopathy treated by "infiltration of this area."

Barr and colleagues (2000) reported a review of 47 consecutive patients with 84 treated levels. Thirty-eight patients described had osteoporotic fractures, one had a hemangioma, and eight had malignancies. Although 95% of the patients with osteoporosis had significant initial pain relief that lasted at least 18 months, only 50%, or four of the eight patients with malignancies had pain relief. One patient had T3 dermatome radicular neuritis that resolved slowly with oral steroids. Another patient developed a new fracture immediately inferior to the treated level, requiring additional vertebroplasty. The authors reported an evolution in their practice, changing from computed tomography (CT) guidance to fluoroscopic guidance for routine procedures, reserving combined CT and fluoroscopic guidance for complex and higher risk procedures.

Moreland and colleagues (2001) published a study of 35 patients with treatment for osteoporotic compression fractures at 53 levels. They had a success rate of 89% with a 6% complication rate, including a patient with an "impressive epidural collection of PMMA" which, while asymptomatic, was surgically removed, and another with radicular pain following extravasation in the lateral recess along the medial aspect of the L4 pedicle, which also underwent surgical removal.

Garfin and colleagues (2001) reviewed the literature in 2001 and provided an illustration of the method of vertebroplasty and kyphoplasty, as well as a summary of results and complications. Data from an ongoing clinical trial of kyphoplasty involving 340 patients was reported with "90% symptomatic and functional improvement rate." The authors reported four complications from kyphoplasty: an epidural hematoma requiring surgical evacuation; spinal canal placement of PMMA requiring surgical evacuation; transient fever and hypoxia (believed to be a systemic response to liquid PMMA); and anterior cord syndrome (possibly from vascular compromise during needle placement). The authors emphasized that complications from kyphoplasty were related to needle placement rather than kyphoplasty itself and emphasized the relative advantages of kyphoplasty, including reduction of kyphosis and controlled introduction of thicker PMMA reducing control of filling and lessening the chances of migration of the material (and hence neurologic compromise).

Kaufmann and colleagues (2001) studied 75 patients (122 vertebrae treated) with a logistical regression analysis and found no independent effect of age of the fracture on pain relief. Kim and colleagues (2002) compared unipedicular and bipedicular approaches for vertebroplasty and found no statistically significant difference in clinical outcomes, including pain relief and change in pain medication requirements. It should be noted that these findings in addition to the lack of correlation of pain relief with degree of lesion filling (Cotten 1996) indicate that at least part of the pain relief forthcoming from vertebroplasty could be secondary to a placebo effect. In this regard, Jarvik and Deyo (Jarvik 2000) have called for a randomized trial of vertebroplasty.

Rationale for Procedure

Vertebroplasty and kyphoplasty are performed for pain relief and fracture stabilization. In a retrospective review of 245 patients, Evans and colleagues (2003) reported significant improvement in pain, ambulatory status, and the ability to perform activities of daily living following vertebroplasty. Tumor necrosis, destruction of sensitive nerve endings, stabilization of microfractures, and reduction of mechanical forces have all been offered as putative mechanisms of pain reduction (Cotten et al, 1996), but as noted by Kaufmann and colleagues (2001), "the mechanism from pain relief remains uncertain." With vertebroplasty, introduction of PMMA into a malignancy that has destroyed cancellous bone will enhance the mechanical stability of the

---

[1]This section is virtually identical to the Equipment and Supplies section in Chapter 2 and can be skipped if the reader is already familiar with this material.

TABLE 8–1. Equipment and Supplies for Vertebroplasty

C-arm fluoroscope and/or helical computed tomography scanner
Surgical scrub solution
Needles for local anesthesia
Needles and instrumentation for vertebral body access
Small mallet
Syringes
Connecting tubing
Nonionic contrast material
Local anesthetic agent and medications for conscious sedation
Polymethylmethacrylate and sterile barium sulfate

---

segment. With kyphoplasty, reduction of kyphosis may be achieved if the procedure is done within 3 months of the injury (Garfin et al, 2001).

Equipment and Supplies

Tables 8–1 and 8–2 list equipment required for vertebroplasty and kyphoplasty.

A high-quality C-arm device is necessary for vertebroplasty and kyphoplasty, and biplane fluoroscopy or dual C-arms are even better. A laser aiming device (an attachment that shows a cross-hair on the fluoroscopic screen corresponding in position to a red dot on the skin surface) is also helpful for proper needle placement. Many manufacturers produce kits for percutaneous vertebroplasty that include the requisite items (Fig. 8–1).

The KyphX Inflatable Bone Tamp (balloon) (Fig. 8–2) for the kyphoplasty technique is a patented device manufactured by Kyphon Inc. of Sunnyvale, California. The balloons come in kits containing all supplies necessary to do the procedure except for sterile drapes, a scalpel, a mallet, PMMA, and barium powder. The balloons come in two sizes, 15 mm and 20 mm in length, two of the same size in each kit. Kyphon controls the use of the KyphX Inflatable Bone Tamp. Only physicians who have completed a company-sponsored course and received certification are allowed to use the device.

In addition to the equipment listed in Table 8–1, a crash cart should be readily available to handle medical emergencies (e.g., contrast media and drug reactions).

Informed Consent Issues

Informed consent issues may be divided into a description of the procedure, warning the patient about a flare in pain

TABLE 8–2. Equipment and Supplies for Kyphoplasty

C-arm fluoroscope
Surgical scrub solution
Needles for local anesthesia
KyphX balloon tamp kit
Small mallet
Syringes
Nonionic contrast material
General anesthetic or local anesthetic agents and medications for conscious sedation
Polymethylmethacrylate and barium sulfate powder
Sterile tape and final dressing

FIGURE 8–1

Percutaneous Vertebroplasty Equipment. **A**, Basic 11-gauge needle system (Cook Incorporated, Bloomington, IN) used for vertebral body access and bone cement delivery. This needle design contains both diamond-tip (arrow 1) and beveled (arrow 2) stylets that are interchangeable with the cannula (arrow 3). The bone cement can be delivered with multiple 1 mL or 3 mL syringes. A number of delivery systems are also available to provide greater control and ease of use. **B**, The PCD Precision System (Stryker Instruments, Kalamazoo, MI) offers the operator the ability to both mix and deliver the bone cement within the same system. The cartridge and delivery tubing (arrow) reduce radiation exposure to the operator's hands.

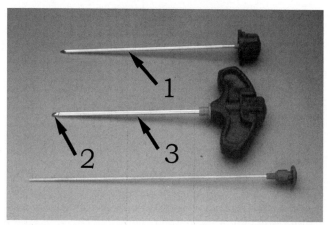

A

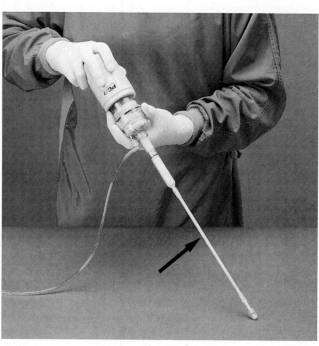

B

following the procedure, and delineation of material risks. The risks, benefits, and alternatives to the procedure should be addressed, particularly the alternative of doing nothing (particularly for osteoporotic compression fractures, which have a generally benign course).

For complications, Moreland and colleagues (2001) list "death, bleeding, major vascular injury, transfusion, infec-tion, pneumothorax, hemothorax, permanent neurologic injury, paralysis, need for an operation, pulmonary embolus of PMMA, no relief of pain, further compression fractures, and risks of anesthesia."

The physician may also elect to inform the patient that the use of PMMA and barium sulfate for these procedures is an off-label use and has not been specifically approved by the

FIGURE 8–2

KyphX Inflatable Bone Tamp (balloon). See text for description.

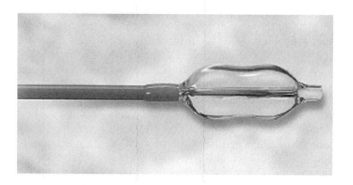

United States Food and Drug Administration (FDA) for percutaneous vertebroplasty or kyphoplasty. Currently, only one bone cement preparation (Simplex P, Stryker-Howmedica-Osteonics, Rutherford, NJ) is approved for use in pathologic fractures, including the spine (Mathis et al 2001).

Patient Selection

Pain secondary to osteoporotic compression fractures is the dominant indication for the procedure. Patients with painful or aggressive vertebral hemangiomas and painful malignancies may also benefit. Vertebroplasty also provides mechanical stabilization in patients with extensive malignant destruction of the vertebral body.

As noted by Murphy and Deramond (2000), although the procedure was initially developed in Europe to treat vertebral angiomas and malignancies, "North American physicians have experienced a growth in this procedure that is patient-driven, resulting from motivated, internet savvy osteoporotic patients referring themselves directly." As Moreland and colleagues (2000), have noted, "Recent articles in such main-stream periodicals as *The Wall Street Journal* and *Readers Digest* promoting the benefits of vertebroplasty will, no doubt, increase public knowledge and demand for this procedure." Moreland and colleagues caution, however, that "minimally invasive does not imply minimal complications" and state, "It is important for surgeons to prepare themselves as well as their patients" for significant complications, including pulmonary emboli and PMMA leakage with neural sequelae.

Although some papers report positive results up to 1 year after the onset of the fracture, vertebroplasty and kyphoplasty appear to have a superior result in fractures of more recent onset. In the case of kyphoplasty, improvement in the fracture deformity is usually achieved in fractures of 3 months' duration or less.

Proper patient selection is critical to the success of these procedures. Therefore, one should carefully assess the patient to ensure that the pain is in fact related to the compression fracture. Unfortunately, given the patient population, many other conditions may be present that produce axial back pain, complicating the evaluation. Pain originating from a compression fracture should be most severe with weight-bearing and exacerbated with twisting or arising from a recumbent position. The pain often completely disappears with recumbency. Compression fracture pain is usually localized and, while referred pain may be present, it should not be radicular in nature. History and physical examination findings, along with plain film localization, are limited, however, in cases in which there is more than one level of compression deformity. Therefore, magnetic resonance imaging (MRI) is the procedure of choice for the initial evaluation of almost all patients who are being considered for internal fracture stabilization. The MRI scans should show both vertebral collapse and loss of normal bone marrow signal intensity, indicating edema within the marrow space of the vertebral body. These findings are best demonstrated with sagittal T1-weighted images (Fig. 3), in which the abnormal bone marrow will be dark relative to the bright, fat-containing marrow within normal vertebra, or chronic compression fractures that have healed. T2-

weighted images using fat-suppression techniques will show bright signal within the affected vertebral body, also indicating marrow edema. If the patient is unable to undergo MRI, then a radionuclide bone scan with single photon emission computed tomography imaging can be substituted for patient evaluation. In the authors' experience, bone scanning has the disadvantages of reduced anatomical localization, limited information regarding other spinal abnormalities, and the presence of increased activity long after there has been substantial healing of the fracture. A negative MRI scan and a negative or "weakly positive" bone scan indicate a low likelihood of success with percutaneous vertebroplasty.

In cases in which the patient has a pathologic fracture or severe back pain related to known or suspected metastatic disease, myeloma, or lymphoma, vertebroplasty can be combined with biopsy of the vertebral body. Before proceeding, however, a CT scan of the treatment level is indicated to determine the extent of bone destruction. If there is destruction of the posterior cortex of the vertebral body, then vertebroplasty is contraindicated in almost all instances, owing to the high risk of cement leakage or posterior tumor displacement into the spinal canal.

Procedure Descriptions

Table 8–3 describes and Figures 8–4, 8–5, and 8–6 illustrate the procedure for vertebroplasty. Table 8–4 describes and Figures 8–7 and 8–8 illustrate the procedure for kyphoplasty.

Text continued on page 149

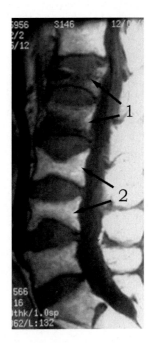

FIGURE 8–3

Magnetic Resonance Imaging (MRI) Study Demonstrating Compression Fractures. T1-weighted sagittal MRI scan of the lumbar spine demonstrates multiple compression fractures. The L1 and L2 compression fractures (arrow 1) reveal low signal intensity within the marrow space indicating active, unhealed fractures. The high signal intensity within the L3 and L4 vertebral bodies (arrow 2) is secondary to fat content within the bone marrow, indicating chronic, healed fractures. Therefore, only the L1 and L2 vertebrae would be appropriate for treatment with vertebroplasty in this patient.

TABLE 8–3. Step-by-Step Description of Vertebroplasty

1. Percutaneous vertebroplasty is most commonly performed in a special procedures suite with high-quality C-arm or biplane fluoroscopy. Computed tomography (preferably with fluoroscopy) may be necessary for cervical and high thoracic cases or in cases in which there is considerable bone destruction related to malignant disease. The patient is placed on the table in the prone position and made comfortable with appropriate arm support and table padding as needed. Anesthesia most commonly consists of conscious sedation with intravenous midazolam and fentanyl, in conjunction with local anesthesia using buffered lidocaine or bupivacaine. General anesthesia is seldom necessary. Patient monitoring should include blood pressure, oxygen saturation, and electrocardiographic monitoring. Preoperative intravenous antibiotics are routinely administered 15 to 20 minutes prior to initiation of the procedure. In selected cases, such as in patients who are immunosuppressed, tobramycin 1.2 g may be mixed in with the bone cement.

2. Two general approaches can be employed to access the vertebral body: the transpedicular approach and the extrapedicular approach (see Fig. 8–4). Each approach has its own advantages and disadvantages, and selection is largely dependent on physician preference. The transpedicular approach is the most common technique and can be used anywhere in the thoracic and lumbar spine. This approach is generally easy to learn and is dependable. However, it often requires bilateral needle placement for adequate filling of the vertebral body. Furthermore, this technique may be quite challenging, or impossible, if the pedicle is extremely small, difficult to visualize secondary to osteoporosis, or destroyed from tumor involvement.

   The advantage of the extrapedicular approach is that the technique is not dependent on the size, axial orientation, or visibility of the vertebral pedicle. Therefore, this approach may be preferable in the upper thoracic spine, where the pedicles tend to be smaller. As a result of the angle of approach to the vertebral body (see Fig. 8–4), the end of the injection cannula is reliably positioned in the anterior-central aspect of the vertebral body for injection of the bone cement, avoiding the necessity of a second needle placement. This technique can also be successfully employed in cases of extreme collapse or "vertebra plana."

   For illustrations of the technique described below, see Figure 8–5. Following introduction of local anesthesia in the skin, soft tissues, and periosteum, a small skin incision in made and the needle is advanced to the target point on the vertebra, depending on the approach that is selected. For the transpedicular technique, 10-, 11-, or 13-gauge needles are typically used. Larger injection cannulas may be used with the extrapedicular technique, if desired. The needle is advanced through the cortex using either a drilling motion or with the use of a small mallet. With the transpedicular technique, the needle is then carefully advanced, using fluoroscopic guidance, across the articular pillar and pedicle to the posterior aspect of the vertebral body. Great care must be taken to ensure that the needle does not deviate medially through the cortex of the pedicle into the spinal canal or neural foramen. This usually requires visualization of the needle in multiple projections during advancement.

   Once the needle has been safely advanced to the junction of the pedicle and vertebral body, biopsy of the vertebra can be performed, if indicated, by advancing a second biopsy needle using coaxial technique through the injection cannula, or by using the injection cannula itself, and simply reintroducing it through the same posterior cortical hole. The needle is then advanced to the anterior-central aspect of the vertebral body. With the extrapedicular approach, once the needle tip has been placed through the vertebral body cortex, a biopsy is performed, if indicated, and the injection cannula is advanced to the desired position.

3. Prior to performing vertebroplasty, many authors advocate vertebral venography before proceeding with injection of the bone cement. This is done by injecting a small amount of nonionic contrast material (typically 3–5 mL) through the needle and performing a digital subtraction angiogram. The vertebrogram is performed to exclude needle placement directly into the basivertebral plexus and to outline the trabecular venous drainage pattern of the vertebral body. The basivertebral vein exits through a small depression within the posterior wall of the vertebral body and communicates with the epidural venous plexus. Therefore, the venogram is performed to assess for risk of cement leakage during vertebroplasty. However, since contrast material and bone cement have different viscosities, it is unknown whether there is accurate correlation between the flow of the two agents. In addition, if contrast material leaks into a nonvascular space, such as leakage through an end-plate fracture into the disc space or leakage into an internal cavity, the contrast material may actually inhibit visualization of cement leakage and interfere with the procedure.

4. A variety of polymethylmethacrylate (PMMA) preparations are available on the market for use with vertebroplasty. These preparations all vary in some degree in their behavior regarding strength and hardening times. PMMA is not intrinsically radiopaque. Therefore, an opacifying agent must be added to the bone cement for adequate visualization with fluoroscopy. This includes those bone cements that already contain barium in the preparation. To achieve adequate visualization with fluoroscopy, the bone cement should contain at least 25% barium by weight. This can be achieved by adding 5 to 6 g of a sterile barium preparation to 20 g of the PMMA copolymer (powder) prior to mixing. Fortunately, several commercially available sterile barium sulfate preparations can be used.

   A variety of mixing techniques are used, depending on the type of bone cement selected. A closed container or sterile vacuum-mixing device is suggested to limit spread of the fumes in the working environment. The monomer and copolymer are then mixed together until the powder is completely liquefied. Alteration of the polymer to monomer ratios is not recommended. Cooling of the preparation before and after mixing can prolong the working time and may be necessary with some of the PMMA preparations. Although the intrinsic strength and stiffness of the commercially available PMMA preparations varies somewhat in the laboratory, no difference in strength has been observed from a clinical standpoint. The viscosity of the different types of PMMA will vary, both initially and over time. The type of cement and the viscosity selected to begin the injection will vary with physician preference and the injection system being utilized. It is recommended that the initial consistency resemble that of toothpaste prior to initiation of delivery.

5. Once the acrylic bone cement has been mixed, a variety of techniques can be used for delivery into the vertebral body. Several commercially available delivery systems have been developed for injection, including one system that allows for mixture of the PMMA and delivery with the same device, eliminating the need for cement transfer. Alternatively, the PMMA can be loaded into a 1.0 mL syringe for direct injection into the cannula. When larger caliber injection cannulas are used, the cannula may be filled with the PMMA and then manually delivered with a blunt-tipped "pusher" or stylet. The closed delivery systems have the advantage of keeping the hands of the operator farther away from the x-ray beam during injection.

Table continued on following page

TABLE 8–3. Continued

Prior to injection of the PMMA, the injection cannula is filled with saline to prohibit injection of significant amounts of air into the venous system. The "dead space" of the needle/cannula may vary from 0.4 mL to 3.5 mL, depending on the system that is used. The C-arm should be positioned so that the vertebral body is profiled in the lateral projection. It is *extremely important* to deliver the cement while viewing the vertebra in this projection to detect early extravasation into the epidural space posteriorly or into the paravertebral veins, both of which could have adverse consequences if unrecognized.

The delivery of the bone cement should proceed very slowly and with caution initially, since the reduced viscosity makes early venous extravasation or cement leakage more likely. As filling continues, assuming satisfactory trabecular filling takes place, the speed of delivery may be slightly increased, depending on the type of PMMA used. At *no* time, however, should the material be delivered in a rapid manner. Periodic visualization in the anterior-posterior projection is also necessary to detect lateral leakage. If cement leakage occurs, the injection should be immediately halted, the needle repositioned either anteriorly or posteriorly, and the injection carefully restarted. If the injection is halted for more than 20 to 30 seconds, the cement may polymerize within the needle, requiring replacement with a second needle. End points for PMMA delivery include adequate filling for fracture stabilization, persistent cement leakage not amenable to needle repositioning and time, and polymerization of the bone cement, prohibiting further injection. Even though very small amounts of PMMA leakage may be tolerated without sequelae, every effort should be made to avoid extravasation.

After completion of the injection, the cannula is withdrawn and pressure is held over the incision for local hemostasis, and a small bandage is applied. Unless the stylet is used to deliver the remaining cement within the cannula, several complete rotations of the cannula should be performed to separate the residual cement within the needle from the cement within the vertebral body. Failure to perform this simple maneuver may result in a cement "spike" projecting through the bone puncture site into the posterior soft tissues. Inadequate filling of the vertebral body may require a contralateral puncture and a second injection. Alternatively, the operator may choose to place two needles at the outset of the procedure. The cannulas may then be injected simultaneously or sequentially, depending on the fill pattern as the cement is injected. Multiple levels may require injection (see Fig. 8–6).

6. Vertebroplasty is routinely performed as an outpatient procedure. For the first 2 hours, the patient is observed in a full supine position. Over the next 1 to 2 hours, the patients are allowed to gradually sit up or stand under nursing supervision. Patients are typically discharged to the care of an adult by 4 hours postprocedure. Since focal pain may be present at the operative site, mild narcotic medication or nonsteroidal anti-inflammatory agents may be necessary for 1 to 3 days. Postprocedural plain radiographs of the appropriate area to serve as a new baseline and to compare with subsequent follow-up studies should be obtained.

Before discharge, the patients are evaluated for new back pain, chest pain, or neurologic dysfunction. Since significant complications are manifest early, prompt recognition is crucial so that early evaluation and treatment, if needed, can be instituted.

Patients are contacted by telephone at 24 to 48 hours and return for follow-up at 10 to 14 days postprocedure. The patients are urged to restrict activity until they are seen for follow-up, since most patients have had their activity status severely restricted as a result of the fracture(s). In selected instances, a short course of bracing may be appropriate in high-risk patients. A physical therapy program to help strengthen the back muscles may also be very helpful in this population. Finally, in patients with osteoporosis who have not been on medical therapy, appropriate referral and aggressive treatment should be implemented to prevent subsequent fractures.

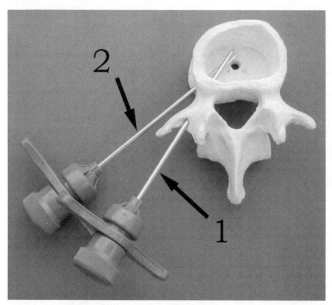

A

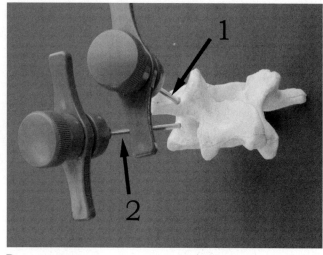

B

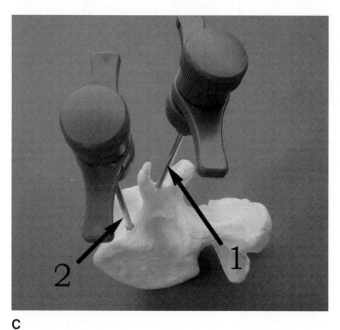

C

FIGURE 8–4

Model Demonstrating Transpedicular and Extrapedicular Approach to Vertebroplasty. **A,** Photograph of a model vertebral body from above with two needles in position. The transpedicular needle (arrow 1) takes a more sagittal course and the needle tip projects slightly anterior and lateral to the extrapedicular needle (arrow 2). The extrapedicular approach enables the operator to reliably place the cannula tip in the midline, usually resulting in adequate vertebral filling with a single injection. **B,** Photograph of a model vertebral body from slightly oblique and posterior position demonstrates the transpedicular needle (arrow 1) entering the pedicle at the groove formed at the base of the transverse process and superior articular process. The extrapedicular needle (arrow 2) enters the dorsolateral vertebral body. **C,** Photograph of a model vertebral body from slightly below also demonstrates the transpedicular needle (arrow 1) entering the pedicle at the groove formed at the base of the transverse process and superior articular process, with the extrapedicular needle (arrow 2) entering the dorsolateral vertebral body. The vertebral body entry point for the extrapedicular approach is anterior and superior to the exiting segmental nerve.

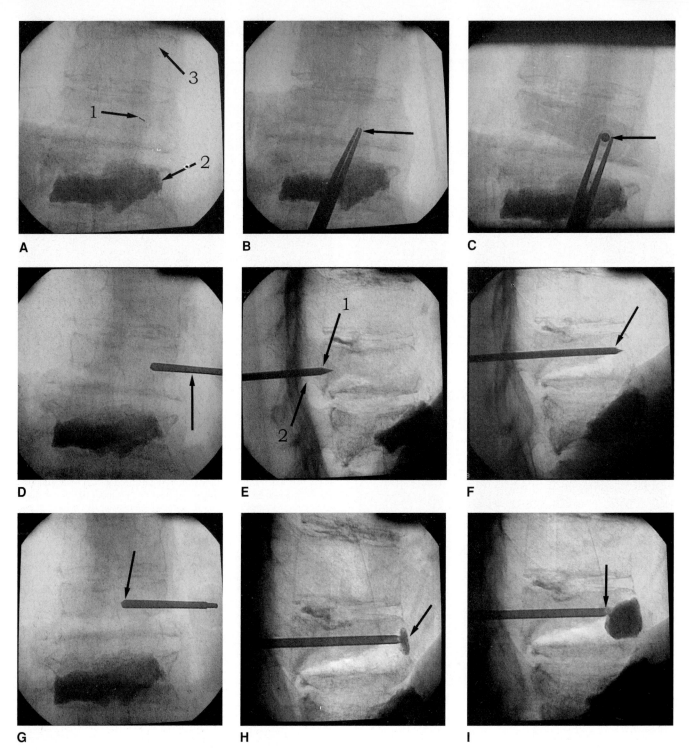

FIGURE 8–5

Step-by-Step Vertebroplasty Procedure. A, Slightly oblique radiograph aligned along the pedicle axis demonstrates a needle in place at the target location of the right pedicle (arrow 1). Note that vertebroplasty has already been performed at the next lower level (arrow 2). Because of marked osteoporosis (typical in cases of vertebroplasty), landmarks such as vertebral body margins and pedicles are difficult to discern with confidence. For example, the pedicle at the next higher vertebral level (arrow 3) is much more easily visualized than the pedicle at the target level. **B,** Slightly oblique radiograph aligned along the right pedicle axis demonstrates that the anesthesia needle has been removed and a clamp has been placed so that its tip (arrow) is at the inferior margin of the right pedicle. **C,** Slightly oblique radiograph aligned along the right pedicle axis demonstrates that the injection needle (arrow) has been placed so that it aligns with the right pedicle. **D,** Frontal radiograph after needle advancement into the pedicle, directed from posterolateral to anteromedial. The tip appears to "contact" the medial aspect of the pedicle. One should not advance the needle from this location without viewing the lateral projection to ensure that the tip overlies the body-pedicle junction, to avoid violation of the medial cortex of the pedicle. **E,** Lateral radiograph with the needle unchanged in position from part D, demonstrates that the injection needle (arrow 1) is at the posterior margin of the vertebral body, through the lower aspect of the pedicle (arrow 2). It is now safe to advance the injection needle into the vertebral body. **F,** Lateral radiograph demonstrates that the injection needle (arrow) has been advanced so that its tip is at the anterior aspect of the vertebral body. Note the large gas-containing cleft inferior to the anterior aspect of the needle within the lower portion of the vertebral body. **G,** Frontal radiograph with the needle in the same position as in part F demonstrates that the tip of the needle is at the midline (arrow). **H,** Lateral radiograph demonstrates a small amount of barium-impregnated polymethylmethacrylate (PMMA) collecting at the needle tip, in the anterior aspect of the vertebral body (arrow). **I,** Lateral radiograph demonstrates a larger amount of barium-impregnated PMMA in the anterior aspect of the vertebral body. The injection needle has been withdrawn slightly, and its tip (arrow) is now more posteriorly located.

Continued.

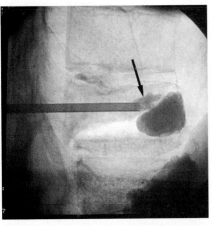

J

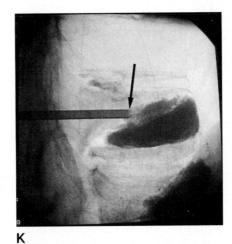

K

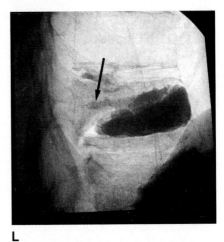

L

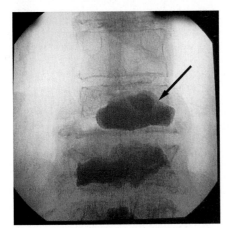

M

FIGURE 8–5 CONTINUED

J, Lateral radiograph demonstrates additional barium-impregnated PMMA (arrow) in a somewhat more superior position. K, Lateral radiograph demonstrates that the needle tip (arrow) has been further withdrawn. Additional barium-impregnated PMMA is seen in the anterior vertebral body, with excellent filling of the previously gas-containing cavity. L, Lateral radiograph demonstrates that the needle has been removed. Additional barium-impregnated PMMA (arrow) is seen along the course of the needle track. This was deposited during needle withdrawal to form a plug in the needle track. M, Frontal radiograph at the end of the procedure demonstrates barium-impregnated PMMA (arrow) spread through much of the vertebral body and crossing the midline.

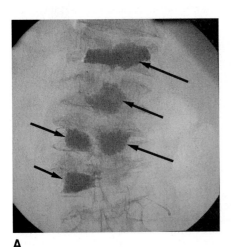

A

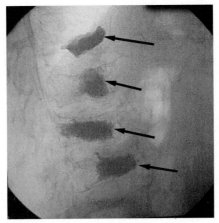

B

FIGURE 8–6

Radiographs following Multilevel Vertebroplasty. A, Frontal radiograph of the thoracolumbar spine following percutaneous vertebroplasty of T12 through L3. Note the variable fill pattern at each level (arrows). The patient had excellent pain relief following the procedure. B, Lateral radiograph of the thoracolumbar spine in the same patient, again demonstrating a variable fill pattern (arrows). Note that the volume of bone cement injected into the vertebral body does not necessarily correlate with clinical success. Nevertheless, the operator should attempt to achieve endplate-to-endplate filling, if possible, to ensure fracture stabilization.

Table 8–4. Step-by-Step Description of Kyphoplasty

1. Kyphoplasty is performed most commonly under general anesthesia with the patient prone and on chest rolls. Prior to beginning the procedure, the size of the vertebra is measured in the anterior-posterior dimension and a balloon size that will fill approximately the anterior two thirds of the vertebra is selected. The fractured vertebra is visualized with image intensifier and the position of the patient or the x-ray beam adjusted to achieve square orientation of the vertebra in anterior-posterior and lateral planes. The medial wall of the pedicles, anterior and posterior cortical margins, and the vertebral end plates must be visualized to safely perform the procedure.

   As with vertebroplasty, there are two approaches to the vertebral body (see Fig. 8–4). The transpedicular approach is most commonly used in the lower lumbar and lower thoracic spines, whereas the extrapedicular approach may be necessary in the upper lumbar and thoracic spine. The diameter of the pedicles and their orientation in the axial plane dictate which approach is appropriate to achieve final placement of the balloon tip sufficiently medial in the body.

   A 5-mm skin incision is made, usually superior and lateral to the pedicle. Trial placement of a 22-gauge spinal needle is helpful in determining appropriate placement of the incision to allow a straight trajectory from the skin through the fascia, the pedicle, and into the midline of the vertebra. The 11-gauge needle is then advanced to the posterior vertebra. For the transpedicular approach, the needle is advanced through the pedicle and into the posterior body. A guide wire is passed through the needle, the needle removed, and the Osteo Introducer (cannula and stylet, see Fig. 8–7) is passed over the guide wire. A mallet may be necessary to penetrate the cortical wall. The tip of the cannula is advanced to 3 mm anterior to the posterior cortical wall. The stylet is now removed from the cannula.

   The technique is similar for the extrapedicular approach, but the entry site into the vertebral body is at the junction of the superior articular facet and the transverse process (see Fig. 8–4). In most cases, bilateral access is desired to achieve optimal reduction and filling of the vertebra with PMMA. On occasion in a small thoracic vertebra, central placement of a single balloon is sufficient.

2. Holes are drilled in the body, with care taken not to penetrate the anterior cortex while attempting to get within 3 to 5 mm of the anterior cortex. Also, at this point, a biopsy sample may be obtained either by saving the bone that remains in the drill flutes or passing one of the bone filler tubes through the cannula and harvesting a core of bone.

3. A collapsed balloon with an attached inflation syringe is passed through the cannula and seated in the hole prepared in the vertebral body. Radiographic markers in the balloon allow determination of balloon position. For most fractures, this position will be 5 mm from the anterior cortex and centered between the endplates on the lateral view, with the anterior-posterior view showing the distal tip of the balloon appearing to touch the image of the cortex of the spinous process. A dose of 1 mL of contrast material is injected into the balloon to hold it in position. The contralateral side is then done in the same manner.

4. Balloon inflation is performed to reduce the fracture kyphosis and created a void in the body for placement of the PMMA.

   Contrast material is added to the balloons while one observes them with the C-arm and watches the pressure monitor on the inflation syringe. The balloons should be seen to enlarge within the vertebral body and flatten out smoothly against the endplates as the vertebral height is restored and/or the kyphosis is reduced (see Fig. 8–8). The pressure with the balloon should not exceed 300 psi. As the fracture reduces, the pressure will initially peak and then gradually degrade as the bone moves. Asymmetric inflation of the balloon or a sudden drop in resistance to injection may indicate a cortical breech that will allow PMMA extravasation and must be watched for carefully. If the balloon is placed properly in the vertebra, lateral or anterior cortical wall breech is rarely a problem. Therefore, the operator will need to observe balloon inflation mainly on the lateral view. However, if the balloon is placed too lateral within the body, the lateral cortex may be breached by the balloon, creating a large defect that is very difficult to salvage.

   The end points of inflation are reduction of the fracture or pressures of up to 300 psi with no significant degradation of the pressure over time or cortical wall contact by the balloon.

5. PMMA is now mixed to a liquid state. The standard formulation is to use half the powder of a standard batch mixed with 6 g of barium sulfate powder. The full amount of liquid monomer is then added and the mixture stirred until it liquefies. This is then drawn into 10-mL syringes and injected into the bone filler devices, with care taken to avoid injecting air bubbles into the tubes. Each tube contains 1.5 mL of PMMA. The cement is allowed to set up until it reaches a more viscous state. The consistency should be somewhat like soft-serve ice cream, allowing both controlled fill of the cavity created in the bone and interdigitation with the cancellous bone but resisting extravasation through small openings or passage out small vessels.

   The balloons are deflated and removed. A bone filler device containing PMMA is inserted into the cavity. Under continuous fluoroscopic monitoring, the PMMA is injected into the cavity while the operator watches for any leakage of cement. If the lateral cortex has not been violated, the lateral projection is viewed while one injects the cement, with occasional anterior-posterior views. The volume of cement injected is usually similar to or slightly less than the volume of inflation of the balloons. Adequate fill of the vertebra is achieved once the cavity is filled and cement is seen to infiltrate the cortical bone. Injection is stopped if any extravasation of cement is seen. Cement should not be allowed to progress into the posterior one quarter of the body because this risks cement leakage into the spinal canal.

   A spent bone filler device and plunger should be inserted into the cannula until the PMMA becomes firm, to prevent tails of cement extending up the path of the cannula.

6. Once the cement has cured, the cannulas are removed and the incisions closed, usually with a butterfly type strip, and a dressing applied. The patient is allowed to ambulate normally after recovery with no bracing required.

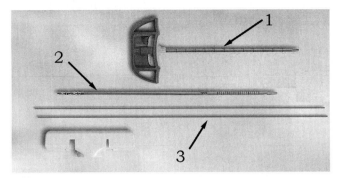

FIGURE 8-7

Osteo Introducer Cannula and Stylet. The kit includes the Osteo Introducer (arrow 1), a stylet (arrow 2), and wires (arrow 3).

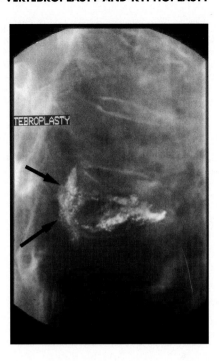

FIGURE 8-9

Leakage of Polymethylmethacrylate (PMMA) into the Spinal Canal after Vertebroplasty. A, Lateral radiograph of the thoracic spine reveals substantial leakage of PMMA into the spinal canal (arrows). The leakage occurred during injection of bone cement while the spine was being viewed in the anteroposterior projection. Magnetic resonance imaging and computed tomography of the thoracic spine (not shown) demonstrated mild to moderate compression of the spinal cord and leakage of PMMA into the right neural foramen. The patient experienced transient radicular pain that resolved following therapeutic nerve block. It is imperative that the operator inject the bone cement into the vertebral body while viewing the spine in the lateral projection to avoid this complication.

Complications

The complication rate from vertebroplasty and kyphoplasty is fortunately low, ranging from 1% to 10% (Jensen 2000). Reported complications include transient fever, transient worsening of pain, rib fracture, infection, and complications related to cement extravasation. Complications of cement leakage include bone cement pulmonary embolism, radiculitis related to foraminal extravasation, and cord compression from extravasation into the spinal canal (Figs. 8-9). The complication rate can be expected to be higher for patients with malignancy and osteolytic metastases (Cotten 1996) secondary to underlying bone destruction. Symptomatic pulmonary embolism may be the result of both PMMA emboli and fat emboli, displaced from the marrow space from injection of the PMMA. Therefore, many authors advocate limiting treatment to two of three levels at one setting. Excellent understanding of fluoroscopic spinal anatomy and fluoroscopic triangulation skills, meticulous technique, and adequate visualization of the bone cement at the time of delivery into the vertebral body will minimize complications from these procedures.

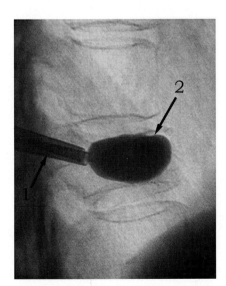

FIGURE 8-8

Lateral Radiograph after Balloon Dilatation and Cement Placement. The cannula extends down the pedicle (arrow 1), and the balloon is dilated and filled with radiopaque cement (arrow 2).

References

Barr JD, Barr MS, Lemley TJ, McCann RM. Percutaneous vertebroplasty for pain relief and spinal stabilization. Spine 2000; 25:923–928.

Cotten A, Dewatre F, Cortet B, Assaker R, Leblond D, Duquesnoy B, Chastanet P, Clarisse J. Percutaneous vertebroplasty for osteolytic metastases and myeloma: effects of the percentage of lesion filling and leakage of methyl methacrylate at clinical follow-up. Radiology 1996; 200:525–530.

Deramond H, Depriester C, Galibert P, Le Gars D. Percutaneous vertebroplasty with polymethylmethacrylate: technique, indications, and results. Radiol Clin North Am 1998; 36:533–546.

Evans AJ, Jensen ME, Kip KE, DiNardo AJ, Lawler GL, Negrin GA, Remley KB, Boutin SM, Dunnagan SA. Vertebral compression fractures: pain reduction and improvement in functional mobility after percutaneous polymethylmethacrylate vertebroplasty—retrospective review of 245 cases. Radiology 2003; 226:366–372.

Galibert P, Deramond H, Rosat P, Le Gars D. Note preliminaire sur le traitment des angiomas vertebraux par vertebroplastie acrilique percutanee. Neurochirurgie 1987; 233:166–168.

Garfin SR, Yuan HA, Reiley MA. New technologies in spine: kyphoplasty and vertebroplasty for the treatment of painful osteoporotic compression fractures. Spine 2001; 26:1511–1515.

Jarvik JG, Deyo RA. Cementing the evidence: time for a randomized trial of vertebroplasty. Am J Neuroradiol 2000; 21:1373–1374.

Jensen ME, Dion JE. Percutaneous vertebroplasty in the treatment of osteoporotic compression fractures. Neuroimag Clin North Am 2000; 10:547–568.

Kaufmann TJ, Jensen ME, Schweickert PA, Marx WF, Kallmes DF. Age of fracture and clinical outcomes of percutaneous vertebroplasty. Am J Neuroradiol 2001; 22:1860–1863.

Kim AK, Jensen ME, Dion JE, Schweickert PA, Kaufmann TJ, Kallmes DF. Unilateral transpedicular percutaneous vertebroplasty: initial experience. Radiology 2002; 222:737–741.

Martin JB, Jean B, Sugiu K, San Millan Ruiz D, Piotin M, Murphy K, Rufenacht B, Muster M, Rufenacht DA. Vertebroplasty: clinical experience and follow-up results. Bone 1999; 25:11S–15S.

Mathis JM, Barr JD, Belkolff SM, Barr MS, Jensen ME, Deramond H. Percutaneous vertebroplasty: a developing standard of care for vertebral compression fractures. Am J Neuroradiol 2001; 22:373–381.

Moreland DB, Landi MK, Grand W. Vertebroplasty: techniques to avoid complications. Spine Journal 2001; 1:66–71.

Murphy KJ, Deramond H. Percutaneous vertebroplasty in benign and malignant disease. Neuroimag Clin North Am 2000; 10:535–545.

9 Intradiscal Electrothermal Annuloplasty

DONALD L. RENFREW • MARK BECKNER

Definition

Intradiscal electrothermal annuloplasty (IDET) involves "introducing into the disc a flexible electrode that is threaded from within the nucleus to engage the annulus from the inside and pass circumferentially around the lateral and posterior annulus. The electrode is used to heat the annulus, ostensibly to coagulate the collagen of the annulus and any nociceptive nerve fibers in it." (Karasek 2000).

Literature Review

The first description of the IDET procedure was published in 2000 by Saal and Saal (Saal 2000a), followed by the first case series in the same year (Saal 2000b). In the prospective case series, 62 patients with chronic back pain underwent the procedure and were subsequently followed for a mean of 16 months and a minimum of 1 year. Patients had an average pain reduction of 3 points on a 10-point visual analogue scale, a difference that was statistically significant. Similarly, the patients demonstrated improvement according to scores on patient questionnaires (Short Form-36 Health Status Questionnaire Physical Function subscale and Short Form-26 Bodily Pain subscale). The same authors (Saal 2002) published an additional study in 2002 reporting the results of follow-up through a minimum of 2 years, with similar results. Karasek and Bogduk (2000) published a case-control study of 35 patients (with 17 control subjects) with improvements of disability and drug use and a return to work rate of 53%. A follow-up study of the same patients (Bogduk 2002) demonstrated that, by and large, patients maintained improvement at 2 years, with approximately half of the patients achieving at least 50% pain reduction and 20% achieving complete pain relief.

Kleinstueck and colleagues (2001) published a cadaver study in 2001 that demonstrated, according to their analysis, that the temperatures developed during IDET were insufficient to alter collagen architecture or stiffen the disc. However, Shah and colleagues (2001) did find collagen denaturation and coalescence in similarly treated discs; the authors of the latter study suggest in a letter (Hong 2002) that the reason for the variance was the use of higher-power magnification for histologic examination in the study that showed histologic changes with IDET temperatures.

Controversy continues regarding this procedure. In a critical clinical review paper published in 2001, Heary noted that the IDET procedure lacked animal experimentation data, peer-reviewed journal evidence for its mechanism of action, and randomized well-controlled studies to demonstrate its efficacy. For supporters, the work of Shah and colleagues (2001), showing collagen denaturation and coalescence in cadaver discs, may be taken as evidence for its mechanism of action, while the last of Heary's objections (the lack of randomized studies) has been at least partially addressed by Pauza and colleagues (2003): these authors showed a statistically significant improvement of pain in a blinded randomized controlled trial of the procedure. Note, however, that the degree of pain relief in this randomized controlled trial was not as dramatic as was achieved in Karasek and Bogduk's earlier uncontrolled study. Such differences may be attributed to patient selection, technical factors, or an added placebo effect in the earlier, nonblinded study.

Rationale for Procedure

As stated by Shah and colleagues (2001), "The therapeutic mechanism may be a combination of effects including destruction of annular nociceptive fibers, cauterization of vascular ingrowth, or induction of healing of annular tears." These authors also go on to state, however, that "the precise mechanism is unknown and further studies are required."

Equipment and Supplies[1]

Table 9-1 lists equipment required for IDET.

---

[1]This section is similar to the Equipment and Supplies section in Chapter 2 and can be skipped if the reader is already familiar with this material.

TABLE 9–1. Equipment and Supplies for IDET

C-arm fluoroscope
Surgical scrub
Needles for local anesthesia
Syringes
Connecting tubes
Nonionic contrast material
Anesthetic
Special proprietary equipment including needle and heating
   catheter

A C-arm device is necessary for IDET. A laser aiming device (an attachment that shows a cross-hair on the fluoroscopic screen corresponding in position to a red dot on the skin surface) is extremely helpful for proper needle placement. Manufacturers produce kits for these procedures that include the requisite items.

In addition to the equipment listed in Table 9–1, a crash cart should be readily available to handle medical emergencies (e.g., contrast media and drug reactions).

Informed Consent Issues

Informed consent issues can be divided into a description of the procedure, warning the patient about a flare in pain following the procedure, and delineation of material risks. The risks, benefits, and alternatives to the procedure should be addressed, including continued conservative management on the one hand and fusion surgery on the other.

Complications appear to be very rare. Heary (2001) states that virtually no published complications have occurred but notes "anecdotal reports" of bacterial discitis, thermal nerve root injury, and catheter breakage. In addition, Hsia and colleagues (2000) have reported a case of apparently permanent cauda equina syndrome following IDET, wherein the catheter was mistakenly placed through a posterior annular fissure and into the spinal canal.

Patient Selection

The IDET procedure was designed to treat "internal disc derangement." Criteria for selection of patients are relatively strict in published trials (Saal 2000b) and include the following:

1. Unremitting, persistent back pain for at least 6 months' continuous duration
2. No satisfactory improvement with nonoperative care
3. Normal neurologic examination findings
4. Negative straight-leg raising test result
5. No neurologically compressive lesion on magnetic resonance imaging
6. Positive discogram with negative control level

Karasek and Bogduk (2000) also noted of the patients in their series that "the majority of patients treated had single-level discogenic pain, and all had preserved disc heights. No patients with severe disc degradation were treated." Additional applicable criteria may also include a lack of magnetic resonance imaging findings for specific pathologic conditions known to cause low back pain (e.g., disc herniation, spinal stenosis, spondylolisthesis) and psychological criteria such as a lack of psychological barriers to recovery and presence of motivation to recover with realistic expectations (Karasek 2002).

Note that the same comments regarding the entity of "internal disc disruption" presented in Chapter 6 apply here.

Procedure Description

Table 9–2 describes and Figures 9–1, 9–2, and 9–3 illustrate the IDET procedure.

Several problems or pitfalls may be encountered during the IDET procedure. Table 9–3 lists these problems and possible solutions. Note that fluid within the disc may act as a "heat sink" during heating and prevent effective disc treatment. Therefore, it is best to wait for at least 2 weeks after discography to perform the IDET procedure, and that injection of contrast material, antibiotics, or other fluids should not be done prior to performance of the procedure (although antibiotics should be injected following the procedure). Furthermore, the tip of the catheter should not be close to the introducer needle, or improper heating may also result.

TABLE 9–2. Step-by-Step Description of Intradiscal Electrothermal Annuloplasty

1. Prior to the procedure, plan the route of approach (right- or left-sided) using the patient's disco-CT. It is usually best to enter the disc on the side opposite the patient's pain and/or annular fissure.
2. Place the patient prone on the procedure table. Prepare and drape the patient in sterile fashion. Depending on the patient's body habitus, a bolster under the patient may be necessary to straighten lumbar lordosis.
3. Test the catheter/generator system.
    a. The actual temperature should equal room temperature.
    b. The impedence should measure between 85 and 230 ohms.
4. Align the C-arm fluoroscope as if performing discography on the disc to be treated. See Chapter 6 for procedural details. Thorough familiarity with discography is a prerequisite for performance of IDET.
5. Anesthetize a tract from the skin surface to the disc margin, using a 25-gauge needle. Anesthetize either "on the way in" or "on the way out," depending on the method chosen for placing the introducer needle (see the next step).
6. Place the introducer needle from the IDET kit to the disc margin. This may be done via one of three methods:
    a. Remove the 25-gauge needle, infiltrating with anesthetic as you withdraw the needle, and raising a skin wheal. The patient must remain in exactly the same position. Place the introducer needle along the same path as that taken by the anesthesia needle.
    b. Place the introducer needle directly alongside the 25-gauge needle. If using this method, be sure to anesthetize the skin surface and other structures duing introduction of the 25-gauge needle.
    c. Put a guide wire through the 25-gauge needle and use this to guide the introducer needle along the identical path to the disc margin. In this case, it is also necessary to anesthetize the needle track "on the way in."
7. Enter the disc with the introducer needle, passing through the annulus and into the nucleus. Ideally, the needle tip should be at the midpoint of the disc in the anterior-to-posterior direction, and slightly lateral to midline (toward the side of disc entry). See Figure 9–1.
8. Turn the introducer needle so that the directional indicator on the needle hub faces posterior.
9. Thread the heating catheter through the introducer needle so that it reaches the opposite, anterior margin of the disc, then coils around the nuclear/annular junction or within the inner annulus to pass along the opposite, posterior margin of the disc and then the same side, posterior margin of the disc. Use the radiopaque markers on the catheter to ensure that the heating element of the catheter is along the posterior margin of the disc, or at least that the heating element crosses the patient's annular fissure. Note that the heating element is contained between the radiopaque markers. See Figures 9–2 and 9–3.
10. Once the catheter has achieved an acceptable position, heat the disc.
    a. Verify correct generator settings. Consult the generator manual.
    b. Verify impedence range is acceptable (85–230 ohms).
    c. Choose heating program. The manufacturers supply these. In general, the catheter needs to reach one of the following end-points: 80 degrees held for 6 minutes, 85 degrees held for 5 minutes, or 90 degrees (the maximum temperature) held for 4 minutes.
    d. Activate the thermal generator.
    e. After heating the disc (total time is usually 14–20 minutes), the generator will automatically stop.
11. Disconnect the catheter from the generator.
12. Remove the heating catheter. Inspect the catheter for damage. In general, it is a good idea to indicate in the procedure description (if appropriate) that the catheter was removed intact with no damage to the wire coating.
13. If administering antibiotics, place them through the introducer needle into the disc at this point of the procedure.
14. Remove the introducer needle.
15. If necessary, repeat the process at the same level from the opposite side or at a second level.
16. Ensure that appropriate postprocedure care is performed.
    a. Give the patient and/or an individual responsible for the patient's care contact information if any questions or concerns arise. Reasons for concern include fever or chills, neurologic symptoms, and exacerbation of existing pain.
    b. Narcotic analgesics will most likely be required for, at minimum, several days and often several weeks following the procedure.
    c. Prescribe a lumbosacral corset to be worn while upright for the first 6 weeks after the procedure.
    d. Instruct the patient to avoid bending or twisting at the waist for at least 6 weeks.
    e. Instruct the patient to limit sitting to 30 to 60 minutes at a time for the first 6 weeks.
    f. Instruct the patient that light to sedentary work can normally be resumed in 1 to 3 weeks if the patient adheres to proper body mechanics.
    g. At 6 weeks, prescribe starting (or resuming) spine stabilization exercises.

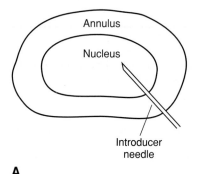
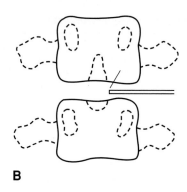
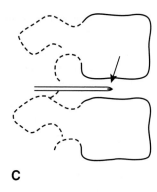

A B C

FIGURE 9–1

Ideal Position of Introducer Needle. A, Axial view of the disc as seen from above with the introducer needle entering the posterior, right side of the disc. The needle is in good position for threading of the heating catheter. **B,** Frontal view of the disc and adjacent vertebrae demonstrates that the introducer needle tip (arrow) is to the right of midline, about one third the way across the intervertebral disc. **C,** Lateral view of the disc and adjacent vertebrae demonstrates that the introducer needle tip (arrow) is just slightly posterior to the anterior-to-posterior midpoint of the intervertebral disc. (Modified from a drawing provided by Smith-Nephew, Memphis, TN.)

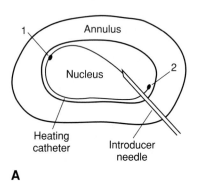
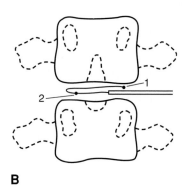
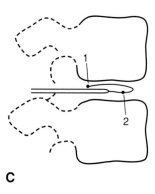

A B C

FIGURE 9–2

Drawing of Ideal Position of Introducer Needle and Heating Catheter. A, Axial drawing of the disc as seen from above with the introducer needle entering the posterior, right side of the disc. The heating catheter is coiled along the nucleus/annulus interface. The portion of the catheter between the distal (arrow 1) and proximal (arrow 2) radiopaque markers denotes the active portion of the catheter (which will be heated). **B,** Frontal drawing of the disc and adjacent vertebrae shows the active portion of the heating catheter (between the distal [arrow 1] and proximal [arrow 2] markers crossing the midline). Note that from this projection alone, it is not possible to say whether the active portion of the catheter is across the posterior or anterior aspect of the intervertebral disc. **C,** Lateral drawing of the disc and adjacent vertebrae shows the active portion of the catheter (between the distal [arrow 1] and proximal [arrow 2] markers along the posterior aspect of the intervertebral disc). (Modified from a drawing provided by Smith-Nephew, Memphis, TN.)

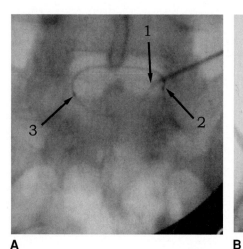
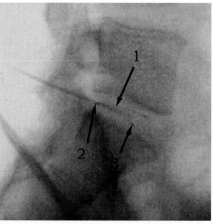

A B

FIGURE 9–3

Radiographs of Ideal Position of Introducer Needle and Heating Catheter. A, Frontal radiograph demonstrates the introducer needle tip (arrow 1) lateral to the midline. The active portion of the heating catheter between the distal (arrow 1) and proximal (arrow 2) radiopaque markers crosses the midline. **B,** Lateral radiograph demonstrates the introducer needle tip (arrow 1) slightly posterior to the anterior-to-posterior midpoint of the disc. The distal (arrow 2) and proximal (arrow 3) radiopaque markers indicate that the active portion of the heating catheter lies along the posterior disc margin.

TABLE 9–3. Problems Encountered during Intradiscal Electrothermal Annuloplasty

Problem	Possible Solution
Introducer needle placement is incorrect. If the needle tip is medial and posterior (see Fig. 9–4) or if it is lateral and anterior (see Fig. 9–5), the catheter may not feed freely around the inner margin of the annulus.	As noted in Table 9–2, the needle tip should be at the midpoint of the disc in the anterior-to-posterior direction, and slightly lateral to midline (toward the side of disc entry). Repositioning the introducer needle to a more optimal position should be done. Be sure to remove the catheter from the introducer needle before making any major changes in the introducer needle's position.
The heating catheter won't feed through the tip of the introducer needle.	This may result from an incorrect introducer needle placement adjacent to or within the annulus. Repositioning of the introducer needle is usually necessary.
Even though it leaves the introducer needle tip, the heating catheter won't feed along the inner margin of the annulus. For example, the catheter may bow or even kink when fed through the introducer needle (see Fig. 9–6).	As the catheter follows the path of least resistance, the tip may become lodged in annular fibers or otherwise positioned so that it will not feed appropriately. In this case, gentle to-and-fro motions and rotations of the catheter are usually effective at getting the catheter to advance. Occasionally, it is necessary to reposition the introducer needle in order to get the catheter to follow the correct path. It may help to reposition the introducer needle and heating catheter as a unit, but this should be done very cautiously, because such movement runs the risk of kinking or even shearing off the catheter. If acceptable catheter position cannot be obtained, it may be necessary to discontinue the procedure from the current side and attempt to position the catheter via a contralateral approach.
The heating catheter fails to reach ideal position (see Fig. 9–7).	Attempt to reposition the catheter so that it does reach ideal position. Remember that if the heating element crosses the annular fissure and the patient's pain lateralizes to the side of the annular fissure, this may represent an acceptable position. However, if the pain is bilateral or on the side opposite the portion of the annulus that has been treated, proceeding with a contralateral procedure may be necessary to treat the remaining (and presumably symptomatic) portion of the annulus.
The heating catheter leaves the disc margin (see Figs. 9–8 and 9–9).	*Do not heat the catheter if this has happened.* The catheter must be repositioned prior to heating.
The patient complains of radicular pain, or unfamiliar and intense pain, upon heating of the catheter.	*Immediately stop heating the catheter if this happens.* The catheter needs to be moved. Assess catheter position carefully in multiple fluoroscopic planes, and reposition catheter to a different position. If acceptable catheter position cannot be obtained, it may be necessary to discontinue the procedure from the current side and attempt to position the catheter via a contralateral approach.
The heating catheter won't withdraw through the introducer needle.	Gently roll and wiggle the catheter and attempt to withdraw it again. If after repeated manipulations with gentle withdrawal tension the catheter still will not slide out of the introducer needle, it is possible to slowly withdraw the introducer needle and catheter as a unit. Note that the disc may be punctured with another needle for instillation of antibiotics if necessary.

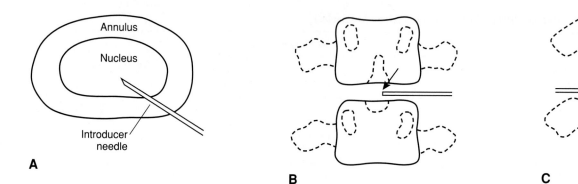

FIGURE 9–4

Suboptimal Position of Introducer Needle, with the Needle Tip Located Too Far Posteriorly. A, Axial view of the disc as seen from above with the intro-ducer needle entering the posterior, right side of the disc. If the catheter is advanced through the introducer needle with the needle in this position, it may deviate anteriorly when it reaches the opposite side of the nucleus. **B,** Frontal view of the disc and adjacent vertebrae demonstrates that the introducer needle tip (arrow) is at the midline, rather than to the right of midline (compare to Figure 9–1). **C,** Lateral view of the disc and adjacent vertebrae demon-strates that the introducer needle tip (arrow) is at about the midpoint of the intervertebral disc. (Modified from a drawing provided by Smith-Nephew, Memphis, TN.)

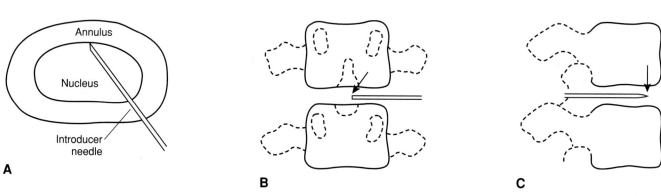

FIGURE 9–5

Suboptimal Position of Introducer Needle, with the Needle Tip Located Too Far Anteriorly. A, Axial view of the disc as seen from above with the intro-ducer needle entering the posterior, right side of the disc. If the catheter is advanced through the introducer needle with the needle in this position, it may not advance because of the needle tip position against the annulus. **B,** Frontal view of the disc and adjacent vertebrae demonstrates that the introducer needle tip (arrow) is at the midline. **C,** Lateral view of the disc and adjacent vertebrae demonstrates that the introducer needle tip (arrow) is too far ante-riorly within the intervertebral disc. Compare to Figure 9–1. (Modified from a drawing provided by Smith-Nephew, Memphis, TN.)

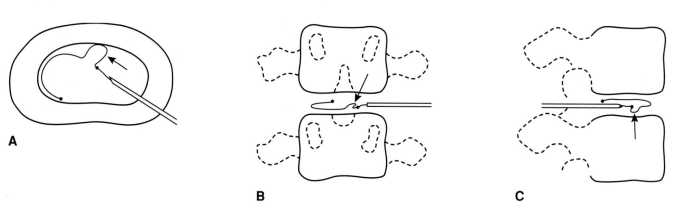

FIGURE 9–6

Failure of Heating Catheter to Advance. A, Axial view of the disc as seen from above with the introducer needle entering the posterior, right side of the disc. Although the heating catheter has advanced along the interface between the annulus and the nucleus, it has apparently encountered resistance at the tip, with a bow (arrow) forming along the more proximal aspect of the catheter where it leaves the introducer needle. **B,** Frontal view of the disc and adja-cent vertebrae shows the bow (arrow) of the catheter as it leaves the introducer needle. **C,** Lateral view of the disc and adjacent vertebrae shows the bow (arrow) of the catheter as it leaves the introducer needle. (Modified from a drawing provided by Smith-Nephew, Memphis, TN.)

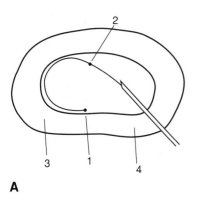
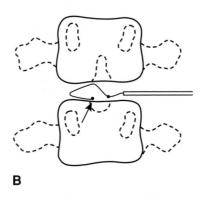
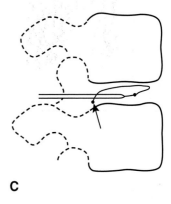

A   **B**   **C**

FIGURE 9–7

Possibly Inappropriate Catheter Position. A, Axial view of the disc as seen from above with the introducer needle entering the posterior, right side of the disc. The heating element will treat the area from the distal radiopaque marker (1) to the proximal radiopaque marker (2). The heating catheter is in an acceptable position to treat an annular fissure in the posterior side opposite the side of entry (3), but not an annular fissure on the side ipsilateral to the side of entry (4). B, Frontal view of the disc and adjacent vertebrae shows that the distal radiopaque marker (arrow) of the heating catheter, marking the distal tip, has not passed back to cross the midline but remains on the side opposite the introducer needle. C, Lateral view of the disc and adjacent vertebrae shows the heating catheter with its distal tip (arrow) located posteriorly. Note that from only this position, it would not be possible to confirm that the heating catheter was in a possibly unacceptable position. (Modified from a drawing provided by Smith-Nephew, Memphis, TN.)

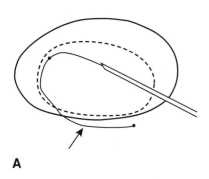
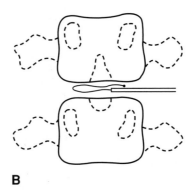
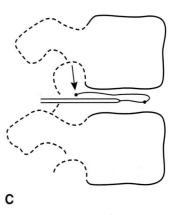

A   **B**   **C**

FIGURE 9–8

Definitely Inappropriate Catheter Position, with the Catheter out of the Disc. A, Axial view of the disc as seen from above with the introducer needle entering the posterior, right side of the disc. The end of the catheter (arrow) has left the disc and is in a dangerous position outside the posterior aspect of the intervertebral disc. *The heating catheter should never be activated in this position.* Neurologic damage could result from heating nerve roots within the spinal canal. B, Frontal view of the disc and adjacent vertebrae shows the heating catheter to project within the intervertebral disc. Note that from this projection alone, it would not be possible to recognize the dangerous position of the catheter. This emphasizes the critical importance of multiple views when performing intradiscal electrothermal annuloplasty. C, Lateral view of the disc and adjacent vertebrae shows the heating catheter with the end of the catheter (arrow) posterior to the intervertebral disc. (Modified from a drawing provided by Smith-Nephew, Memphis, TN.)

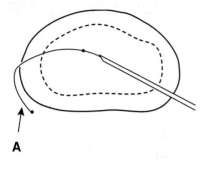

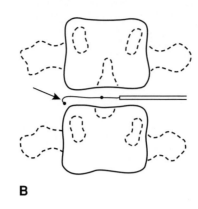

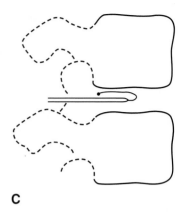

FIGURE 9–9

Definitely Inappropriate Catheter Position, with the Catheter out of the Disc. A, Axial view of the disc as seen from above with the introducer needle entering the posterior, right side of the disc. The end of the catheter (arrow) has left the disc and is in a dangerous position lateral to the intervertebral disc. *The heating catheter should never be activated in this position.* Neurologic damage could result from heating the spinal segmental nerve. **B,** Frontal view of the disc and adjacent vertebrae shows the end of the heating catheter (arrow) projecting out of the intervertebral disc. **C,** Lateral view of the disc and adjacent vertebrae shows that the heating catheter projects within the intervertebral disc. Note that from this projection alone, it would not be possible to recognize the dangerous position of the catheter. This emphasizes the critical importance of multiple views when performing intradiscal electrothermal annuloplasty. (Modified from a drawing provided by Smith-Nephew, Memphis, TN.)

References

Bogduk N, Karasek M. Two-year follow-up of a controlled trial of intradiscal electrothermal anuloplasty for chronic low back pain resulting from internal disc disruption. Spine J 2002; 2:343–350.

Heary RF. Intradiscal electrothermal annuloplasty: the IDET procedure. J Spinal Disord 2001; 14:353–360.

Hsia AW, Isaac K, Katz JS. Cauda equina syndrome from intradiscal electrothermal therapy. Neurology 2000; 55:320.

Hong HM, Lutz GE. Letter. Spine 2002; 27:1248–1250.

Karasek ME, Bogduk N. Twelve month follow-up of a controlled trial of intradiscal thermal anuloplasty for back pain due to internal disc disruption. Spine 2000; 25:2601–2607.

Karasek ME, Carragee EJ (Discussants). Curve/countercurve: intradiscal electrothermal therapy. SpineLine 2002; March/April:12–18.

Kleinstueck FS, Diederich CJ, Nau WH, Puttlitz CM, Smith JA, Bradford DS, Lotz JC. Acute biomechanical and histologic effects of intradiscal electrothermal therapy on human lumbar discs. Spine 2001; 26:2198–2207.

Pauza K, Howell S, Dreyfuss P, Peloza J, Dawson K, Park K, Bogduk N. Randomized placebo-controlled trial of intradiscal electrothermal therapy for chronic low back pain. Presented at the 2003 Annual Scientific Conference of the Spine Society of Australia, April 25–27, 2003.

Saal JS, Saal JA. Management of chronic discogenic low back pain with a thermal intradiscal catheter: a preliminary report. Spine 2000a; 25:382–388.

Saal JA, Saal JS. Intradiscal electrothermal treatment for chronic discogenic low back pain: a prospective outcome study with minimum 1-year follow-up. Spine 2000b; 25:2622–2627.

Saal JA, Saal JS. Intradiscal electrothermal treatment for chronic discogenic low back pain. Prospective outcome study with a minimum 2 year follow-up. Spine 2002; 27:966–974.

Shah RV, Lutz GE, Lee J, Doty SB, Rodeo S. Intradiskal electrothermal therapy: a preliminary histologic study. Arch Phys Med Rehabil 2001; 82:1230–1237.

10 Myelography

DONALD L. RENFREW

This chapter emphasizes the technical, rather than the interpretive, factors involved in myelography.

Definition

Myelography is the introduction of contrast material into the thecal sac for diagnostic purposes.

Literature Review

Oil-based contrast material began to be supplanted in the 1970s by the water-based contrast material metrizamide (Amundsen 1975, Gonsette 1973, Skalpe 1975) and subsequently by alternate water-based contrast materials iopamidol and iohexol (Elkin 1986, Floras 1990). Water-based contrast materials allowed myelography to be wedded to computed tomography (CT), and this marriage resulted in the best imaging option until supplanted by magnetic resonance imaging (MRI). Magnetic resonance imaging, supplemented on occasion by "magnetic resonance myelography" (Nagayama 2002) has largely supplanted both myelography and CT-myelography in most institutions; interestingly, Zeng and colleagues (Zeng 1999) report the use of intrathecal gadopentetate dimeglumine (gadolinium) with subsequent MRI, a technique that may result in a return to intrathecal injection. In addition, a recent article by Bartynski and Lin (2003) suggests that myelography may better assess nerve root compression compared with MRI.

Two topics merit review from the technical aspect: placement of contrast material and prevention and treatment of "post-tap headaches."

Placement of Contrast Material

Oil-based contrast materials had many disadvantages and were justifiably replaced; however, one of their strengths was that they allowed a "complete" myelogram to be performed by movement of the contrast material from the lumbar to the thoracic and then the cervical region. When first introduced, water-based contrast material did not share this feature, because it became too dilute to visualize (at least without CT). Myelographers employed two methods to overcome this difficulty: instillation of contrast material in

C1-2 puncture and lumbar puncture procedures with subsequent manipulation of the patient to "run the contrast up."

Kelly and Alexander first described lateral C1-2 puncture for oil-based myelography in 1968 as a problem-solving technique when lumbar puncture was difficult (Kelly 1968). In 1972, Heinz and Goldman described C1-2 puncture for gas myelography (Heinz 1972), and in 1975 Amundsen and Skalpe described C1-2 puncture for water-soluble contrast material (Amundsen 1975). Lateral fluoroscopy was used to direct a spinal needle into the subarachnoid space between the posterior arch of C1 and the lamina of C2. Interestingly, the initial papers described a needle position in the anterior one third of the canal (Kelly 1968), an approach modified by Rice and Bathia in 1979 (Rice 1979) to avoid injury to the cord and vertebral artery. Because of the generous anteroposterior dimension of the subarachnoid space relative to the anteroposterior dimension of the spinal cord at this level, this lateral C1-2 approach usually succeeded in producing subarachnoid puncture and myelography. Unfortunately, unless MRI has been done, it is difficult to be certain that a spinal needle directed toward this space will not encounter low-lying cerebellar tonsils or an aberrant vertebral artery. Furthermore, variation in the cord diameter and in the position of the posterior margin of the subarachnoid space may make it difficult to simultaneously avoid the spinal cord and obtain access to the subarachnoid space. For these reasons, significant complications of C1-2 puncture have been reported, including subarachnoid hematoma with neurologic deficit (Abla 1986) and spinal cord injection resulting in permanent neurologic damage (Johansen 1983) and death (Rogers 1983). The most severe complications follow puncture of the vertebral artery, which may be unavoidable in certain cases despite excellent needle position: Katoh and colleagues (Katoh 1990) reported that 2% of reviewed arteriograms demonstrated that the vertebral artery lies in the posterior one third of the canal at the C1-2 level.

Lumbar puncture with manipulation of the patient to move the contrast material from the lumbar to the cervical position has been advocated as an alternative to C1-2 puncture for cervical myelography. Sortland (1977) advocated a head-down position with cervical extension by using a tilting table; Tamura (1991) accomplished the same goal on a flat table by placing the patient in a "knee-chest" position (Fig. 10–1). Although transport of the contrast material results in some compromise of image quality for the plain film myelography portion of the examination (Sortland

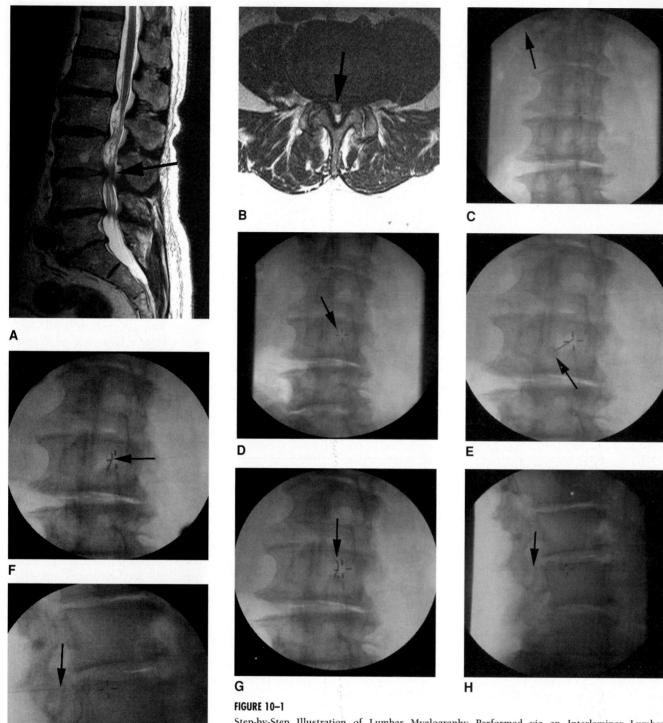

FIGURE 10–1

Step-by-Step Illustration of Lumbar Myelography Performed via an Interlaminar Lumbar Approach. This 70-year-old man had progressive lower extremity weakness and numbness. *A*, Sagittal T2-weighted magnetic resonance imaging (MRI) study demonstrates multilevel degenerative disc disease with disc bulging and spinal stenosis, most severe at the L3-4 level (arrow). *B*, Axial T2-weighted MRI study at the L3-4 level demonstrates narrowing of the spinal canal (arrow) secondary to a combination of degenerative disc bulging and facet arthropathy. *C*, Frontal fluoroscopic view obtained for evaluation of levels in the lumbar spine demonstrates a rib at the top of the field of view (arrow). The cross-hairs of the laser aiming device are therefore at the L2-3 level. *D*, Oblique view after adjusting the C-arm so that the cross-hairs of the laser aiming device are directed at the left L2-3 interlaminar space. The laser is inferior to the inferior margin (arrow) of the inferior articular process of L2. *E*, Oblique view after anchoring a 25-gauge needle in the skin. The hub of the needle (arrow) is inferior and lateral to the tip (located in the central portion of the cross-hairs of the laser aiming device). Thus, the bevel should be directed superior and to the right as the needle is advanced to enter the spinal canal through the L2-3 interlaminar space. *F*, Oblique view following advancement of the needle with the bevel directed superiorly and to the right demonstrates that the needle has altered course (arrow). The bevel should be directed superiorly and laterally to bring the needle to the middle of the left L2-3 interlaminar space. *G*, Oblique view following further advancement of the needle. Although the needle tip continued along the same line following bevel adjustment, a distinct change of resistance was palpated. The needle tip projects just at or above the inferior articular margin of the left L2 inferior articular process, indicating that the needle is either posterior to the laminae (and will encounter bone soon) or that it is anterior to the laminae (and thus in the spinal canal). The C-arm fluoroscope should be turned to lateral position at this time. *H*, Lateral view demonstrates the needle with the tip apparently in the middle of the spinal canal (arrow). However, the needle tip is somewhat difficult to identify. *I*, Lateral view with magnification better demonstrates the needle tip (arrow). The stylus was removed and no cerebrospinal fluid was forthcoming, indicating that the needle tip was probably slightly posterior to ideal position.

Continued

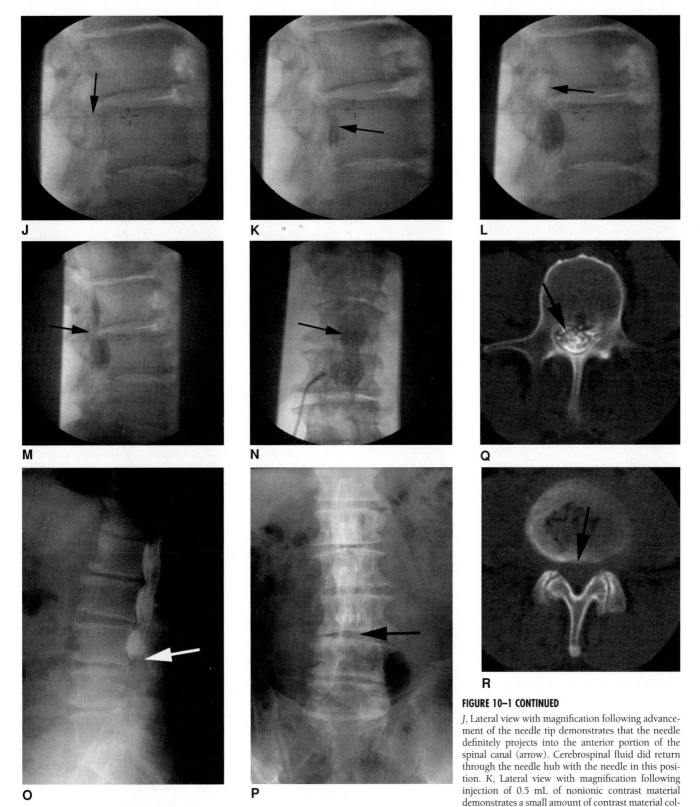

FIGURE 10–1 CONTINUED

J, Lateral view with magnification following advancement of the needle tip demonstrates that the needle definitely projects into the anterior portion of the spinal canal (arrow). Cerebrospinal fluid did return through the needle hub with the needle in this position. *K*, Lateral view with magnification following injection of 0.5 mL of nonionic contrast material demonstrates a small amount of contrast material collecting along the posterior surface of the L3 vertebral body (arrow). Although appearances in this regard may sometimes be deceiving, the contrast material appears to be intrathecal. *L*, Lateral view with magnification following injection of an additional 1.0 mL of nonionic contrast material demonstrates contrast along the posterior L2-3 intervertebral disc margin and along the posterior aspect of the L2 vertebral body (arrow), with a thin line of contrast highly characteristic of intrathecal injection. *M*, Lateral view without magnification following injection of an additional 1.0 mL of nonionic contrast material shows further spread of material in the thecal sac (arrow). *N*, Frontal view following injection of an additional 1.0 mL of nonionic contrast material shows further, superior spread of contrast material in the thecal sac (arrow). A total of 10.0 mL of Omnipaque 240 mg/mL was injected and plain films were taken. *O*, Lateral myelogram demonstrates complete block to flow at the L3-4 level (arrow). Note multilevel degenerative disc disease. *P*, Frontal view from the myelogram again demonstrates complete block to flow at L3-4 (arrow). *Q*, Axial computed tomographic (CT) scan following myelography at the level of the L3 pedicles. There is contrast in the thecal sac (arrow) surrounding nerve roots. *R*, Axial CT scan following myelography at the level of the L3-4 intervertebral disc. No contrast is seen within the spinal canal, consistent with severe stenosis. This CT study was actually the second CT study done following contrast injection: the first study was done approximately 1 hour after injection, and this study was performed after an additional hour in which the patient was upright for the duration, despite which no contrast flowed through the level of stenosis (lower levels had no contrast either). Note that the bony margins of the canal underestimate the degree of stenosis, as does the MRI examination. On the basis of the myelogram, the patient's scheduled stenosis surgery was moved to an earlier date.

1977), the CT portion is generally equally diagnostic using either method.

Post-Myelography Headaches

Post-myelography headaches may occur because of a "nocebo" effect (Hahn 1997), because of neural irritation of the contrast material, or because of the spinal tap performed. The first two effects generally abate in a relatively short period, whereas spinal tap headaches may persist and often require specific treatment. Usually, spinal tap headaches are positional, with the headache being severe when the patient is in an upright position and much milder or absent when the patient is supine (Raskin 1990). Awwad and colleagues (Awwad 1995) showed that the presence of epidural contrast "leaking" through the puncture site on the post-myelogram CT scan is predictive of development of a post-procedure headache: 57% of such patients got a headache, compared with only 20% of patients without such leakage.

Sand, in a 1989 meta-analysis of headaches following myelography, found that larger (20-gauge or larger) needles were more frequently associated with headache than smaller (22-gauge or smaller) needles (Sand 1989), a finding supported by a study by Wilkinson and Sellar in 1991 (Wilkinson 1991). In addition to needle size, the type of needle seems to play a role in headache causation: Braune and Huffman (Braune 1992) found that use of the usual sharp Quincke needle resulted in post-puncture headache in 36% of cases, whereas use of an "atraumatic" (pencil-point, Sprotte) needle reduced this percentage to 4%. Similarly, Prager and colleagues (Prager 1996) found a reduction of post-puncture headaches from 25% to 8% when comparing Sprotte and Quincke needles.

In a 1990 review article on myelography, Raskin proposed that changes in cerebrospinal fluid volume "may be the signal closest to the headache mechanism." He postulated that adenosine receptor activation following volume loss was the cause of post-tap headaches, and noted that intravenous caffeine (500 mg, followed by an additional 500 mg in 2 hours if the first dose was unsuccessful) or theophylline (300 mg three times daily) were both effective in headache relief even though these drugs could not "patch" the hole in the dura created by lumbar puncture. If drug treatment is undesirable or unsuccessful, epidural injection of saline (20 mL/hr for 48 to 72 hours) or blood (single injection of 12 mL) can be used. Occasionally, the blood patch required repetition for success in treatment of the headache.

TABLE 10–1. Equipment and Supplies for Myelography

C-arm fluoroscope
Surgical scrub solution
Needles
Syringes
Connecting tube
Nonionic contrast material
Anesthetic agent (if desired for skin anesthetization)

Rationale for Procedure

Myelography and myelo-CT examinations provide diagnostic information regarding the spine.

Equipment and Supplies[1]

Table 10–1 lists equipment required for myelography. A standard fluoroscope can be used for myelography, but it is generally much more difficult to obtain ideal positioning than with a C-arm device. A laser aiming device (an attachment that shows a cross-hair on the fluoroscopic screen corresponding in position to a red dot on the skin surface) is extremely helpful for proper needle placement. Selection of needle type varies with the operator; generally speaking, a pencil-point 22- or 25-gauge needle is preferable, as these seem to result in the fewest headaches (see under Literature Review). In addition to the equipment listed in Table 10–1, a crash cart should be readily available to handle medical emergencies (e.g., contrast media reactions).

Informed Consent Issues

Informed consent issues can be divided into two topics: a description of the procedure and delineation of material risks. Informed consent also implies that alternatives to the proposed diagnostic method have been described. MRI has largely supplanted myelography and myelo-CT, and if MRI can be done but has not been, then performing MRI is probably preferable to performing myelo-CT. If MRI is not a good alternative, no other imaging method really offers comparable information, and treatment would need to be based on other data.

Either the performing physician or a trained subordinate should completely explain the entire procedure in detail to the patient prior to performance of the procedure. Patients who know what to expect are much less anxious than those who do not. A step-by-step description, including reassurance that the procedure takes only a few minutes, that many patients undergo a similar procedure every day, and that the amount of pain caused by needle insertion is similar to that caused by drawing blood or starting an intravenous access line, provides a considerable calming effect in most patients. Many patients may have heard "horror stories" regarding myelography because of the pain and complications of oil-based myelography: the procedure was typically done with larger needles and almost inevitably resulted in post-tap headaches. These patients need reassurance that technology has changed considerably and that modern myelography is much less traumatic than the myelography of 20 or 30 years ago.

Complications can be subdivided into two categories: occasional (but inevitable) and rare but reported or theoretical. Occasional complications include exacerbation of pain, vasovagal reactions, and spinal tap headaches. Exacerbation of pain occurs more frequently in patients

---

[1]This section is virtually identical to the Equipment and Supplies section in Chapter 2 and can be skipped if the reader is already familiar with this material.

TABLE 10–2. Step-by-Step Description of Lumbar Interlaminar Myelography

1. Position the C-arm fluoroscope so that a clear view of the appropriate interlaminar space is identified. Generally, the L2-3 space is a good level. This is below the spinal cord but superior enough to be away from the disc disease and spinal stenosis in most patients. In postoperative patients, it may be advisable to inject through the laminectomy defect.
2. Insert needle along the course of the x-ray beam far enough so that it is anchored.
3. Check position of the needle with a C-arm fluoroscope.
4. Adjust needle position as necessary while advancing in 3 to 5 mm increments.
5. Advance needle until it feels as if the needle has entered the thecal sac, or until the needle is clearly on a course to enter the thecal sac. Go to the lateral position.
6. If the needle tip is posterior to the spinal canal, advance until it projects within the spinal canal. Pay special attention to any "dural pop" or change in resistance as the needle is advanced.
7. When the needle appears to be in appropriate location, remove the stylus and assess for cerebrospinal fluid (CSF) return through the needle. With small needles, only a tiny amount of CSF may return. Adjust needle until CSF return is identified.
8. Inject 0.1 to 0.2 mL of nonionic contrast material and document an intrathecal position of the injected material. Reposition if not intrathecal.
9. Inject 8.0 to 12.0 mL of nonionic contrast material under fluoroscopic visualization.
10. Perform plain film radiography and CT myelography.
11. Release patient when stable. Advise patient to remain relatively horizontal for a 24-hour period. Provide patient with a telephone number to call if there is persistent or increased pain or numbness or if fever, swelling, or redness develops. Advise patient to call if a headache (particularly a positional headache worse when upright and at least partially relieved when horizontal) occurs.

with severe spinal stenosis and can be treated with pain medication. Vasovagal reactions are usually best treated with time, intravenous fluids, and atropine as necessary. Spinal tap headaches are reviewed in the section Literature Review; treatment includes bedrest, intravenous caffeine or oral theophylline, or epidural saline or blood patch.

Rare but potential complications of myelography depend on the site of injection. Cervical injections should be undertaken with great caution given the rare but serious nature of complications at this level. As noted earlier, these complications include epidural hematoma formation with neurologic deficit (Abla 1986), cord injection with neurologic deficit (Johansen 1983), and death (Rogers 1983). It should be noted that not all instances of cord injection are associated with permanent neurologic sequelae (Farese 1990, Nakstad 1988, Servo 1985). Other serious complications include contrast reaction and infection.

Patient Selection

Myelography and myelo-CT examinations have been largely supplanted by MRI. In some cases, implanted devices within the patient preclude MRI (e.g., cardiac pacers, certain aneurysm clips, certain otologic implants). In some cases, additional and complementary information is provided even after magnetic resonance myelography has been performed.

Procedure Description

Table 10–2 describes and Figures 10–1, 10–2, and 10–3 illustrate myelography performed via an interlaminar, lumbar approach. The following is the report associated with the case illustrated in Figure 10–1:

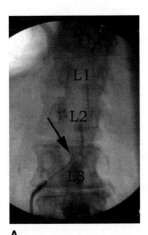
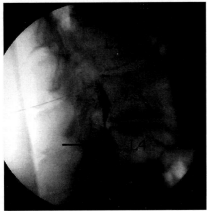
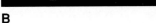
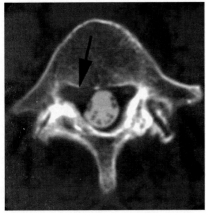

A **B** **C**

FIGURE 10–2

Lumbar Myelography in a Patient with a Pacer. This 78-year-old woman had chronic low back pain with the recent onset of right leg pain radiating into her lateral ankle. The patient had an indwelling cardiac pacer, precluding magnetic resonance imaging examination. *A,* Frontal view of myelogram demonstrating a 25-gauge needle in place beneath the left L2 laminae (arrow). Note that the lamina projects lower than the L2-3 intervertebral disc, and that contrast flows inferiorly from the level of injection. *B,* Lateral view during performance of the myelogram demonstrates the needle tip in the spinal canal at the L2-3 intervertebral disc level. Note that the contrast/cerebrospinal fluid interface forms a discrete horizontal "fluid-fluid" layer. This is the usual appearance on the lateral when performing myelography; in Figure 10–1, the patient's spinal stenosis prevented this appearance. *C,* Axial computed tomography study done following myelography demonstrates a right-sided cranially dissecting disc extrusion along the medial margin of the right L5 pedicle (arrow). The patient had excellent relief of pain following subsequent epidural steroid injection.

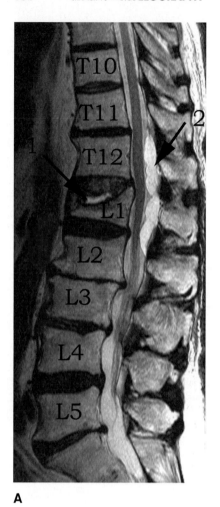

A

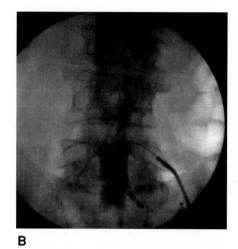

B

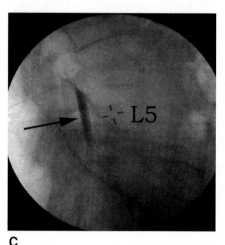

C

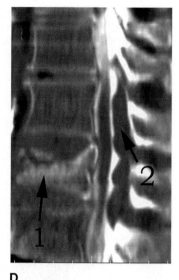

D

FIGURE 10–3

Injection Level Altered to Avoid a Known Tumor. This 84-year-old man had midback pain following yard work. He had no known primary malignancy. *A,* Sagittal T2-weighted magnetic resonance imaging scan demonstrates an L1 deformity with T2 prolongation (arrow 1) consistent with an acute or subacute compression fracture. There is multilevel degenerative disc disease. In addition, there is a posterior extradural multilevel fusiform tumor demonstrating relatively uniform T2 prolongation (arrow 2). Injection at the usual L2-3 level would result in puncture of the tumor, so a lower injection site was used. *B,* Frontal view obtained during myelography. The needle has been placed beneath the right L4 lamina and the needle tip is centered in the spinal canal (arrow). Contrast flows freely superiorly and inferiorly from the needle tip. *C,* Lateral view taken during myelography demonstrates the needle at the L4-5 level. The contrast forms a sharp "fluid-fluid" level with the cerebrospinal fluid (arrow). *D,* CT reconstruction done following myelography demonstrates the L1 compression fracture (arrow 1) as well as the posterior tumor (arrow 2).

INTRODUCTION

Back and leg pain. Leg weakness and numbness, with MRI examination demonstrating spinal stenosis.

The procedure and possible complications as well as alternatives to the procedure were discussed with the patient. Informed consent was obtained.

TECHNICAL INFORMATION

Using sterile technique and fluoroscopic guidance, a 3.5-inch 25-gauge spinal needle was placed in the subarachnoid space at the L2-3 level using a posterolateral, interlaminar approach, and 10 mL of iohexol (Omnipaque) 240 mg/mL was injected. Fluoroscopic spot films documented needle tip position and contrast flow. There were no immediate complications. Films were obtained and CT was subsequently performed (see separate report).

INTERPRETATION

The patient has extensive, multilevel degenerative disc disease. At L3-4, there is a complete block to contrast flow. This is persistent on the CT examination, even when one repeats the CT examination approximately 2 hours after original injection and has the patient ambulate and sit in the interim.

CONCLUSION

1. Complete block to flow of contrast material at the L3-4 level due to severe spinal stenosis secondary to degenerative changes.
2. Multilevel degenerative disc disease with vacuum phenomenon seen at multiple levels.
3. See CT-myelography report for further morphologic details.

When multilevel decompression surgery has been performed, there may be no interlaminar space left. In this case, placing the needle through the dorsal defect into the thecal sac is generally the best method of completing the examination (Figs. 10–4 and 10–5). This method of needle insertion is rarely associated with a post-tap headache, probably because scar formation prevents dural leakage. Note that epidural injections are difficult or impossible to perform at such levels. Intrathecal injections may also be difficult or impossible if there is arachnoiditis of the region

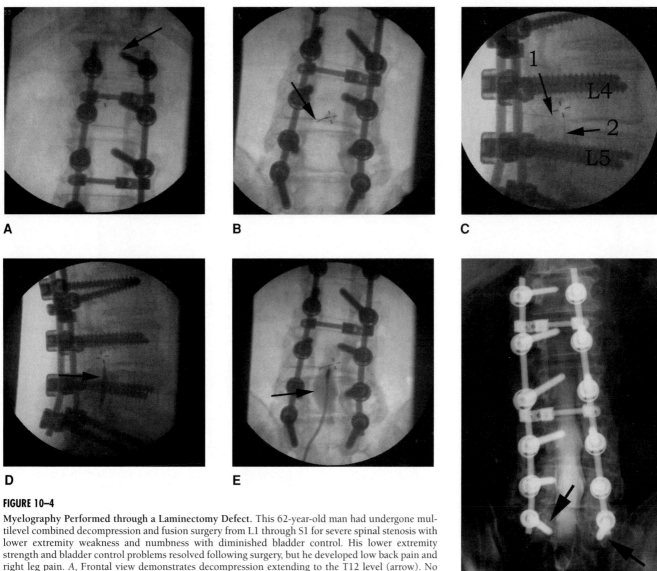

A

B

C

D

E

F

FIGURE 10–4

Myelography Performed through a Laminectomy Defect. This 62-year-old man had undergone multilevel combined decompression and fusion surgery from L1 through S1 for severe spinal stenosis with lower extremity weakness and numbness with diminished bladder control. His lower extremity strength and bladder control problems resolved following surgery, but he developed low back pain and right leg pain. *A*, Frontal view demonstrates decompression extending to the T12 level (arrow). No interlaminar space exists for needle placement. Note multilevel hardware. The level of spinal canal entry should be chosen so that the needle can be easily seen on the lateral examination; this is usually best accomplished by placing the needle approximately midway (from superior to inferior) between two sets of pedicle screws. *B*, Frontal view with a spinal needle in place through the laminectomy defect at the L4-5 level. The tip (arrow) projects approximately in the midline and about halfway between the L4 and L5 pedicle screws. The needle path may be difficult to control because of dense scar tissue, and the usual "dural pop" encountered as the needle passes through the dorsal dura will rarely be felt. *C*, Magnified lateral view during myelography. The needle tip (arrow 1) projects between the L4 and L5 pedicle screws. There was return of cerebrospinal fluid with the needle tip in this position, and 0.1 mL of contrast material was injected. This flows along the anterior spinal canal (arrow 2) in a thin, linear configuration typical of intrathecal injection. *D*, Lateral view following injection of an additional 0.5 mL of contrast material, demonstrating free flow in the anterior thecal sac (arrow). *E*, Frontal view following injection of an additional 1.0 mL of contrast material demonstrates flow away from the needle tip and into the spinal canal (arrow). *F*, Frontal view following completion of injection demonstrates lucency around the S1 pedicle screws (arrows) consistent with motion at the L5-S1 level. Computed tomographic examination (not shown) confirmed this lucency but demonstrated no significant neural compression. The patient's ongoing pain may have been due at least partly to persistent motion (pseudarthrosis) at the L5-S1 level.

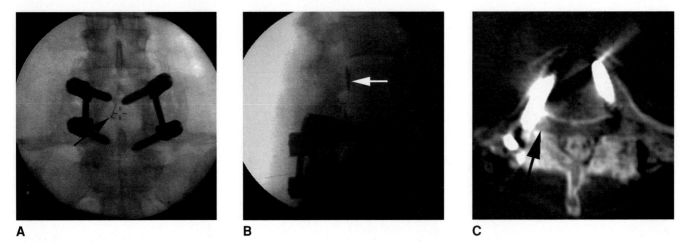

A   B   C

FIGURE 10–5

Myelography Performed through a Laminectomy Defect. This 63-year-old woman had low back pain and underwent decompression and fusion surgery. Following surgery, she developed new right hip pain radiating along the lateral thigh and to the lateral ankle and foot. *A,* Frontal view taken during myelography demonstrates L4 and L5 pedicle screws with lateral fusion graft material. The needle has a distal angle secondary to difficulty in advancing through scar tissue (arrow). *B,* Lateral view taken during myelography. Note that the hardware obscures the needle tip. However, cerebrospinal fluid flowed freely through the needle and it was believed to be safe to inject. Injection of 2.0 mL of nonionic contrast material resulted in contrast material accumulating along the ventral aspect of the thecal sac (arrow), typical of intrathecal injection. *C,* Axial computed tomography at the level of the L5 pedicles following myelography. The right L5 pedicle screw contacts the preganglionic L5 nerve root sleeve in the lateral recess (arrow) and may be the source of right lower extremity pain.

(Fig. 10–6). Even with no arachnoiditis, stenosis may complicate intrathecal injection (Fig. 10–7). Mixed epidural and intrathecal injections may be difficult to identify (see Fig. 10–7); occasionally, the examination may contin-ue, despite a mixed injection, with diagnostic results (Fig. 10–8).

Table 10–3 describes and Figure 10–9 illustrates myelography performed via a C1-2 cervical approach.

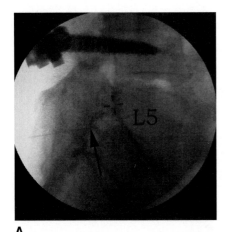

A

B

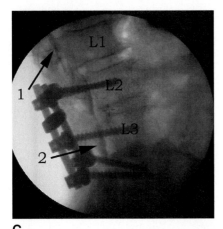

C

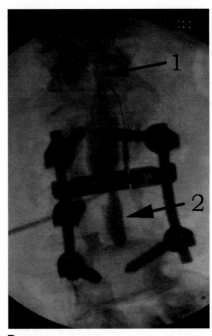

D

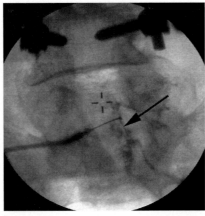

E

FIGURE 10–6

Myelography Attempted through a Laminectomy Defect which Failed, Followed by Successful Interlaminar Myelography. This 70-year-old man had undergone remote spinal fusion surgery with moderately good relief of low back pain, but with a gradual return of severe low back and bilateral leg pain. The patient had L2, L3, and L4 pedicle screws with dorsal interconnecting hardware. *A*, Lateral view taken during myelography demonstrates that the spinal needle projects within the spinal canal at the L5 level (arrow). A minimal amount of cerebrospinal fluid returned through the needle tip. *B*, Frontal view taken during myelography following injection of 1.0 mL of nonionic contrast material demonstrates contrast collecting in an irregular appearance along the right side of the spinal canal (arrow). The appearance is not convincing for an intrathecal location and may be epidural. Injection was discontinued at this level and the needle was removed. *C*, Lateral view following introduction of another 25-gauge needle at the T12-L1 level demonstrates the needle tip (arrow 1) in the posterior spinal canal. Contrast flows freely into the lower spinal canal (arrow 2). Note that injection at this level must be done with great caution and with close attention to any symptoms, since inadvertent injection into the distal spinal cord may occur. *D*, Frontal view demonstrates the needle tip at the T12-L1 level (arrow 1) with flow of contrast inferiorly. Filling is somewhat irregular at the inferior L3 level (arrow 2). *E*, Frontal view following completion of the injection and following ambulation. The contrast column ends at the top of the L4 vertebral body (arrow), consistent with severe adhesive arachnoiditis. Computed tomography study (not shown) confirmed complete lack of flow into the lower spinal canal, again indicative of adhesive arachnoiditis.

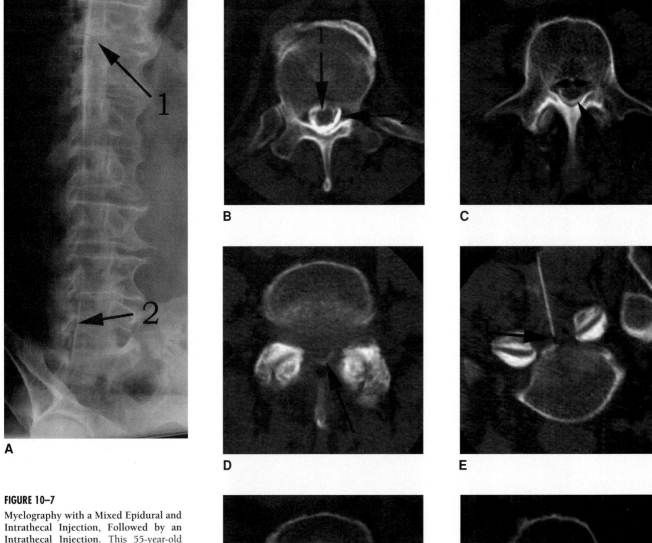

FIGURE 10-7

Myelography with a Mixed Epidural and Intrathecal Injection, Followed by an Intrathecal Injection. This 55-year-old patient had chronic low back and bilateral leg pain with a more recent onset of perineal pain, with suspected spinal stenosis. *A*, Oblique view following injection of 10.0 mL of nonionic contrast material demonstrates the spinal cord (arrow 1) at the lower thoracic level. There is a paucity of contrast material in the midlumbar region, with a thin band of contrast material in the lower lumbar spine (arrow 2). *B*, Axial computed tomographic (CT) scan at the bottom of the T12 pedicle following myelography. The spinal cord (arrow 1) is clearly seen, with intrathecal contrast surrounding it. There also may be some denser, posterolateral material suggesting a combined intrathecal/epidural injection (arrow 2). *C*, Axial CT scan at the level of the L3 pedicle demonstrates dense, peripheral contrast (arrow) in the spinal canal consistent with epidural placement. *D*, Axial CT scan at the level of the L4-5 intervertebral disc again demonstrates a small amount of peripheral contrast (arrow) consistent with epidural placement. Note degenerative disc bulging, severe bilateral facet arthropathy, and spinal stenosis. It was felt that the contrast injection pattern might be secondary to spinal stenosis but could also represent a combined intrathecal/epidural injection. The patient returned at a later date for puncture at the L5-S1 level. This was done under fluoroscopic control, but no cerebrospinal fluid was forthcoming. The patient was therefore transported to the CT scanner with the needle in place. *E*. Axial CT at the L5 level demonstrates the needle in place, with the tip (arrow) projecting within the spinal canal. No cerebrospinal fluid was forthcoming with the needle in this position, but injection of 0.5 mL of contrast material resulted in opacification of the thecal sac. *F*, Axial CT scan at the L4-5 level following contrast injection demonstrates a typical myelographic appearance, with the nerve roots seen as filling defects in the contrast column (arrow). Again seen is severe facet arthropathy and degenerative disc bulging. *G*, Axial CT scan at the L3 pedicle level also demonstrates the nerve roots as filling defects within the contrast column (arrow). Compare with image C, in which the contrast is in the epidural location.

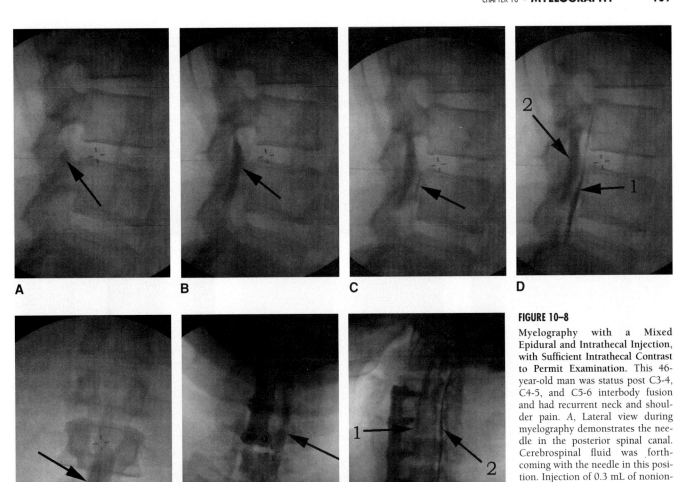

A   B   C   D

E   F   G

FIGURE 10–8

Myelography with a Mixed Epidural and Intrathecal Injection, with Sufficient Intrathecal Contrast to Permit Examination. This 46-year-old man was status post C3-4, C4-5, and C5-6 interbody fusion and had recurrent neck and shoulder pain. A, Lateral view during myelography demonstrates the needle in the posterior spinal canal. Cerebrospinal fluid was forthcoming with the needle in this position. Injection of 0.3 mL of nonionic contrast material resulted in contrast material pooling around the needle tip (arrow), strongly suggesting an epidural injection. B, Lateral view following injection of an additional 1.5 mL of nonionic contrast material confirms an extrathecal injection pattern (arrow). C, Lateral view following advance of the needle 2 mm with injection of an additional 0.2 mL of nonionic contrast material shows flow along the ventral aspect of the thecal sac (arrow), typical of an intrathecal injection. D, Lateral view following injection of an additional 1.0 mL of nonionic contrast material demonstrates continued accumulation, with additional contrast seen anteriorly (arrow 1), consistent with intrathecal injection, but also some additional contrast posteriorly (arrow 2), consistent with an epidural location and a mixed injection. E, Frontal view demonstrates contrast within the spinal canal. It is difficult to separate epidural from intrathecal contrast on this view (arrow). A total of 10.0 mL of nonionic contrast material was injected into the thecal sac. The patient was placed in a head-down position and the contrast material moved to the cervical spine. F, Frontal view following movement of contrast material. The majority of contrast material appears to be in the thecal sac (arrow). Note the fixation hardware. G, An oblique view demonstrates a combination of intrathecal (arrow 1) and epidural (arrow 2) contrast. The epidural contrast material flowed freely all the way from the lumbar injection point to the cervical spine. Computed tomographic examination followed (not shown) and was diagnostic despite some epidural contrast material.

TABLE 10–3. Step-by-Step Description of Cervical Approach C1-2 Myelography

1. Position the C-arm fluoroscope so that a clear view of the posterior C1-2 interspace is visualized.
2. Insert needle along the course of the x-ray beam far enough so that it is anchored.
3. Check position of the needle with the C-arm fluoroscope.
4. When the needle is well anchored, switch to the frontal view and check whether the needle has reached midline position. Advance the needle until it is approximately midline, paying close attention to whether needle placement is causing any symptoms of cord irritation (sudden, sharp sensations coming from the arms or legs).
5. When the needle appears to be in an appropriate location, remove the stylus and assess for cerebrospinal fluid (CSF) return through the needle. With small needles, only a tiny amount of CSF may return. Adjust the needle until CSF return is identified.
6. Inject 0.1 to 0.2 mL of nonionic contrast material and document an intrathecal position of the injected material. Reposition if not intrathecal.
7. Inject 8.0 to 12.0 mL of nonionic contrast material under fluoroscopic visualization.
8. Perform plain film radiography and myelography.
9. Release patient when stable. Advise patient to remain relatively horizontal for a 24-hour period. Provide patient with a telephone number to call if there is persistent or increased pain or numbness or if fever, swelling, or redness develops. Advise patient to call if a headache (particularly a positional headache worse when upright and at least partially relieved when horizontal) occurs.

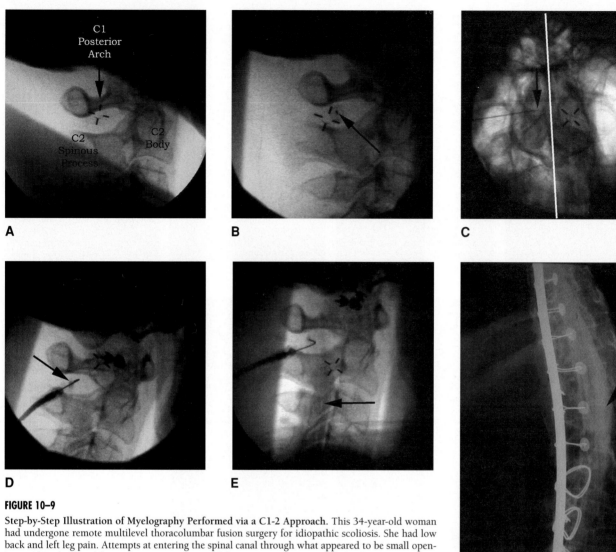

A   B   C

D   E

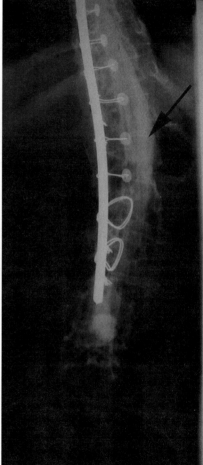

F

FIGURE 10–9

Step-by-Step Illustration of Myelography Performed via a C1-2 Approach. This 34-year-old woman had undergone remote multilevel thoracolumbar fusion surgery for idiopathic scoliosis. She had low back and left leg pain. Attempts at entering the spinal canal through what appeared to be small openings within the dorsal fusion mass were unsuccessful, as were attempts to reach the thecal sac through the caudal hiatus. Therefore, a C1-2 puncture was performed. *A,* Lateral view with magnification demonstrates the posterior arch of C1 (arrow) and spinous process of C2. The cross-hairs of the laser aiming device are located in the appropriate place along the dorsal aspect of the spinal canal at C1-2. *B,* Lateral view following insertion of a 25-gauge needle. The needle tip (arrow) projects at the posterior aspect of the spinal canal at the C1-2 level. *C,* Frontal view demonstrates that the needle tip (arrow) is not yet at a midline position (marked by a white line). The needle was advanced 3 mm and the C-arm fluoroscope returned to a lateral position. Cerebrospinal fluid returned through the needle. *D,* Lateral view following injection of 0.1 mL of nonionic contrast material. Contrast material is collecting at the needle tip (arrow). The needle was advanced 1 mm and more cerebrospinal fluid returned through the needle. *E,* Lateral view following injection of an additional 8.0 mL of nonionic contrast material demonstrates opacification of the thecal sac (arrow). *F,* Frontal view of the lumbar spine demonstrates an intrathecal location of contrast material (arrow). Note extensive postoperative changes with fixation rods and interlaminar wires. Computed tomographic examination (not shown) demonstrated possible pseudarthrosis at L5-S1 with subarticular recess narrowing and compression of the traversing left S1 nerve root. The patient underwent a series of caudal epidural steroid injections, with partial pain relief.

References

Abla AA, Rothfus WE, Maroon JC, Deeb ZL. Delayed spinal subarachnoid hematoma: a rare complication of C1-2 cervical myelography. AJNR 1986; 7:526–528.

Amundsen P, Skalpe IO. Cervical myelography with a water-soluble contrast medium (Metrizamide). Neuroradiology 1975; 8:209–212.

Awwad EE, Martin DS, Klein J. Predictive value of postmyelographic computed tomography for patients with severe postmyelographic headache. Sout Med J 1995; 88:944–946.

Bartynski WS, Lin L. Lumbar root compression in the lateral recess: MR imaging, conventional myelography, and CT myelography comparison with surgical confirmation. Am J Neuroradiol 2003; 24:348–360.

Braune H-J, Huffman G. A prospective double-blind clinical trial, comparing the sharp Quincke needle (22G) with an "atraumatic" needle (22G) in the induction of post-lumbar puncture headache. Acta Neurol Scand 1992; 86:50–54.

Elkin CM, Levan AMT, Leeds NE. Tolerance of iohexol, iopamidol, and metrizamide in lumbar myelography. Surg Neurol 1986; 26:524–526.

Farese MG, Martinez CR, Fisher CH. Inadvertent cervical cord puncture during myelography via C1-C2 approach. J Fla Med Assoc 1990; 77:91–93.

Floras P, Gross C, Paty J, Caille JM. Neurotoxicity of iohexol vs iopamidol in lumbar myelography. J Neuroradiol 1990; 17:190–200.

Gonsette RE. Metrizamide as contrast medium for myelography and ventriculography. Acta Radiol (Suppl) 1973; 335:346–358.

Hahn RA. The nocebo phenomenon: scope and foundations. In Harrington A (ed). The Placebo Effect. Cambridge, MA, Harvard University Press, 1997.

Heinz ER, Goldman RL. The role of gas myelography in neuroradiologic diagnosis: comments on a new and simple technique. Radiology 1972; 102:629–634.

Johansen JG, Orrison WW, Amundsen P. Lateral C1-2 puncture for cervical myelography. Part I. Report of a complication. Radiology 1983; 146:391–393.

Katoh Y, Itoh T, Tsuji H, Matsui H, Hirano N, Kitagawa H. Complications of lateral C1-2 puncture myelography. Spine 1990; 15:1085–1087.

Kelly DL, Alexander E. Lateral cervical puncture for myelography. J Neurosurg 1968; 29:106–110.

Nagayama M, Watanabe Y, Okumura A, Amoh Y, Nakashita S, Dodo Y. High-resolution single-slice MR myelography. AJR 2002; 179:515–521.

Nakstad PH, Kjartansson O. Accidental spinal cord injection of contrast material during cervical myelography with lateral C1-2 puncture. Am J Neuroradiol 1988; 9:410.

Prager JM, Roychowdhury S, Gorey MT, Lowe GM, Diamond CW, Ragin A. Spinal headaches after myelograms: comparison of needle types. Am J Radiol 1996; 167:1289–1292.

Raskin NH. Lumbar puncture headache: a review. Headache 1990; 30:197–200.

Rice JF, Bathia AL. Lateral C1-2 puncture for myelography: posterior approach. Radiology 1979; 132:760–762.

Rogers LA. Acute subdural hematoma and death following lateral cervical spinal puncture: case report. J Neurosurg 1983; 58:284–286.

Sand T. Which factors affect reported headache incidences after lumbar myelography? A statistical analysis of publications in the literature. Neuroradiology 1989; 31:55–59.

Servo A, Laasonen EM. Accidental introduction of contrast medium into the cervical spinal cord. Neuroradiology 1985; 27:80–82.

Skalpe IO, Amundsen P. Thoracic and cervical myelography with metrizamide. Radiology 1975; 116:101–106.

Sortland O, Skalpe IO. Cervical myelography by lateral cervical and lumbar injection of metrizamide. Acta Radiol (Suppl) 1977; 355:154–163.

Tamura T. A simple technique for cervical myelography. Spine 1991; 16:1267–1268.

Wilkinson AG, Sellar RJ. The influence of needle size and other factors on the incidence of adverse effects caused by myelography. Clin Radiol 1991; 44:338–341.

Zeng Q, Xiong L, Jinkins JR, Fan Z, Liu Z. Intrathecal gadolinium-enhanced MR myelography and cisternography: a pilot study in human patients. AJR 1999; 173:1109–1115.

Calls and Concerns Following Procedures

DONALD L. RENFREW

Patients undergoing the procedures described in this book may later call because of side effects or complications of the injections. Most of these side effects and complications are covered in the chapters on the individual injections, but patients frequently forget what they are told just prior to the examination and do not read the handouts given them. When a patient calls with concerns following the procedure, a few specific points need to be established, and appropriate treatment given. Following the general rule that "if it's not documented, it didn't happen," it is good policy to make a permanent record regarding these conversations.

The first order of business when answering a phone call from a patient who has undergone a procedure is to determine the date, time, and type of procedure, as complications vary according to the type of procedure. It is then usually best to allow the patient to explain in his or her own words the nature of the difficulty. Once these two goals have been accomplished, a few specific points need to be established:

1. **Does the patient have any symptoms to suggest neurologic compromise?** You should ask patients whether they have had any new loss of control of their bowel or bladder function or new extremity weakness. If they indicate that they have, and if there is any chance that the needle has entered or approached the spinal canal, then epidural hematoma and epidural abscess are both considerations, and the patient should probably undergo immediate diagnostic imaging to exclude these possibilities. Depending on the results, surgical or neurologic consultation may be in order.

2. **Does the patient have symptoms to suggest an infection?** Fever and chills strongly suggest this possibility, but it should be noted that half of patients who have infectious discitis do not have these symptoms (Carragee 1997, Hadjipavlou 2000, Hitchon 1992). New severe, unremitting backache unrelieved by rest or position should also suggest this possibility. Immediate imaging to evaluate morphologic findings of abscess or infectious spondylitis should be considered, with treatment based on the results of the imaging. Imaging results are sometimes equivocal, and evaluation of erythrocyte sedimentation rate (ESR) may be helpful, since it is virtually always elevated in nonimmunocompromised patients with infectious spondylitis (Carragee 1997, Hadjipavlou 2000, Hitchon 1992); C-reactive protein measurement may be more sensitive and specific (Fouquet 1992, Grane 1998).

3. **Does the patient have a post-procedure headache?** Patients may have headache following spine procedures for a number of reasons, including the "nocebo" effect, wherein the suggestion of the possibility triggers a headache; side effect of steroids; and a "post-tap headache" from puncture of the dura. The first two can be treated with time or oral analgesics. Post-tap headaches may be more difficult to treat and are recognized by their striking positional component: the headache will go away, or nearly go away, when the patient is supine but be quite severe when the patient is upright. Such headaches usually accompany myelograms but may also follow epidural steroid injections with either recognized or unrecognized dural puncture. Generally the headache is noticeable the day of or the day after the procedure, but occasionally post-tap headaches develop several days after a procedure. Initial treatment consists of a recumbent position; analgesics are generally ineffective at headache relief but theophylline 300 mg tid may be of benefit (Raskin 1990). Often, a blood patch (or, occasionally, two) is required for benefit; usually, dramatic relief follows immediately after this procedure.

4. **Does the patient have a pain flare from a procedure?** Epidural steroid injection may be accompanied by a pain flare, and patients after discography and rhizotomy may have ongoing pain for 2 or 3 days after the procedure. Indeed, after discography and rhizotomy, it is generally wise to prescribe a short course of hydrocodone or other analgesic. If the patient seems to be having significant pain following a procedure and does not already have such medications, oral naproxen or hydrocodone can be prescribed for pain relief.

5. **Does the patient have steroid side effects?** Insomnia can be treated with reassurance or medication; anxiety and/or hiccups (which seem to follow betamethasone

injection more frequently than they do the other steroids) can be treated with diazepam. Diabetic patients may have marked changes in blood sugar levels and should be warned about this and told to monitor their blood sugar and consult with their internist regarding blood sugar control. Other steroid side effects include changes in mood or appetite (either up or down), steroid rash, and gastrointestinal upset (reflux symptoms or diarrhea). The best treatment for these is usually reassurance that they will pass in a few days.

The exercise of answering these five questions will usually take care of most patient calls, although patients occasionally either manifest very unusual complications of procedures or have unrelated symptoms fortuitously arise following the injection.

References

Carragee EJ. Pyogenic vertebral osteomyelitis. J Bone Joint Surg Am 1997; 79:874–880.

Fouquet B, Goupile P, Jattiot F, Cotty P, Lapierre F, Valat JP, Amouroux J, Benatre A. Discitis after lumbar disc surgery: features of "aseptic" and "septic" forms. Spine 1992; 17:356–358.

Grane P, Josephsson A, Seferlis A, Tullberg T. Septic and aseptic post-operative discitis in the lumbar spine: evaluation by MR imaging. Acta Radiol 1998; 39:108–115.

Hadjipavlou AG, Mader JT, Necessary JT, Muffoletto AJ. Hematogenous pyogenic spinal infections and their surgical management. Spine 2000; 25:1668–1679.

Hitchon PW, Osenbach RK, Yuh WTC, Menezes AH. Spinal infections. Clin Neurosurg 1992; 38:373–387.

Raskin NH. Lumbar puncture headache: a review. Headache 1990; 30:197–200.

2 Medications, Contrast Material, and Needles

DONALD L. RENFREW

Certain common items are used in virtually all of the procedures discussed in this book. Rather than repeating the same discussion in each chapter, some concise comments regarding medications, contrast material, and needles are given here.

Medications

The following comments are meant as brief introduction to the medications alluded to elsewhere in this textbook. These descriptions are by no means exhaustive, and the reader is urged to review current pharmacology textbooks and the package inserts of any substance he or she intends to inject into or prescribe for a patient.

ANESTHETICS

Lidocaine and bupivacaine are excellent local anesthetics in widespread use. Injection of 2.0 to 3.0 mL of these agents into the epidural space generally results in relief of low back and leg pain and occasionally numbness in the buttocks and perineum. Injection of the same amount of material into the thecal sac may be associated with a spinal block and associated loss of bladder control and lower extremity strength and sensation. These substances therefore help differentiate where an injection has occurred. When used in nerve blocks or transforaminal injections, even small amounts (0.5–1.0 mL) may result in lower extremity paralysis and loss of sensation. For medial branch blocks, 0.5 to 1.0 mL at each level is sufficient, resulting in a total dose of 100 mg or less. Most adverse reactions are dose related and, given the small amounts of total anesthetic used for the procedures discussed in this book, should virtually never be encountered. Allergic reactions, of course, may occur after injection of even very small amounts of an anesthetic agent but are fortunately extremely rare. Allergic reactions to anesthetic agents, as allergic reactions to other substances, manifest as urticaria, edema, or anaphylactoid reactions and

are treated as other allergic reactions. The duration of drug effect varies greatly between individuals. As a generalization, bupivacaine lasts approximately three times longer than lidocaine.

STEROIDS

Until it became virtually unavailable in 2001, the betamethasone-containing product Celestone was the steroid of choice for epidural injection. At present, it does not appear that Celestone will be commercially available anytime soon. Therefore, alternatives to Celestone have been used for epidural injection. These include methylprednisolone and triamcinolone. Dosage is generally 40 to 80 mg in the epidural space and 20 to 40 mg within facet joints.

ANALGESICS

During rhizotomy or immediately following discography (or, occasionally, other procedures) acute pain management may be necessary. There are a number of possible ways to deal with this problem. One helpful drug is meperidine, administered as a 50 mg intramuscular injection.

Patients may have a pain flare following virtually any procedure involving the spine and a needle. These pain flares usually subside but may be quite uncomfortable. Again, there are many ways to deal with such a problem and a wide variety of non-narcotic and narcotic medications can be employed in the treatment of such pain flares. Naproxen (550 mg q 8 hours), a nonsteroidal anti-inflammatory, may be helpful. A more powerful drug is hydrocodone (5 mg), which is usually compounded with acetaminophen (500 mg).

SLEEP AIDS

Following steroid injection, many people suffer from insomnia for one or two nights. Zolpidem tartrate (5 mg) may be prescribed in limited supply with instructions to take one or two doses at bedtime for insomnia.

Contrast Material

Nonionic contrast material safe for intrathecal injection should be used routinely when performing the procedures described in this book. Iohexol is available in 200 mg/mL, 240 mg/mL, and 300 mg/mL concentrations. The total injection of nonionic contrast material should be limited to 3 g of iodine, so up to 10 mL of the most concentrated form may be used, which is more than adequate for myelography. Other procedures require far less contrast material.

Needles

Most procedures performed in this book can be done with 22- or 25-gauge Quincke point "spinal" needles. These nee-dles are readily available, inexpensive, and relatively easy to direct. Note, however, that manufacturers' products vary. The characteristics of how the needle moves through tissue are very important, particularly when it is necessary (as it often is) to adjust needle direction during a procedure.

Performance of myelography with Sprotte tip needles results in fewer headaches (see Chapter 10). These needles have a pencil point and use a side-hole for injection. Epidural needles can be used for epidural injection, but these needles are generally of greater bore and are used as part of the procedure of epidural catheter placement. Biopsy needles are larger and come in a variety of shapes, sizes, and tip designs. Specialized equipment is generally required for vertebroplasty and kyphoplasty; manufacturers provide kits with the requisite supplies and needles.

Index